Evidence-Based Clinical Practice in Otolaryngology

Evidence-Based Clinical Practice in Otolaryngology

LUKE RUDMIK, MD, BSC, MSC (HEALTH ECON), FRCSC
Clinical Associate Professor
Endoscopic Sinus & Skull Base Surgery
Section of Otolaryngology/Head and Neck Surgery
Department of Surgery
Department of Community Health Sciences
University of Calgary
Calgary, AB, Canada

ELSEVIER

ELSEVIER

3251 Riverport Lane
St. Louis, Missouri 63043

Content Strategist: Jessica McCool
Content Development Manager: Taylor Ball
Content Development Specialist: Meredith Madeira
Publishing Services Manager: Deepthi Unni
Project Manager: Janish Ashwin Paul
Designer: Gopalakrishnan Venkatraman

Working together
to grow libraries in
developing countries

www.elsevier.com • www.bookaid.org

Printed in United States of America

Last digit is the print number: 9 8 7 6 5 4 3 2 1

List of Contributors

Editor

Luke Rudmik, MD, BSc, MSc (Health Econ), FRCSC
Clinical Associate Professor
Endoscopic Sinus & Skull Base Surgery
Section of Otolaryngology/Head and Neck Surgery
Department of Surgery
Department of Community Health Sciences
University of Calgary
Calgary, AB, Canada

Contributors

Martyn L. Barnes, FRCS-ORL (Ed), MD
Consultant Rhinologist
Southend University Hospital
Southend On Sea, United Kingdom

Pete S. Batra, MD, FACS
Stanton A. Friedberg, MD, Chair in Otolaryngology
Professor and Chairman
Department of Otorhinolaryngology, Head and Neck
    Surgery
Rush University Medical Center
Chicago, IL, United States

Daniel F. Brasnu, MD
Department of Otolaryngology, Head & Neck Surgery
Fondation A. de Rothschild
University René Descartes, Paris Sorbonne Cité
Paris, France

Ingrid Breuskin, MD, PhD
Department of Head and Neck Oncology
Gustave Roussy
Villejuif, France

Daniel J. Cates, MD
Department of Otolaryngology, Head & Neck
    Surgery
University of California – Davis
Sacramento, CA, United States

Katie de Champlain, MSc
Foothills Medical Centre
Calgary, AB, Canada

Justin Chau, MD, FRCSC
Section of Otolaryngology, Head and Neck Surgery
Department of Surgery
University of Calgary
Calgary, AB, Canada

David Conrad, MD, FAAP
Assistant Professor - Otolaryngology - Head and Neck
    Surgery
University of California, San Francisco
San Francisco, CA, United States

John M. DelGaudio, MD
Professor
Department of Otolaryngology, Head and Neck
    Surgery
Sinus, Nasal, and Allergy Center
Emory University
Atlanta, GA, United States

Charles S. Ebert, MD, MPH
Associate Professor
Department of Otolaryngology, Head and Neck
    Surgery
University of North Carolina at Chapel Hill
Chapel Hill, NC, United States

Matthew G. Ewend, MD
Professor and Chairman
Department of Neurosurgery
University of North Carolina at Chapel Hill
Chapel Hill, NC, United States

Zachary Farhood, MD
Resident Physician
Saint Louis University
Department of Otolaryngology, Head and Neck
    Surgery
Saint Louis, MO, United States

Dana M. Hartl, MD, PhD
Department of Head and Neck Oncology
Gustave Roussy
Villejuif, France

Euna Hwang, MD, FRCSC
Clinical Lecturer
Section of Otolaryngology, Head and Neck Surgery
Department of Surgery
University of Calgary
Calgary, AB, Canada

Danny Jandali, MD
Department of Otorhinolaryngology, Head and Neck
    Surgery
Rush University Medical Center
Chicago, IL, United States

Cristine N. Klatt-Cromwell, MD
Rhinology and Skull Base Fellow
Department of Otolaryngology, Head and Neck Surgery
University of North Carolina at Chapel Hill
Chapel Hill, NC, United States

Joshua M. Levy, MD, MPH
Assistant Professor
Department of Otolaryngology, Head and Neck Surgery
Sinus, Nasal & Allergy Center
Emory University
Atlanta, GA, United States

Justin Lui, MD
Foothills Medical Centre
Calgary, AB, Canada

Lauren J. Luk, MD
Orange County Sinus Institute
Department of Otolaryngology, Head and Neck Surgery
Southern California Permanente Medical Group
Irvine, CA, United States

Alison Maresh, MD
Assistant Professor
Department of Otolaryngology, Head & Neck Surgery
Weill Cornell Medicine/NewYork-Presbyterian
    Hospital
New York, NY, United States

Sean T. Massa, MD
Resident Physician
Saint Louis University
Department of Otolaryngology, Head and Neck
    Surgery
Saint Louis, MO, United States

Albert L. Merati, MD, FACS
Professor and Chief, Laryngology
Department of Otolaryngology, Head & Neck Surgery
School of Medicine
Adjunct Professor, School of Music
Adjunct Professor, Speech & Hearing Sciences
College of Arts and Sciences
University of Washington
Seattle, WA, United States

Stephanie Misono, MD, MPH
Assistant Professor
Department of Otolaryngology, Head and Neck
    Surgery
University of Minnesota
Minneapolis, MN, United States

Vikash K. Modi, MD, FAAP
Associate Professor
Division Chief of Pediatric Otolaryngology
Department of Otolaryngology, Head & Neck
    Surgery
Weill Cornell Medicine/NewYork- Presbyterian
    Hospital
New York, NY, United States

Lourdes Quintanilla-Dieck, MD
Assistant Professor
Otolaryngology Head & Neck Surgery
Oregon Health & Science University
Portland, OR, United States

Derrick R. Randall, MD, MSc, FRCSC
Section of Otolaryngology, Head & Neck Surgery
Department of Surgery
University of Calgary
Calgary, AB, Canada

Kristina Rosbe, MD, FAAP
Professor of Otolaryngology and Pediatrics
Chief, Division of Pediatric Otolaryngology
Benioff Children's Hospitals
University of California, San Francisco
San Francisco, CA, United States

Deanna M. Sasaki-Adams, MD
Assistant Professor
Department of Neurosurgery
University of North Carolina at Chapel Hill
Chapel Hill, NC, United States

Theodore A. Schuman, MD
Department of Otolaryngology, Head & Neck Surgery
Virginia Commonwealth University Richmond
VA, United States

Angus Shao, FRACS-ORLHNS
Rhinology Fellow
Southend University Hospital
Southend On Sea, United Kingdom

Maisie Shindo, MD, FACS
Professor
Otolaryngology Head & Neck Surgery
Director
Thyroid & Parathyroid Center
Oregon Health & Science University
Portland, OR, United States

Patrick M. Spielmann, FRCS-ORL (Ed)
Consultant Otolaryngologist
Ninewells Hospital and Medical School
Dundee, United Kingdom

Michael G. Stewart, MD, MPH
Chairman
Professor
Department of Otolaryngology, Head & Neck Surgery
Weill Cornell Medicine/NewYork-Presbyterian
    Hospital
New York, NY, United States

Bobby A. Tajudeen, MD
Department of Otorhinolaryngology
Head and Neck Surgery and Rush Sinus Program
Rush University Medical Center
Chicago, IL, United States

Brian D. Thorp, MD
Assistant Professor
Department of Otolaryngology, Head and Neck
    Surgery
University of North Carolina at Chapel Hill
Chapel Hill, NC, United States

Darren Tse, BMBS, MRCS (Eng), FRCSC
Assistant Professor
Department of Otolaryngology, Head and Neck
    Surgery
University of Ottawa
Ottawa, ON, Canada

Scott G. Walen, MD
Assistant Professor
Saint Louis University
Department of Otolaryngology, Head and Neck
    Surgery
Saint Louis, MO, United States

Paul S. White, FRACS, FRCS (Ed), MBChB
Consultant Rhinologist
Ninewells Hospital & Medical School
Dundee, United Kingdom

Sarah K. Wise, MD, MSCR
Associate Professor
Department of Otolaryngology, Head and Neck
    Surgery
Sinus, Nasal & Allergy Center
Emory University
Atlanta, GA, United States

Adam M. Zanation, MD
Associate Professor
Department of Otolaryngology, Head and Neck
    Surgery
Department of Neurosurgery
University of North Carolina at Chapel Hill
Chapel Hill, NC, United States

Contents

CHAPTER 1

Evidence-Based Practice: Management of Acute Vertigo

EUNA HWANG, MD, FRCSC • DARREN TSE, BMBS, MRCS(ENG), FRCSC

Vertigo is a form of dizziness. The American Academy of Otolaryngology-Head and Neck Surgery (AAO-HNS) has defined vertigo as "an illusory sensation of motion of either the self or the surroundings in the absence of true motion" and "the sensation of motion when no motion is occurring relative to earth's gravity."[1,2] In other words, it is a symptom of perceived movement. Vertigo is caused by asymmetric inputs from the vestibular system following damage or perturbation to the peripheral vestibular apparatus (inner ear and vestibular nerve) or the central vestibular apparatus (brainstem and cerebellum). Vertigo is frequently experienced by the general population, accounting for a quarter of dizziness complaints, with a 12-month prevalence of 5% and an annual incidence of 1.4%.[3] Vertigo can result in significant disability, including loss of work time and disruption of daily activities.[4] As the prevalence of vertigo increases with age, it is also associated with an increased risk of fall and injury in the elderly population. This article focuses on the evidence-based practice in the management of the two most common diagnoses of acute vertigo: benign paroxysmal positional vertigo (BPPV) and vestibular neuritis (VN).[5,6]

BENIGN PAROXYSMAL POSITIONAL VERTIGO

Introduction

BPPV is a disorder of the inner ear in which episodic vertigo is elicited by changes in the head position relative to gravity.[1] Although these episodes of positional vertigo are rather short in duration, they can cause remarkable acute vertigo and persist for weeks to months, leading to distress and restricted movements and activities. BPPV had a lifetime prevalence of 2.4%, a 1-year prevalence of 1.6%, and a 1-year incidence of 0.6% in a population-based neurotologic survey.

The 1-year prevalence of BPPV increased significantly with age, as it was seven times higher in the group aged above 60 years (3.4%), compared with the group aged 18–39 years (0.5%). The cumulative incidence of BPPV was near 10% by the age of 80 years.[7] The peak age of onset appears to be in the sixth decade for idiopathic BPPV, and the mean age of onset is lower for secondary BPPV.[8] About 17% of patients were found to have BPPV in one large dizziness clinic that evaluated more than 15,000 patients over almost 23 years.[9] In addition to being reported as the most frequent cause of acute, recurrent vertigo, BPPV is typically treated successfully by noninvasive and inexpensive particle-repositioning maneuvers (PRMs).[10] Hence, proper recognition and timely management of this peripheral vestibular disorder are paramount for adequate patient care in both primary care and subspecialty settings.

Pathophysiology

BPPV is generally accepted as the result of the abnormal presence of heavy calcium carbonate debris in a semicircular canal. These loose particles are otoconia (otoliths) that have been displaced from their original location in the utricle to a canal, where they provoke abnormal movement of the endolymph and cupula after reaching a critical mass when the head moves in the plane of the affected canal, resulting in abnormal nystagmus and vertigo. BPPV is thought to be caused by either canalithiasis (particles in a canal itself) or cupulolithiasis (particles adherent to the cupula of a canal) and can involve any of the three semicircular canals, whereas the superior (anterior) canal is rarely affected.[11,12] The underlying reasons for the dislodgement of otoliths from the vestibule remain unclear. Head trauma or whiplash injuries (15%), as well as other inner ear pathologies, such as Meniere disease (30%), VN (15%), otologic surgery, or sudden sensorineural hearing loss, are associated with secondary BPPV. The most common cause of secondary BPPV is head trauma. BPPV is primary or idiopathic in most cases (35%–70%).[8,9,12–16] The above-mentioned mechanism of canalithiasis leading to posterior canal BPPV and nystagmus was explained by Epley.[17,18] Free-floating particles have indeed been confirmed intraoperatively in patients with refractory posterior canal BPPV.[11,19,20] Lateral (horizontal) canal BPPV is also believed to be caused by the abnormal presence of debris in the lateral canal, which has not been demonstrated in vivo. Its pathophysiology is not as well understood as that of posterior canal BPPV, but the presence of particles in the lateral canal is supported by the phenomenon of canal conversion when a PRM to treat posterior canal BPPV results in lateral canal BPPV or vice versa.[1,21,22] Cupulolithiasis is thought to be more relevant in lateral canal BPPV than in posterior canal BPPV. The vertigo and nystagmus associated with the lateral canal variant are typically strong and last as long as the head is in the provocative position as debris adhere to the cupula.[12] The literature on superior canal BPPV is rather sparse because of its rarity from the anatomy of the superior canal that renders it difficult for debris to enter and stay. Its pathophysiology and findings are poorly understood and debated.[23–26]

Posterior canal BPPV is the most common type, accounting for 60%–90% of BPPV diagnoses.[27–30] Lateral canal BPPV is present in 10%–20% of BPPV cases.[30] However, it may be underestimated in most reports as a large case series of 589 patients with BPPV revealed that lateral canal BPPV occurred in 40% of patients examined within 24 h of vertigo onset, as opposed to 26% when patients presented after 7 days of onset, which is consistent with the high natural remission rate of this type.[27,31] Superior canal BPPV is the rarest type with a reported frequency of 1%–2%.[30] Other infrequent variations comprise ipsilateral multicanal BPPV and bilateral multicanal BPPV.[32]

Diagnosis

The diagnosis of BPPV is supported by a history of repeated episodes of positional vertigo that typically resolve within 1 min. They might be associated with nausea and vomiting. The transient vertigo is positional in that it is triggered by specific head movements, including looking up, bending forward, lying down from the sitting position, sitting up from the supine position, and turning over in bed. Such attacks can recur intermittently for weeks to months.[33] Imbalance may be reported between attacks.[7] Proper examination with provoking maneuvers and adequate analysis of

nystagmus are required to diagnose the type and the side of the BPPV.

Further workup, including audiometric testing, vestibular testing, or neuroimaging, is not required for the diagnosis of typical BPPV, which is made based on history and physical examination with provoking maneuvers. However, these investigations should be considered in the presence of concurrent vestibular or central signs and/or symptoms incompatible with BPPV, or when concomitant vestibular dysfunction, peripheral or central, is suspected.[1] Audiometry is usually normal in BPPV.[34] Positive findings on various vestibular tests are attributed to simultaneous peripheral vestibulopathy.[8,35,36] Neuroimaging, which tends to be normal in the absence of coexisting central signs and/or symptoms, is recommended if the nystagmus is equivocal or atypical (e.g., down-beating nystagmus suggestive of central positional nystagmus) or if the patient does not respond to treatment.[13,37]

Posterior canal benign paroxysmal positional vertigo

The guidelines on BPPV from the AAO-HNS state that the diagnosis of posterior canal BPPV is made by a history of episodic positional vertigo and the finding of characteristic nystagmus elicited by the Dix-Hallpike test. The use of the Dix-Hallpike test as a diagnostic maneuver for posterior canal BPPV was described in 1952.[38] It is conducted by moving the patient from a sitting to supine position with the head turned 45 degrees to one side and neck extended with the tested ear down. It should be performed on both sides, especially if the testing of the first side is negative.[1] The characteristic nystagmus according to the above-mentioned guidelines and other described features of the nystagmus in posterior canal BPPV are outlined in Table 1.1.

The Dix-Hallpike test is accepted as the gold standard test for the diagnosis of posterior canal BPPV.[40] In the absence of another well-established alternative diagnostic test, it is the most used diagnostic criterion in clinical trials and meta-analyses.[41] The side-lying test, which involves brisk side-lying with the nose turned 45 degrees away from the tested side, has been described as a substitute provoking maneuver for patients who are unable to move into the Dix-Hallpike test positions.[42,43] The sensitivity of the Dix-Hallpike test in posterior canal BPPV ranges from 48% to 88%.[43,44] Its diagnostic accuracy is likely variable between specialty and nonspecialty clinicians. Because BPPV is an intermittent condition, the test may also require a repeat execution at a separate visit to avoid missing a diagnosis due to a previously false-negative result. Primarily in

---

TABLE 1.1
Nystagmus During Dix-Hallpike Test in Posterior Canal BPPV

AAO-HNS Diagnostic Criteria[1,a]	Other Classic Features[12,39]
Up-beating and torsional (geotropic, toward dependent ear) nystagmus associated with vertigo	Upon sitting back up and returning to the upright head position, nystagmus and vertigo may recur, with reversed direction of the nystagmus
Latent nystagmus and vertigo (typically 5–20 s, up to 1 min) Nystagmus and vertigo increase and then decrease in intensity before resolving within 60 s of onset	Nystagmus and vertigo fatigue (diminish in intensity and duration) with each repetition of the test

AAO-HNS, American Academy of Otolaryngology-Head and Neck Surgery; BPPV, benign paroxysmal positional vertigo.
[a]All three criteria must be fulfilled for the diagnosis of posterior canal BPPV.

---

the specialty setting, its sensitivity was reported to be 82% and its specificity lower at 71%.[45] In the primary care setting, its positive predictive value was found to be 83% but its negative predictive value was low at 52%.[6] Hence, a negative Dix-Hallpike test should not rule out posterior canal BPPV entirely, although a positive test is considered adequate for diagnosis.

Lateral canal benign paroxysmal positional vertigo

The guidelines on BPPV from the AAO-HNS state that the diagnosis of lateral canal BPPV is made by a history of episodic positional vertigo and confirmation of horizontal nystagmus elicited by the supine roll test after the finding of horizontal or absent nystagmus on the Dix-Hallpike test. The supine roll test is conducted by positioning the patient supine with the head in neutral position at the beginning and then rapidly rotating the head 90 degrees to one side. Once the nystagmus and vertigo subside, if present, the head is returned to the initial supine neutral position. After any additional nystagmus and vertigo have resolved, the head is again rapidly rotated 90 degrees but to the opposite side.[1]

As the horizontal nystagmus is direction changing and observed on both sides during the supine roll test in lateral canal BPPV, the direction and the intensity of the nystagmus determine whether it is caused by canalithiasis or cupulolithiasis and the affected side, respectively.[1,12] Geotropic nystagmus (beating toward the dependent ear) indicates canalithiasis in the long arm of the lateral canal, and it is the most common variant and the most amenable to treatment.[46–48] Apogeotropic nystagmus (beating away from the dependent ear) indicates cupulolithiasis as in debris attached to the cupula or located close to it in the anterior arm of the lateral canal.[49] The side that exhibits stronger nystagmus and vertigo is the affected ear in geotropic nystagmus, whereas the side that exhibits weaker

nystagmus and vertigo is the affected ear in apogeotropic nystagmus.[50–52]

The supine roll test is the diagnostic test of choice for lateral canal BPPV and the most used diagnostic criterion in clinical trials.[46,48,49,53] Clear lateralization is not achieved in about 20% of cases.[54,55] The bow and lean test has been described as an alternative provoking maneuver. The sitting patient starts by bowing the head forward, making the lateral canal vertical, and then leans the head backward, turning over the lateral canal 180 degrees. Right lateral canalithiasis results in right-beating nystagmus during the bow and left-beating nystagmus during the lean.[56,57] It might clarify the side of involvement when it is added to the supine roll test, as it has been reported to be better at lateralizing lateral canal BPPV than the supine roll test. The remission rates of lateral canalithiasis following PRMs were improved when the bow and lean test was combined to the supine roll test during diagnosis, compared with when the supine roll test was performed alone.[57]

Superior canal benign paroxysmal positional vertigo

Again, the entity of superior canalithiasis is debatable and thought to be rare, as the superior semicircular canal is oriented vertically and located high in the labyrinth so it would appear unlikely that otoliths would resist gravitational forces and make their way into it. Nevertheless, there is a general agreement as to its clinical features based on a growing number of case series in the literature. Superior canal BPPV produces down-beating and torsional nystagmus that is elicited by the Dix-Hallpike test or straight head hanging. The positional nystagmus can be present unilaterally or on both sides of the Dix-Hallpike test. The torsional component is directed toward the affected ear.[58–62] Hence, determining the direction of the torsion helps establish the involved side. However, the torsional component is often subtle or absent, so the nystagmus can be observed as purely down-beating.[61,63,64] In a case series of 18 patients with superior canal BPPV, only 33% (six patients) exhibited a torsional component.[58] The clinician should thus be cautious and consider the possibility of a central pathology such as a brainstem or cerebellar lesion in the presence of such positional down-beating nystagmus.[65]

Management

The mainstay of treatment of BPPV is the appropriate use of PRMs after proper diagnosis of the semicircular canal and side that are affected. These physical maneuvers serve to move the ectopic otoconial debris from the semicircular canals and relocate them into the vestibule. As these repositioning methods are usually highly and immediately effective in most patients, they also contribute in confirming the diagnosis. However, they do not prevent recurrences.[66] BPPV also has a natural history of possible spontaneous resolution over time. The time to natural remission is typically longer in the posterior canal type and shorter in the lateral canal type.[31] Various repositioning procedures exist for posterior canal, lateral canal, and superior canal BPPV, with the most evidence available for the treatment of the posterior canal variant. Surgery has been described for refractory posterior canal and superior canal BPPV. Vestibular rehabilitation therapy has a limited role in acute vertigo caused by BPPV.

Physical maneuvers

Posterior canal benign paroxysmal positional vertigo. Two PRMs effectively treat posterior canal BPPV[1]: the Epley maneuver[67] and the Semont liberatory maneuver.[68] There is considerable evidence for the efficacy of both procedures, whereas the Epley maneuver has been more extensively studied. The Epley maneuver utilizes gravity to displace the otoconial debris from the posterior semicircular canal back into the vestibule as the patient is moved successively through a series of head positions (Table 1.2), whereas the Semont liberatory maneuver utilizes both inertial and gravitational forces as the patient is briskly moved down on the involved side (side-lying position) and then brought to the opposite side-lying position on the uninvolved side through a rapid 180-degree arc.[66]

The efficacy of the Epley maneuver has been shown in randomized studies comparing it with a placebo (sham) maneuver.[69–71] Inspection of the nystagmus during Step 3 (Table 1.2) of the Epley maneuver can predict the outcome of the procedure: absent or reversed nystagmus suggests an unsuccessful maneuver.[72] Repetition of the Epley maneuver over multiple sessions is also beneficial when symptoms are not fully cleared after the first session or when there is relapse after the initial treatment. Subsequent therapies seem to have a similar likelihood of benefit as the first therapy.[73] The updated 2014 Cochrane Review on the Epley maneuver included 11 randomized controlled trials for a total of 745 patients and reported that this PRM is a safe and effective treatment for posterior canal BPPV with a high recurrence rate of BPPV following treatment (36%). It concluded that the Epley maneuver was more effective than sham maneuvers or controls and Brandt-Daroff exercises, but its outcomes were comparable with those of the Semont and Gans maneuvers.[41] Other systematic reviews and meta-analyses have supported that PRMs are safe and effective for treating posterior canal BPPV.[40,74–76]

TABLE 1.2
Steps of the Epley Maneuver

Step 1: The patient is sitting with the head turned 45 degrees toward the affected ear (the ear that was positive on the Dix-Hallpike test).

Step 2: The patient is quickly laid back to the supine position with the head hanging at 20 degrees. This position is maintained for 30 s.

Step 3: The head is turned 90 degrees toward the opposite (unaffected) side and held for 30 s.

Step 4: The head is again turned 90 degrees further toward the unaffected side such that the head is essentially facing the ground for 30 s. This step requires the patient to simultaneously move from the supine position to the lateral decubitus position while turning the head.

Step 5: The patient is brought from the lateral decubitus position into the sitting position.

Adapted from Bhattacharyya N, Gubbels SP, Schwartz SR, et al. Clinical practice guideline: benign paroxysmal positional vertigo (update). *Otolaryngol Head Neck Surg*. 2017;156(3S):S1–S47, with permission.

The Semont maneuver is superior to sham maneuvers based on randomized trials.[77,78] The Semont and Epley maneuvers are equally safe and effective based on recent meta-analyses,[79,80] but a multicenter randomized study of 99 patients demonstrated that the Epley maneuver was significantly more effective per maneuver than the Semont or sham maneuvers for the short-term treatment of posterior canal BPPV.[81]

Lateral canal benign paroxysmal positional vertigo. Three PRMs are commonly used to treat lateral canal BPPV: the Lempert ("barbeque" or log) roll,[82] the Gufoni maneuver,[83] and the forced prolonged position.[84] The successful treatment of the lateral canal variant is challenged by the difficulty in accurately identifying the affected side, as there may be no obvious difference in the intensity of the nystagmus between the two sides on examination with the supine roll test. However, as previously explained, correct determination of the problematic side in lateral canal BPPV may be improved by the bow and lean test.[57] The best-studied and most clinically responsive subtype of lateral canal BPPV is the geotropic form.[1]

The Lempert roll is used for the treatment of geotropic lateral canal BPPV. It consists of sequential 90-degree rotations of the head, moving 360 degrees from the head turned on the side of the affected ear (or from the supine position) toward the unaffected side until the head is back to the original position, each position being held for 30 s.[40] It is the better-studied maneuver, as it is the most frequently used procedure in case series and prospective cohorts, several of which have demonstrated response rates from 50% (for the apogeotropic form) to 100% (for the geotropic form) with use of this maneuver.[46,53,85–90]

The Gufoni maneuver can be performed for either geotropic or apogeotropic lateral canal BPPV. For the geotropic form, the sitting patient quickly bends to lie on the unaffected ear for 30 s and the head is then rapidly turned 45 degrees down toward the ground for 2 min before sitting back up.[1,48] For the apogeotropic form, the sitting patient quickly bends to lie on the affected ear for 30 s and the head is then rapidly turned 45 degrees down toward the ground for 2 min before sitting back up for debris thought to be on the utricular side of the cupula, or the head is then rapidly turned 45 degrees up toward the ceiling for 2 min for debris thought to be on the canal side of the cupula.[1,91] The efficacy of the Gufoni maneuver over a sham maneuver[92,93] and the Lempert roll plus forced prolonged position[48] has been demonstrated in randomized trials.

A systematic review of the Gufoni maneuver including three studies for a total of 389 patients found that the Gufoni maneuver was easy to perform and more effective than a sham maneuver or vestibular suppressants for the geotropic form of lateral canal BPPV.[94]

The forced prolonged position designed by Vannucchi requires the patient to lie supine with the healthy ear down (for the geotropic form) or the affected ear down (for the apogeotropic form) for 12 h. It is a simple alternative for patients with severe symptoms who might not tolerate the other maneuvers, but it may also be performed in combination with the other techniques.[48] It is useful in patients with significantly restricted mobility as well. It was significantly more effective than one application of the Lempert roll, and it had an efficacy similar to the Gufoni maneuver in one prospective study.[95] The short-term remission rate based on case series was promising and as high as over 90%.[84,86,88,96]

Superior canal benign paroxysmal positional vertigo. There is paucity in the evidence for the management of superior canal BPPV. There are no clinical trials, and the evidence is based on case reports and case series. The PRMs used for posterior canal BPPV are also employed in the treatment of superior canal BPPV. As a superior semicircular canal is coplanar with the contralateral posterior semicircular canal, a "reverse" Epley maneuver initiated from the unaffected side has been described as a treatment.[97] Further modifications of the "reverse" Epley maneuver were described.[97–99] Therapeutic success has also been reported with the modified Epley maneuver starting from the affected side.[23,26,61,100] According to a systemic review including therapeutic data on 312 patients from 20 studies, the mean success rate was high in all three categories of PRMs for superior canal BPPV: 75.9% for the Epley or reverse Epley maneuver, 78.8% for the Yacovino maneuver, and 92% for the other nonstandard, unique maneuvers.[24] The Yacovino maneuver has the advantage of not requiring identification of the affected side. It comprises four stages with 30-s intervals: the patient is first brought from the sitting position to the supine head-hanging position; the head is then tilted forward so that the chin is in contact with the chest; and finally, the patient returns to the sitting position.[66,101] It was inspired by Crevits who reported successful remission in two patients who were administered a forced prolonged technique for 24 h during which they were in the supine position with the head bent forward and supported by a pulley system.[102]

Surgery for refractory benign paroxysmal positional vertigo

BPPV is intractable in a very small number of patients who do not recover spontaneously or respond to PRMs. If they are debilitated by their symptoms, these patients become candidates for surgical intervention.

For refractory posterior canal BPPV, there are two recognized operations: singular neurectomy and posterior semicircular canal occlusion.[12,103,104] The latter has demonstrated success rates near 90% in uncontrolled reports[20,105–107] and has become the favored procedure, as it is simpler than the former. Nguyen-Huynh summarized the outcomes of both singular neurectomy (six case series) and posterior canal occlusion for refractory posterior canal BPPV (eight case series).[108] For singular neurectomy, the cure rate was 96%, the rate of postoperative hearing loss greater than 10 dB pure tone average was 7%, and 43% of the patients who had a postoperative ENG/VNG electronystagmography/videonystagmography were found to have absent or reduced caloric responses. Singular neurectomy is acknowledged as a technically difficult procedure. For posterior semicircular canal occlusion, the cure rate was 100%, the rate of postoperative hearing loss greater than 10 dB pure tone average was 7%, and 22% of the patients who had a postoperative ENG/VNG were found to have absent or reduced caloric responses.

Successful resolution of refractory cases of lateral canal BPPV[109] and superior canal BPPV with respective semicircular canal plugging has also been reported in case reports.[59,110]

Vestibular rehabilitation therapy

PRMs are more effective at treating BPPV in the short term than vestibular rehabilitation therapy, but a combination of the two therapies is effective for long-term functional recovery[111] and may reduce recurrence while improving balance in the short term.[112,113] However, the addition of vestibular rehabilitation therapy was not found to affect resolution or recurrence in elderly patients with chronic BPPV, but the numbers were small in this randomized trial.[114] There appears to be a small, beneficial effect on balance, but no effect on vertigo intensity, of vestibular rehabilitation in addition to a PRM.[115]

VESTIBULAR NEURITIS

Introduction

VN is an acute vestibular syndrome and is the second most common cause of acute vertigo after BPPV, with an estimated incidence at approximately 3.5 per 100,000 population.[5,116] VN typically presents as a spontaneous, sudden onset of vertigo that can persist for hours to days. The severe constant nature of the vertigo (present even without head motion), along with the extended duration, is what differentiates VN from other causes of acute vertigo (Table 1.3). There are often other associated symptoms, including tinnitus and aural fullness, nausea and vomiting, headache, and other autonomic symptoms. Hearing loss is not typical for VN; presence of objective hearing loss should make the clinician consider other diagnoses such as acute labyrinthitis or idiopathic sudden sensorineural hearing loss with vertigo.

Pathophysiology

VN results from unilateral sudden loss of afferent neuronal input from the vestibular nerve. It predominantly affects the superior division but can affect the inferior division or both.[117] In the same vein that idiopathic sudden sensorineural hearing loss is thought to result from acute loss of cochlear nerve function, VN can be

TABLE 1.3 Common Causes of Vertigo Classified by Duration of Symptoms	
Duration of Vertigo	**Differential Diagnosis**
Seconds to minutes	Benign paroxysmal positional vertigo Superior semicircular canal dehiscence Perilymph fistula Dynamic symptoms from previously uncompensated vestibulopathy Vestibular paroxsmia Vertebrobasilar insufficiency Cardiovascular cause
Minutes to hours	Meniere disease Vestibular migraine Autoimmune inner ear disease
Hours to days	Vestibular neuritis Vestibular migraine Labyrinthitis Functional dizziness (anxiety, stress related)
Chronic	Bilateral vestibular hypofunction Functional dizziness (anxiety, stress related) Persistent postural perceptual dizziness

thought of as acute sensorineural vestibular loss. Given that vestibular neurons have a resting firing rate, loss of unilateral input leads to a sudden imbalance in afferent input, causing vertigo. The etiology of this sudden vestibular loss is controversial; however, the likeliest pathophysiology is related to reactivation of herpes simplex virus type I (HSV-1).[117-121] Rarely, patients with a schwannoma arising from the cochlear nerve or cochlea may present with acute vertigo.[122] There may be small branch vessel occlusion causing ischemia of the vestibular nerve.[123] The lifetime recurrence rate of VN is estimated at between 2% and 11%, with a small proportion of patients being more at risk of developing BPPV as well.[124-126]

Diagnosis

Patients with VN usually present with a spontaneous, sudden onset of acute vertigo and nystagmus. There is usually no clear inciting event or precipitating activity nor is it brought on by specific body or head movements. However, prodromal symptoms, consisting of nonvertiginous dizziness, nausea, vomiting, or viral illness-type symptoms, may be reported.[127,128] Severe vertigo typically lasts from hours to days and is present even at rest. There are commonly associated nausea and vomiting and other autonomic symptoms. On examination, patients have nystagmus in a direction corresponding to the semicircular canals that have been affected. Horizontal nystagmus is observed for the lateral semicircular canals, whereas mixed vertical and torsional nystagmus is observed for the superior or posterior semicircular canals. Most commonly, the superior vestibular nerve, which innervates the lateral and superior semicircular canals, is affected, so the most common pattern of nystagmus is horizontal combined with up-beating and torsional, beating away from the side of the lesion. This nystagmus obeys Alexander's

law in that it becomes more intense when looking in the direction of the fast phase of nystagmus and is direction fixed.

The diagnostic priority in the acutely vertiginous patient is to differentiate VN from a central cause of acute vertigo, such as cerebellar infarction. This can be done by applying a battery of clinical examinations called the HINTS examination (Table 1.4). When applied to the acutely vertiginous patient who has nystagmus, the HINTS examination is highly sensitive and specific for stroke.[131-133] Initial diffusion-weighted magnetic resonance imaging, the current gold standard imaging study for stroke, has a false-negative rate of up to 20% in patients with stroke in the first 48 h.[131,133]

Management

The management of VN starts with symptom management. Patients should be stabilized if there has been a significant history of fluid loss from vomiting. Commonly used pharmacologic agents in VN include vestibular suppressants, antiemetics, and steroids. It should be noted that pharmacologic therapy in VN is most appropriate during the acute phase. Many of these medications can hamper central compensation and result in prolonged or incomplete recovery over time.[134]

Vestibular suppressants

The intense vertigo and nystagmus resulting from acute unilateral vestibular loss (and resultant vestibular imbalance) can be reduced by the use of vestibular suppressants. These medications also aim to decrease symptoms of motion sensitivity and motion sickness. As such, they are commonly used medications in the treatment of VN. Most agents can also be given by injection because patients with VN are

---

	TABLE 1.4 Clinical Examinations in the HINTS Examination		
	Examination	**Findings in Vestibular Neuritis**	**Findings in Cerebellar Stroke**
HI	Head Impulse test	Saccadic eye correction toward the visual target when the head is thrust toward the side of the lesion; no saccadic eye correction when the head is thrust toward the contralateral side	Saccadic eye correction toward the visual target when the head is thrust in either direction may be seen (depending on the location of the stroke), but more commonly, the head impulse test is negative[129,130]
N	Nystagmus type	Spontaneous jerk nystagmus, beating away from the side of the lesion, direction fixed	Direction-changing or gaze-evoked nystagmus
TS	Test of Skew	No skew deviation	Positive vertical skew deviation

often extremely nauseated and might not tolerate oral medication.

Benzodiazepines are commonly used as vestibular suppressants in the acute setting. Examples of benzodiazepines used in VN include diazepam, clonazepam, and lorazepam. This group of medications suppresses vestibular responses by centrally potentiating inhibitory γ-aminobutyric acid receptors. They also have the added effect of being anxiolytic, which helps to minimize the panic associated with acute vertigo. They are used in small doses and can be effective in the acute phase of VN and should be stopped as soon as severe vertigo and spontaneous nystagmus have subsided. Common side effects include sedation, habituation, impaired memory, increased risk of falls, and poor vestibular compensation.[134]

Antihistamines act by reducing the symptoms of motion sickness associated with acute vertigo.[135] They are often also antiemetic in action. The exact mechanism of their action on the vestibular system is unknown, but it is thought to revolve around modification of cochlear blood flow.[136] Common antihistamines in use for VN include meclizine, dimenhydrinate, and diphenhydramine. Scopolamine is an anticholinergic alkaloid that exerts its effects by blocking cholinergic transmission between vestibular nuclei and higher centers. It is commonly used in patch form for reducing the effects of motion sickness.[137]

Antiemetics
The vestibular suppressants described in the previous section also act as antiemetics. Dimenhydrinate and scopolamine are commonly used to treat the nausea and vomiting associated with VN. Metoclopramide works by speeding up gastric emptying and may have some benefits in acute vertigo.[138] Ondansetron is a powerful serotonin antagonist that has proven efficacy in chemotherapy-induced nausea and vomiting. Early studies show this benefit may extend to acute vertigo.[139] Dexamethasone is commonly used as an antiemetic agent in postoperative recovery, but its use in VN is still under investigation.[140]

Betahistine
The mechanism of action of betahistine is thought to be via vasodilation of cochlear blood vessels through agonist action on H1-receptors and antagonist action on H3-receptors.[136] Its use in Meniere disease is widespread, but there is lack of strong evidence to support its efficacy.[141,142] However, it is an extremely commonly prescribed medication by primary care physicians in the emergency care setting. More controlled trials are needed to determine the true effects of betahistine before it can be recommended as an appropriate treatment in VN.[143]

Antivirals
Although there is evidence that VN is caused by the reactivation of HSV-1 in the vestibular nerve,[121] there is lack of evidence to support the use of antivirals for initial management.[144] This would be consistent with other disease processes that are thought to be caused by viral reactivation (for example, Ramsay-Hunt syndrome) where antivirals have proven to be ineffective.[145]

Steroids
Steroids have shown efficacy in returning nerve function in disorders such as idiopathic sudden sensorineural hearing loss[146] and idiopathic facial nerve paralysis (Bell palsy).[147] Despite similarities in pathophysiology between these conditions and VN, evidence has not been convincing thus far on the benefits of steroids, whether in oral, intravenous, or intratympanic form, for patient symptoms or eventual vestibular function in VN.[148-154] More controlled trials are still needed to determine the true efficacy of steroids in VN.

Vestibular rehabilitation therapy
Physiotherapy after acute vestibulopathy aims to rebuild the vestibuloocular reflex function and postural control through the use of active head and eye movement exercises and goal-directed postural training.[155] There is now strong evidence that vestibular rehabilitation therapy should be offered to patients recovering from all forms of acute or chronic unilateral or bilateral vestibular hypofunction.[156-165] In VN, patients can be started on vestibular rehabilitation therapy once the acute phase is resolved. More recently, there is work being done on how to effectively perform vestibular rehabilitation using common electronic gaming devices,[166-169] or even remotely via mobile applications.[170]

REFERENCES

1. Bhattacharyya N, Gubbels SP, Schwartz SR, et al. Clinical practice guideline: benign paroxysmal positional vertigo (update). *Otolaryngol Head Neck Surg.* 2017;156(3S):S1–S47.
2. American Academy of Otolaryngology-Head and Neck Foundation, Inc., Committee on hearing and equilibrium guidelines for the diagnosis and evaluation of therapy in Menière's disease. *Otolaryngol Head Neck Surg.* 1995;113(3):181–185.

3. Neuhauser HK. The epidemiology of dizziness and vertigo. In: Furman JM, Lempert T, eds. *Handbook of Clinical Neurology (3rd Series)*. vol. 137. Elsevier; 2016:67–82.

4. Neuhauser HK, Radtke A, von Brevern M, Lezius F, Feldmann M, Lempert T. Burden of dizziness and vertigo in the community. *Arch Intern Med*. 2008;168(19):2118–2124.

5. Jeong SH, Kim HJ, Kim JS. Vestibular neuritis. *Semin Neurol*. 2013;33(3):185–194.

6. Hanley K, O'Dowd T. Symptoms of vertigo in general practice: a prospective study of diagnosis. *Br J Gen Pract*. 2002;52(483):809–812.

7. von Brevern M, Radtke A, Lezius F, et al. Epidemiology of benign paroxysmal positional vertigo: a population based study. *J Neurol Neurosurg Psychiatry*. 2007;78(7):710–717.

8. Baloh RW, Honrubia V, Jacobson K. Benign positional vertigo. Clinical and oculographic features in 240 cases. *Neurology*. 1987;37(3):371–378.

9. Katsarkas A. Benign paroxysmal positional vertigo (BPPV): idiopathic versus post-traumatic. *Acta Otolaryngol*. 1999;119(7):745–749.

10. Neuhauser HK, Lempert T. Vertigo: epidemiologic aspects. *Semin Neurol*. 2009;29(5):473–481.

11. Parnes LS, McClure JA. Free-floating endolymph particles: a new operative finding during posterior semicircular canal occlusion. *Laryngoscope*. 1992;102(9):988–992.

12. Parnes LS, Agrawal SK, Atlas J. Diagnosis and management of benign paroxysmal positional vertigo (BPPV). *CMAJ*. 2003;169(7):681–693.

13. Hughes CA, Proctor L. Benign paroxysmal positional vertigo. *Laryngoscope*. 1997;107(5):607–613.

14. Dispenza F, De Stefano A, Mathur N, Croce A, Gallina S. Benign paroxysmal positional vertigo following whiplash injury: a myth or a reality? *Am J Otolaryngol*. 2011;32(5):376–380.

15. Lee NH, Ban JH, Lee KC, Kim SM. Benign paroxysmal positional vertigo secondary to inner ear disease. *Otolaryngol Head Neck Surg*. 2010;143(3):413–417.

16. Kim MB, Ban JH. Benign paroxysmal positional vertigo accompanied by sudden sensorineural hearing loss: a comparative study with idiopathic benign paroxysmal positional vertigo. *Laryngoscope*. 2012;122(12):2832–2836.

17. Epley JM. New dimensions of benign paroxysmal positional vertigo. *Otolaryngol Head Neck Surg*. 1980;88(5):599–605.

18. Epley JM. Human experience with canalith repositioning maneuvers. *Ann NY Acad Sci*. 2001;942:179–191.

19. Welling DB, Parnes LS, O'Brien B, Bakaletz LO, Brackmann DE, Hinojosa R. Particulate matter in the posterior semicircular canal. *Laryngoscope*. 1997;107(1):90–94.

20. Agrawal SK, Parnes LS. Human experience with canal plugging. *Ann NY Acad Sci*. 2001;942:300–305.

21. Herdman SJ, Tusa RJ. Complications of the canalith repositioning procedure. *Arch Otolaryngol Head Neck Surg*. 1996;122(3):281–286.

22. Yimtae K, Srirompotong S, Srirompotong S, Sae-Seaw P. A randomized trial of the canalith repositioning procedure. *Laryngoscope*. 2003;113(5):828–832.

23. Imbaud-Genieys S. Anterior semicircular canal benign paroxysmal positional vertigo: a series of 20 patients. *Eur Ann Otorhinolaryngol Head Neck Dis*. 2013;130(6):303–307.

24. Anagnostou E, Kouzi I, Spengos K. Diagnosis and treatment of anterior-canal benign paroxysmal positional vertigo: a systematic review. *J Clin Neurol*. 2015;11(3):262–267.

25. Kim J-S, Zee DS. Clinical practice: benign paroxysmal positional vertigo. *N Engl J Med*. 2014;370(12):1138–1147.

26. Jackson LE, Morgan B, Fletcher JC, Krueger WW. Anterior canal benign paroxysmal positional vertigo: an underappreciated entity. *Otol Neurotol*. 2007;28(2):218–222.

27. Chung KW, Park KN, Ko MH, et al. Incidence of horizontal canal benign paroxysmal positional vertigo as a function of the duration of symptoms. *Otol Neurotol*. 2009;30(2):202–205.

28. Babac S, Djeric D, Petrovic-Lazic M, Arsovic N, Mikic A. Why do treatment failure and recurrences of benign paroxysmal positional vertigo occur? *Otol Neurotol*. 2014;35(6):1105–1110.

29. De Stefano A, Dispenza F, Suarez H, et al. A multicenter observational study on the role of comorbidities in the recurrent episodes of benign paroxysmal positional vertigo. *Auris Nasus Larynx*. 2014;41(1):31–36.

30. von Brevern M. Benign paroxysmal positional vertigo. *Semin Neurol*. 2013;33(3):204–211.

31. Imai T, Ito M, Takeda N, et al. Natural course of the remission of vertigo in patients with benign paroxysmal positional vertigo. *Neurology*. 2005;64(5):920–921.

32. Tomaz A, Gananca MM, Gananca CF, Gananca FF, Caovilla HH, Harker L. Benign paroxysmal positional vertigo: concomitant involvement of different semicircular canals. *Ann Otol Rhinol Laryngol*. 2009;118(2):113–117.

33. Brandt T, Daroff RB. Physical therapy for benign paroxysmal positional vertigo. *Arch Otolaryngol*. 1980;106(8):484–485.

34. Dorresteijn PM, Ipenburg NA, Murphy KJ, et al. Rapid systematic review of normal audiometry results as a predictor for benign paroxysmal positional vertigo. *Otolaryngol Head Neck Surg*. 2014;150(6):919–924.

35. Kentala E. Characteristics of six otologic diseases involving vertigo. *Am J Otol*. 1996;17(6):883–892.

36. Kentala E, Pyykkö I. Vertigo in patients with benign paroxysmal positional vertigo. *Acta Otolaryngol Suppl*. 2000;543:20–22.

37. Chang MB, Bath AP, Rutka JA. Are all atypical positional nystagmus patterns reflective of central pathology? *J Otolaryngol*. 2001;30(5):280–282.

38. Dix MR, Hallpike CS. Pathology, symptomatology and diagnosis of certain disorders of the vestibular system. *Proc R Soc Med*. 1952;45(6):341–354.

39. Furman JM, Cass SP. Benign paroxysmal positional vertigo. *N Engl J Med.* 1999;341(21):1590–1596.

40. Fife TD, Iverson DJ, Lempert T, et al. Practice parameter: therapies for benign paroxysmal positional vertigo (an evidence-based review). Report of the Quality Standards Subcommittee of the American Academy of Neurology. *Neurology.* 2008;70(22):2067–2074.

41. Hilton M, Pinder D. The Epley (canalith repositioning) manoeuvre for benign paroxysmal positional vertigo. *Cochrane Database Syst Rev.* 2014;(12):CD003162.

42. Cohen HS. Side-lying as an alternative to the Dix-Hallpike test of the posterior canal. *Otol Neurotol.* 2004;25(2):130–134.

43. Halker RB, Barrs DM, Wellik KE, Wingerchuk DM, Demaerschalk BM. Establishing a diagnosis of benign paroxysmal positional vertigo through the Dix-Hallpike and side-lying maneuvers: a critically appraised topic. *Neurologist.* 2008;14(3):201–204.

44. Hoffman RM, Einstadter D, Kroenke K. Evaluating dizziness. *Am J Med.* 1999;107(5):468–478.

45. Lopez-Escamez JA, Lopez-Nevot A, Gamiz MJ, et al. Diagnosis of common causes of vertigo using a structured clinical history. *Acta Otorhinolaryngol Esp.* 2000;51(1):25–30.

46. Nuti D, Agus G, Barbieri MT, Passali D. The management of horizontal-canal paroxysmal positional vertigo. *Acta Otolaryngol.* 1998;118(4):455–460.

47. Steenerson RL, Cronin GW, Marbach PM. Effectiveness of treatment techniques in 923 cases of benign paroxysmal positional vertigo. *Laryngoscope.* 2005;115(2):226–231.

48. Casani AP, Nacci A, Dallan I, Panicucci E, Gufoni M, Sellari-Francheschini S. Horizontal semicircular canal benign paroxysmal positional vertigo: effectiveness of two different methods of treatment. *Audiol Neurootol.* 2011;16(3):175–184.

49. Cakir BO, Ercan I, Cakir ZA, Civelek S, Sayin I, Turgut S. What is the true incidence of horizontal semicircular canal benign paroxysmal positional vertigo? *Otolaryngol Head Neck Surg.* 2006;134(3):451–454.

50. McClure JA. Horizontal canal BPV. *J Otolaryngol.* 1985;14(1):30–35.

51. Pagnini P, Nuti D, Vannucchi P. Benign paroxysmal vertigo of the horizontal canal. *ORL J Otorhinolaryngol Relat Spec.* 1989;51(3):161–170.

52. Baloh RW, Jacobson K, Honrubia V. Horizontal semicircular canal variant of benign positional vertigo. *Neurology.* 1993;43(12):2542–2549.

53. White JA, Coale KD, Catalano PJ, Oas JG. Diagnosis and management of lateral semicircular canal benign paroxysmal positional vertigo. *Otolaryngol Head Neck Surg.* 2005;133(2):278–284.

54. Lee SH, Choi KD, Jeong SH, Oh YM, Koo JW, Kim JS. Nystagmus during neck flexion in the pitch plane in benign paroxysmal positional vertigo involving the horizontal canal. *J Neurol Sci.* 2007;256(1–2):75–80.

55. Hwang M, Kim SH, Kang KW, et al. Canalith repositioning in apogeotropic horizontal canal benign paroxysmal positional vertigo: do we need faster maneuvering? *J Neurol Sci.* 2015;358(1–2):183–187.

56. Choung YH, Shin YR, Kahng H, Park K, Choi SJ. 'Bow and lean test' to determine the affected ear of horizontal canal benign paroxysmal positional vertigo. *Laryngoscope.* 2006;116(10):1776–1781.

57. Lee JB, Han DH, Choi SJ, et al. Efficacy of the "bow and lean test" for the management of horizontal canal benign paroxysmal positional vertigo. *Laryngoscope.* 2010;120(11):2339–2346.

58. Casani AP, Cerchiai N, Dallan I, Sellari-Franceschini S. Anterior canal lithiasis: diagnosis and treatment. *Otolaryngol Head Neck Surg.* 2011;144:412–418.

59. Naples JG, Eisen MD. Surgical management for benign paroxysmal positional vertigo of the superior semicircular canal. *Laryngoscope.* 2015;125(8):1965–1967.

60. Korres SG, Balatsouras DG. Diagnostic, pathophysiologic, and therapeutic aspects of benign paroxysmal positional vertigo. *Otolaryngol Head Neck Surg.* 2004;131(4):438–444.

61. Lopez-Escamez JA, Molina MI, Gamiz MJ. Anterior semicircular canal benign paroxysmal positional vertigo and positional downbeating nystagmus. *Am J Otolaryngol.* 2006;27(3):173–178.

62. Jackson L, Morgan B, Fletcher J, Krueger WW. Anterior canal benign paroxysmal vertigo: an underappreciated entity. *Otol Neurotol.* 2007;28(2):218–222.

63. Bertholon P, Bronstein AM, Davies RS, Rudge P, Thilo KV. Positional down beating nystagmus in 50 patients: cerebellar disorders and possible anterior semicircular canal canalithiasis. *J Neurol Neurosurg Psychiatry.* 2002;72(3):366–372.

64. Ogawa Y, Suzuki M, Otsuka K, et al. Positional and positioning down-beating nystagmus without central nervous system findings. *Auris Nasus Larynx.* 2009;36(6):698–701.

65. Fife TD. Benign paroxysmal positional vertigo. *Semin Neurol.* 2009;29(5):500–508.

66. Nuti D, Masini M, Mandala M. Benign paroxysmal positional vertigo and its variants. In: Furman JM, Lempert T, eds. *Handbook of Clinical Neurology (3rd Series).* vol. 137. Elsevier; 2016:241–256.

67. Epley JM. The canalith repositioning procedure: for treatment of benign paroxysmal positional vertigo. *Otolaryngol Head Neck Surg.* 1992;107(3):399–404.

68. Semont A, Freyss G, Vitte E. Curing the BPPV with a liberatory maneuver. *Adv Otorhinolaryngol.* 1998;42:290–293.

69. von Brevern M, Seelig T, Radtke A, Tiel-Wilck K, Neuhauser H, Lempert T. Short-term efficacy of Epley's manoeuvre: a double-blind randomised trial. *J Neurol Neurosurg Psychiatry.* 2006;77(8):980–982.

70. Seo T, Miyamoto A, Saka N, Shimano K, Sakagami M. Immediate efficacy of the canalith repositioning procedure for the treatment of benign paroxysmal positional vertigo. *Otol Neurotol.* 2007;28(7):917–919.

71. Prokopakis E, Vlastos IM, Tsagournisakis M, Christodoulou P, Kawauchi H, Velegrakis G. Canalith repositioning procedures among 965 patients with benign paroxysmal positional vertigo. *Audiol Neurootol.* 2013;18(2):83–88.

72. Oh HJ, Kim JS, Han BI, Lim JG. Predicting a successful treatment in posterior canal benign paroxysmal positional vertigo. *Neurology.* 2007;68(15):1219–1222.

73. Reinink H, Wegner I, Stegeman I, Grolman W. Rapid systematic review of repeated application of the Epley maneuver for treating posterior BPPV. *Otolaryngol Head Neck Surg.* 2014;151(3):399–406.

74. Woodworth BA, Gillespie MB, Lambert PR. The canalith repositioning procedure for benign positional vertigo: a meta-analysis. *Laryngoscope.* 2004;114(7):1143–1146.

75. Helminski JO, Zee DS, Janssen I, Hain TC. Effectiveness of particle repositioning maneuvers in the treatment of benign paroxysmal positional vertigo: a systematic review. *Phys Ther.* 2010;90(5):663–678.

76. van Duijn JG, Isfordink LM, Nij Bijvank JA, et al. Rapid systematic review of the Epley maneuver for treating posterior canal benign paroxysmal positional vertigo. *Otolaryngol Head Neck Surg.* 2014;150(6):925–932.

77. Chen Y, Zhuang J, Zhang L, et al. Short-term efficacy of Semont maneuver for benign paroxysmal positional vertigo: a double-blind randomized trial. *Otol Neurotol.* 2012;33(7):1127–1130.

78. Mandala M, Santoro GP, Asprella Libonati G, et al. Double-blind randomized trial on short-term efficacy of the Semont maneuver for the treatment of posterior canal benign paroxysmal positional vertigo. *J Neurol.* 2012;259(5):882–885.

79. Zhang X, Qian X, Lu L, et al. Effects of Semont maneuver on benign paroxysmal positional vertigo: a meta-analysis. *Acta Otolaryngol (Stockh).* 2017;137(1):63–70.

80. Liu Y, Wang W, Zhang AB, Bai X, Zhang S. Epley and Semont maneuvers for posterior canal benign paroxysmal positional vertigo: a network meta-analysis. *Laryngoscope.* 2016;126(4):951–955.

81. Lee JD, Shim DB, Park HJ, et al. A multicenter randomized double-blind study: comparison of the Epley, Semont, and sham maneuvers for the treatment of posterior canal benign paroxysmal positional vertigo. *Audiol Neurootol.* 2014;19(5):336–341.

82. Lempert T. Horizontal benign positional vertigo. *Neurology.* 1994;44(11):2213–2214.

83. Gufoni M, Mastrosimone L, Di Nasso F. Repositioning maneuver in benign paroxysmal vertigo of horizontal semicircular canal. *Acta Otorhinolaryngol Ital.* 1998;18(6):363–367.

84. Vannucchi P, Giannoni B, Pagnini P. Treatment of horizontal semicircular canal benign paroxysmal positional vertigo. *J Vestib Res.* 1997;7(1):1–6.

85. Lempert T, Tiel-Wilck K. A positional maneuver for treatment of horizontal-canal benign positional vertigo. *Laryngoscope.* 1996;106(4):476–478.

86. Appiani GC, Gagliardi M, Magliulo G. Physical treatment of horizontal canal benign positional vertigo. *Eur Arch Otorhinolaryngol.* 1997;254(7):326–328.

87. Fife TD. Recognition and management of horizontal canal benign positional vertigo. *Am J Otol.* 1998;19(3):345–351.

88. Casani AP, Vannucci G, Fattori B, Berrettini S. The treatment of horizontal canal positional vertigo: our experience in 66 cases. *Laryngoscope.* 2002;112(1):172–178.

89. Tirelli G, Russolo M. 360-Degree canalith repositioning procedure for the horizontal canal. *Otolaryngol Head Neck Surg.* 2004;131(5):740–746.

90. Prokopakis EP, Chimona T, Tsagournisakis M, et al. Benign paroxysmal positional vertigo: 10-year experience in treating 592 patients with canalith repositioning procedure. *Laryngoscope.* 2005;115(9):1667–1671.

91. Kim JS, Oh SY, Lee SH, et al. Randomized clinical trial for apogeotropic horizontal canal benign paroxysmal positional vertigo. *Neurology.* 2012;78(3):159–166.

92. Kim JS, Oh SY, Lee SH, et al. Randomized clinical trial for geotropic horizontal canal benign paroxysmal positional vertigo. *Neurology.* 2012;79(7):700–707.

93. Mandala M, Pepponi E, Santoro GP, et al. Double-blind randomized trial on the efficacy of the Gufoni maneuver for treatment of lateral canal BPPV. *Laryngoscope.* 2013;123(7):1782–1786.

94. van den Broek EM, van der Zaag-Loonen HJ, Bruintjes TD. Systematic review: efficacy of Gufoni maneuver for treatment of lateral canal benign paroxysmal positional vertigo with geotropic nystagmus. *Otolaryngol Head Neck Surg.* 2014;150(6):933–938.

95. Korres S, Riga MG, Xenellis J, Korres GS, Danielides V. Treatment of the horizontal semicircular canal canalithiasis: pros and cons of the repositioning maneuvers in a clinical study and critical review of the literature. *Otol Neurotol.* 2011;32(8):1302–1308.

96. Chiou WY, Lee HL, Tsai SC, Yu TH, Lee XX. A single therapy for all subtypes of horizontal canal positional vertigo. *Laryngoscope.* 2005;115(8):1432–1435.

97. Rahko T. The test and treatment methods of benign paroxysmal vertigo and an addition to the management of vertigo due to the superior vestibular canal (BPPV-SC). *Clin Otolaryngol Allied Sci.* 2002;27(5):392–395.

98. Kim YK, Shin JE, Chung JW. The effect of canalith repositioning for anterior semicircular canal canalithiasis. *ORL J Otorhinolaryngol Relat Spec.* 2005;67(1):56–60.

99. Park S, Kim BG, Kim SH, Chu H, Song MY, Kim M. Canal conversion between anterior and posterior semicircular canal in benign paroxysmal positional vertigo. *Otol Neurotol.* 2013;34(9):1725–1728.

100. Lopez-Escamez JA, Molina MI, Gamiz M, et al. Multiple positional nystagmus suggests multiple canal involvement in benign paroxysmal vertigo. *Acta Otolaryngol.* 2005;125(9):954–961.

101. Yacovino DA, Hain TC, Gualtieri F. New therapeutic manoeuvre for anterior canal benign paroxysmal positional vertigo. *J Neurol.* 2009;256(11):1851–1855.

102. Crevits L. Treatment of anterior canal benign paroxysmal positional vertigo by a prolonged forced position procedure. *J Neurol Neurosurg Psychiatry.* 2004;75(5):779–781.

103. Gacek RR. Technique and results of singular neurectomy for the management of benign paroxysmal positional vertigo. *Acta Otolaryngol.* 1995;115(2):154–157.

104. Leveque M, Labrousse M, Seidermann L, Chays A. Surgical therapy in intractable benign paroxysmal positional vertigo. *Otolaryngol Head Neck Surg.* 2007;136(5):693–698.

105. Kisilevsky V, Bailie NA, Dutt SN, Rutka JA. Lessons learned from the surgical management of benign paroxysmal positional vertigo: the University Health Network experience with posterior semicircular canal occlusion surgery (1988-2006). *J Otolaryngol Head Neck Surg.* 2009;38(2):212–221.

106. Ahmed RM, Pohl DV, MacDougall HG, Makeham T, Halmagyi GM. Posterior semicircular canal occlusion for intractable benign positional vertigo: outcome in 55 ears in 53 patients operated upon over 20 years. *J Laryngol Otol.* 2012;126(7):677–682.

107. Ramakrishna J, Goebel JA, Parnes LS. Efficacy and safety of bilateral posterior canal occlusion in patients with refractory benign paroxysmal positional vertigo: case report series. *Otol Neurotol.* 2012;33(4):640–642.

108. Nguyen-Huynh AT. Evidence-based practice: management of vertigo. *Otolaryngol Clin North Am.* 2012;45(5):925–940.

109. Zhu Q, Liu C, Lin C, et al. Efficacy and safety of semicircular canal occlusion for intractable horizontal semicircular benign paroxysmal positional vertigo. *Ann Otol Rhinol Laryngol.* 2015;124(4):257–260.

110. Brantberg K, Bergenius J. Treatment of anterior benign paroxysmal positional vertigo by canal plugging: a case report. *Acta Otolaryngol.* 2002;122(1):28–30.

111. McDonnell MN, Hillier SL. Vestibular rehabilitation for unilateral peripheral vestibular dysfunction. *Cochrane Database Syst Rev.* 2015;(1):CD005397.

112. Chang WC, Yang YR, Hsu LC, Chern CM, Wang RY. Balance improvement in patients with benign paroxysmal positional vertigo. *Clin Rehabil.* 2008;22(4):338–347.

113. Toledo H, Cortes ML, Pane C, Trujillo V. Semont maneuver and vestibular rehabilitation exercises in the treatment of benign paroxysmal postural vertigo. A comparative study. *Neurologia.* 2000;15(4):152–157.

114. Ribeiro KM, Ferreira LM, Freitas RV, Silva CN, Deshpande N, Guerra RO. "Positive to negative" Dix-Hallpike test and benign paroxysmal positional vertigo recurrence in elderly undergoing canalith repositioning maneuver and vestibular rehabilitation. *Int Arch Otorhinolaryngol.* 2016;20(4):344–352.

115. van der Scheer-Host E, van Benthem PP, Bruintjes TD, van Leeuwen RB, van der Zaag-Loonen H. The efficacy of vestibular rehabilitation in patients with benign paroxysmal positional vertigo: a rapid review. *Otolaryngol Head Neck Surg.* 2014;151(5):740–745.

116. Kroenke K, Hoffman RM, Einstadter D. How common are various causes of dizziness? A critical review. *South Med J.* 2000;93(2):160–167; quiz 168.

117. Himmelein S, Lindemann A, Sinicina I, et al. Differential involvement during latent HSV-1 infection of the superior and inferior divisions of the vestibular ganglia: implications for vestibular neuritis. *J Virol.* 2017;91.

118. Arbusow V, Schulz P, Strupp M, et al. Distribution of herpes simplex virus type 1 in human geniculate and vestibular ganglia: implications for vestibular neuritis. *Ann Neurol.* 1999;46(3):416–419.

119. Arbusow V, Strupp M, Wasicky R, Horn AK, Schulz P, Brandt T. Detection of herpes simplex virus type 1 in human vestibular nuclei. *Neurology.* 2000;55(6):880–882.

120. Davis LE. Viruses and vestibular neuritis: review of human and animal studies. *Acta Otolaryngol Suppl.* 1993;503:70–73.

121. Esaki S, Goshima F, Kimura H, et al. Auditory and vestibular defects induced by experimental labyrinthitis following herpes simplex virus in mice. *Acta Otolaryngol.* 2011;131(7):684–691.

122. Jiang ZY, Kutz Jr JW, Roland PS, Isaacson B. Intracochlear schwannomas confined to the otic capsule. *Otol Neurotol.* 2011;32(7):1175–1179.

123. Gianoli G, Goebel J, Mowry S, Poomipannit P. Anatomic differences in the lateral vestibular nerve channels and their implications in vestibular neuritis. *Otol Neurotol.* 2005;26(3):489–494.

124. Huppert D, Strupp M, Theil D, Glaser M, Brandt T. Low recurrence rate of vestibular neuritis: a long-term follow-up. *Neurology.* 2006;67(10):1870–1871.

125. Kim YH, Kim KS, Kim KJ, Choi H, Choi JS, Hwang IK. Recurrence of vertigo in patients with vestibular neuritis. *Acta Otolaryngol.* 2011;131(11):1172–1177.

126. Mandala M, Santoro GP, Awrey J, Nuti D. Vestibular neuritis: recurrence and incidence of secondary benign paroxysmal positional vertigo. *Acta Otolaryngol.* 2010;130(5):565–567.

127. Lee H, Kim BK, Park HJ, Koo JW, Kim JS. Prodromal dizziness in vestibular neuritis: frequency and clinical implication. *J Neurol Neurosurg Psychiatry.* 2009;80(3):355–356.

128. Silvoniemi P. Vestibular neuronitis. An otoneurological evaluation. *Acta Otolaryngol Suppl.* 1988;453:1–72.

129. Cnyrim CD, Newman-Toker D, Karch C, Brandt T, Strupp M. Bedside differentiation of vestibular neuritis from central "vestibular pseudoneuritis". *J Neurol Neurosurg Psychiatry.* 2008;79(4):458–460.

130. Kremmyda O, Kirchner H, Glasauer S, Brandt T, Jahn K, Strupp M. False-positive head-impulse test in cerebellar ataxia. *Front Neurol.* 2012;3:162.

131. Kattah JC, Talkad AV, Wang DZ, Hsieh YH, Newman-Toker DE. HINTS to diagnose stroke in the acute vestibular syndrome: three-step bedside oculomotor examination more sensitive than early MRI diffusion-weighted imaging. *Stroke.* 2009;40(11):3504–3510.

132. Newman-Toker DE, Kattah JC, Alvernia JE, Wang DZ. Normal head impulse test differentiates acute cerebellar strokes from vestibular neuritis. *Neurology.* 2008;70(24 Pt 2):2378–2385.

133. Tarnutzer AA, Berkowitz AL, Robinson KA, Hsieh YH, Newman-Toker DE. Does my dizzy patient have a stroke? A systematic review of bedside diagnosis in acute vestibular syndrome. *CMAJ.* 2011;183(9):E571–E592.

134. Baloh RW. Clinical practice. Vestibular neuritis. *N Engl J Med.* 2003;348(11):1027–1032.

135. Takeda N, Morita M, Hasegawa S, Kubo T, Matsunaga T. Neurochemical mechanisms of motion sickness. *Am J Otolaryngol.* 1989;10(5):351–359.

136. Bertlich M, Ihler F, Freytag S, Weiss BG, Strupp M, Canis M. Histaminergic H3-heteroreceptors as a potential mediator of betahistine-induced increase in cochlear blood flow. *Audiol Neurootol.* 2015;20(5):283–293.

137. Renner UD, Oertel R, Kirch W. Pharmacokinetics and pharmacodynamics in clinical use of scopolamine. *Ther Drug Monit.* 2005;27(5):655–665.

138. Stewart IA, Maran AG. The effects of metoclopramide on nystagmus and vertigo. *Postgrad Med J.* 1973;49(suppl 4):19–21.

139. Venail F, Biboulet R, Mondain M, Uziel A. A protective effect of 5-HT3 antagonist against vestibular deficit? Metoclopramide versus ondansetron at the early stage of vestibular neuritis: a pilot study. *Eur Ann Otorhinolaryngol Head Neck Dis.* 2012;129(2):65–68.

140. Kim JC, Cha WW, Chang DS, Lee HY. The effect of intravenous dexamethasone on the nausea accompanying vestibular neuritis: a preliminary study. *Clin Ther.* 2015;37(11):2536–2542.

141. Adrion C, Fischer CS, Wagner J, et al. Efficacy and safety of betahistine treatment in patients with Meniere's disease: primary results of a long term, multicentre, double blind, randomised, placebo controlled, dose defining trial (BEMED trial). *BMJ.* 2016;352:h6816.

142. James AL, Burton MJ. Betahistine for Meniere's disease or syndrome. *Cochrane Database Syst Rev.* 2001;(1):CD001873.

143. Murdin L, Hussain K, Schilder AG. Betahistine for symptoms of vertigo. *Cochrane Database Syst Rev.* 2016;(6):CD010696.

144. Strupp M, Zingler VC, Arbusow V, et al. Methylprednisolone, valacyclovir, or the combination for vestibular neuritis. *N Engl J Med.* 2004;351(4):354–361.

145. Uscategui T, Doree C, Chamberlain IJ, Burton MJ. Antiviral therapy for Ramsay Hunt syndrome (herpes zoster oticus with facial palsy) in adults. *Cochrane Database Syst Rev.* 2008;(4):CD006851.

146. Han X, Yin X, Du X, Sun C. Combined intratympanic and systemic use of steroids as a first-line treatment for sudden sensorineural hearing loss: a meta-analysis of randomized, controlled trials. *Otol Neurotol.* 2017;38(4):487–495.

147. Madhok VB, Gagyor I, Daly F, et al. Corticosteroids for Bell's palsy (idiopathic facial paralysis). *Cochrane Database Syst Rev.* 2016;7:CD001942.

148. Batuecas-Caletrio A, Yanez-Gonzalez R, Sanchez-Blanco C, et al. Glucocorticoids improve acute dizziness symptoms following acute unilateral vestibulopathy. *J Neurol.* 2015;262(11):2578–2582.

149. Fishman JM, Burgess C, Waddell A. Corticosteroids for the treatment of idiopathic acute vestibular dysfunction (vestibular neuritis). *Cochrane Database Syst Rev.* 2011;(5):CD008607.

150. Goudakos JK, Markou KD, Franco-Vidal V, Vital V, Tsaligopoulos M, Darrouzet V. Corticosteroids in the treatment of vestibular neuritis: a systematic review and meta-analysis. *Otol Neurotol.* 2010;31(2):183–189.

151. Goudakos JK, Markou KD, Psillas G, Vital V, Tsaligopoulos M. Corticosteroids and vestibular exercises in vestibular neuritis. Single-blind randomized clinical trial. *JAMA Otolaryngol Head Neck Surg.* 2014;140(5):434–440.

152. Karlberg ML, Magnusson M. Treatment of acute vestibular neuronitis with glucocorticoids. *Otol Neurotol.* 2011;32(7):1140–1143.

153. Shupak A, Issa A, Golz A, Margalit K, Braverman I. Prednisone treatment for vestibular neuritis. *Otol Neurotol.* 2008;29(3):368–374.

154. Wegner I, van Benthem PP, Aarts MC, Bruintjes TD, Grolman W, van der Heijden GJ. Insufficient evidence for the effect of corticosteroid treatment on recovery of vestibular neuritis. *Otolaryngol Head Neck Surg.* 2012;147(5):826–831.

155. Whitney SL, Sparto PJ. Principles of vestibular physical therapy rehabilitation. *NeuroRehabilitation.* 2011;29(2):157–166.

156. Arnold SA, Stewart AM, Moor HM, Karl RC, Reneker JC. The effectiveness of vestibular rehabilitation interventions in treating unilateral peripheral vestibular disorders: a systematic review. *Physiother Res Int.* 2015.

157. Hall CD, Herdman SJ, Whitney SL, et al. Vestibular rehabilitation for peripheral vestibular hypofunction: an evidence-based clinical practice guideline: from the American Physical Therapy Association Neurology Section. *J Neurol Phys Ther.* 2016;40(2):124–155.

158. Hillier S, McDonnell M. Is vestibular rehabilitation effective in improving dizziness and function after unilateral peripheral vestibular hypofunction? An abridged version of a Cochrane review. *Eur J Phys Rehabil Med.* 2016;52(4):541–556.

159. Jeribi S, Yahia A, Achour I, et al. Effect of a vestibular rehabilitation protocol to improve the health-related quality of life and postural balance in patients with peripheral vertigo. *Ann Phys Rehabil Med.* 2016;59S:e125.

160. Lorin P, Donnard M, Foubert F. Vestibular neuritis: evaluation and effect of vestibular rehabilitation. *Rev Laryngol Otol Rhinol (Bord).* 2015;136(1):21–27.

161. Martins ESDC, Bastos VH, de Oliveira Sanchez M, et al. Effects of vestibular rehabilitation in the elderly: a systematic review. *Aging Clin Exp Res.* 2016;28(4):599–606.

162. Porciuncula F, Johnson CC, Glickman LB. The effect of vestibular rehabilitation on adults with bilateral vestibular hypofunction: a systematic review. *J Vestib Res.* 2012;22(5–6):283–298.

163. Ricci NA, Aratani MC, Caovilla HH, Gananca FF. Effects of vestibular rehabilitation on balance control in older people with chronic dizziness: a randomized clinical trial. *Am J Phys Med Rehabil.* 2016;95(4):256–269.

164. Rossi-Izquierdo M, Santos-Perez S, Soto-Varela A. What is the most effective vestibular rehabilitation technique in patients with unilateral peripheral vestibular disorders? *Eur Arch Otorhinolaryngol.* 2011;268(11):1569–1574.

165. Strupp M, Arbusow V, Maag KP, Gall C, Brandt T. Vestibular exercises improve central vestibulospinal compensation after vestibular neuritis. *Neurology.* 1998;51(3):838–844.

166. Meldrum D, Glennon A, Herdman S, Murray D, McConn-Walsh R. Virtual reality rehabilitation of balance: assessment of the usability of the Nintendo Wii((R)) Fit Plus. *Disabil Rehabil Assist Technol.* 2012;7(3):205–210.

167. Meldrum D, Herdman S, Moloney R, et al. Effectiveness of conventional versus virtual reality based vestibular rehabilitation in the treatment of dizziness, gait and balance impairment in adults with unilateral peripheral vestibular loss: a randomised controlled trial. *BMC Ear Nose Throat Disord.* 2012;12:3.

168. Sparrer I, Duong Dinh TA, Ilgner J, Westhofen M. Vestibular rehabilitation using the Nintendo(R) Wii Balance Board – a user-friendly alternative for central nervous compensation. *Acta Otolaryngol.* 2013;133(3):239–245.

169. Verdecchia DH, Mendoza M, Sanguineti F, Binetti AC. Outcomes after vestibular rehabilitation and Wii(R) therapy in patients with chronic unilateral vestibular hypofunction. *Acta Otorhinolaryngol Esp.* 2014;65(6):339–345.

170. Geraghty AWA, Essery R, Kirby S, et al. Internet-based vestibular rehabilitation for older adults with chronic dizziness: a randomized controlled trial in primary care. *Ann Fam Med.* 2017;15(3):209–216.

FURTHER READING

1. Honrubia V, Baloh R, Harris MR, Jacobson KM. Paroxysmal positional vertigo syndrome. *Am J Otol.* 1999;20(4):465–470.

CHAPTER 2

Management of Adult Sensorineural Hearing Loss

DR. JUSTIN T. LUI, MD • KATIE DE CHAMPLAIN, MSC •
DR. JUSTIN K. CHAU, MD

KEY POINTS

- Standard pure-tone audiometry and speech discrimination testing are essential for diagnosing patients with hearing loss (level 1).
- Magnetic resonance imaging (MRI) with gadolinium is a more sensitive diagnostic test in detecting vestibular schwannoma (VS) than auditory brainstem response (ABR) (level 2).
- There is no clear advantage of the bone-anchored hearing aid (BAHA) over the contralateral routing of signals (CROS) hearing aid for use in unilateral sensorineural hearing loss (SNHL) (level 2).
- Extreme variability exists with sudden sensorineural hearing loss (SSNHL) therapy initiation, and current consensus favors prompt initiation of corticosteroid therapy for maximum efficacy and potential benefit sustained up until 6 weeks (level 1).

A previous iteration was published in *Otolaryngologic Clinics of North America*, Vol. 45, No. 5 (October 2012). This manuscript contains updated material not previously published and is not currently under evaluation in any other peer-reviewed publication.

OVERVIEW

Sensorineural hearing loss (SNHL) is a complex disease influenced by interactions between multiple internal and external causative factors. Genetics may dictate one's hearing capacity over a lifetime, and through interaction with numerous external factors, substantial changes may be accelerated over time. SNHL has been well explored in the literature, although the challenge lies in unifying the highest levels of clinical evidence to integrate into daily clinical encounters.

The goal of this article is to present the current best evidence available regarding the diagnostic process and treatments available for the management of hearing loss as it applies to the more controversial aspects of adult SNHL. The levels of evidence proposed by the Oxford Center for Evidence-Based Medicine are used throughout this article.[1]

ETIOLOGIES

Age-Related Hearing Loss (Presbycusis)

As a common chronic condition of the elderly, age-related hearing loss (ARHL) is a result of auditory stresses projected onto a genetically influenced aging process.[2,3] An estimated 63.1% of all-cause-related hearing loss in the US population aged 70 years and older is due to ARHL.[2,3] Its association with hypertension, smoking, diabetes, noise exposure, cardiovascular disease, cerebrovascular disease, and family history has been well documented.[2,3]

ARHL negatively affects mental health, social interactions, and quality of life through sensory deprivation, which may contribute to Alzheimer disease in the elderly.[4,5] ARHL is characterized by the loss of higher frequencies and is caused by the degeneration of the stria vascularis, hair cells, and afferent spiral ganglion neurons.[2,3] Secondary degeneration of central pathways has been identified as well.[6]

Autoimmune

Autoimmune inner ear disease (AIED) is characterized by bilateral SNHL deterioration over weeks to months and was first described by McCabe et al., who suggested a link to a systemic inflammatory disease.[7-9] Autoantibodies that target inner ear-specific antigens have been identified associating SNHL and autoimmune processes, such as Cogan syndrome, rheumatoid arthritis, and systemic lupus erythematosus.[8,10]

In a retrospective review of 908 patients diagnosed with bilateral SNHL, Kishimoto et al. identified AIED in 1.3%.[8] The employed criteria were bilateral SNHL of 50 dB or greater at 500, 1000, and 2000 Hz; hearing difficulty in daily conversations within 4 days to 1 year of onset of awareness; and exclusion of several mimicking diseases for which mixed hearing loss was the result.[8] The 12 AIED cases consisted of an average age of 62 years, and gender preponderance did not exist.[8]

Endolymphatic Hydrops and CNS Disease
Endolymphatic hydrops (EH) is a pathologic anatomic finding that involves an increase in the volume of endolymph causing distention of the surrounding structures.[11] EH has been described in patients with otosclerosis, endolymphatic sac tumors, posttraumatic ears, and AIED.[12–14] Several variables contribute to its pathogenesis in disrupting inner ear homeostasis; however, complete understanding remains uncertain. Primary EH (Meniere disease) presents as recurrent acute attacks of tinnitus, aural fullness, and vertigo superimposed onto deteriorating low-frequency SNHL.[15]

Central nervous system disease, including multiple sclerosis (MS), can produce varying degrees of SNHL. Although SNHL is uncommon in patients with MS, it may be secondary to demyelination of the auditory pathway and has been documented to present as sudden onset.[16] Episodes of hearing loss do demonstrate some recovery.[16,17]

Genetic
Multiple chromosomal loci have been identified in numerous syndromic and nonsyndromic causes of hearing loss. An equal amount of variability in inheritance patterns has been established as well.

Hearing losses caused by developmental disorders of the inner ear have also been linked to spontaneous or inherited genetic abnormalities, such as complete (Michel) aplasia, or cochlear anomalies, such as Mondini malformations, labyrinthine anomalies, and ductal anomalies (enlarged vestibular aqueduct).

Genetic loci predisposing individuals to permanent SNHL from trauma or ototoxic medications have been identified. Mutations of the *SLC26A4* gene increase susceptibility to hearing loss from head trauma or barotrauma.[18] Mitochondrial *MTRNR1* gene mutations have been found in approximately 15% of cases of hearing loss related to aminoglycoside use, suggesting an increased risk of hearing loss from genetic and environmental interactions.[19]

Idiopathic
SSNHL is characterized by a rapid deterioration in hearing perception. The incidence of SSNHL is estimated at 5–30 cases per 100,000/year.[20] Nearly 85%–90% of SSNHL cases lack an identifiable etiology despite thorough evaluation.[21] The most commonly utilized criteria in North America are defined by the National Institute on Deafness and Other Communications Disorders as a loss of at least 30 dB of SNHL across three contiguous frequencies within 72 h.[22] Considerable global variation regarding the definition of SSNHL exists.

Most cases of SSNHL are unilateral, as simultaneous bilateral involvement is extremely rare. Factors that may influence the prognosis for hearing recovery include age over 60 years, the duration of hearing loss, and the presence of vertigo.[23] Moreover, characteristic pure-tone configurations are associated with different recovery rates, although therapy standardization was lacking.[23–26]

Infection
SNHL is a known complication of viral, bacterial, and even fungal otologic and central nervous system infections.[27] With respect to congenital infections, cytomegalovirus is the most common culprit causing hearing loss in 0.2–0.6 per 1000 neonates.[28,29] In addition to TORCH (toxoplasmosis, other (syphillis) rubella, cytomegalovirus, herpes simplex virus) congenital infections, human immunodefi-ciency virus, measles, mumps, and Lyme disease have also been cited as infectious diseases associated with SNHL.[27,29]

Central nervous system infections, such as bacterial meningitis, can lead to SNHL.[30] Labyrinthitis ossificans and permanent SNHL are known sequela of bacterial meningitis, which may influence cochlear implantation (CI) timing.[30]

Neoplasm
VSs are benign neoplasms that account for 10% of all brain neoplasms.[31] With an annual incidence of 10–19 per million per year, VSs most commonly present with asymmetric sensorineural hearing loss (ASNHL) and unilateral tinnitus.[32,33] Various protocols have been published to guide acquisition of MRI with gadolinium to rule out VS.[34]

Noise-Induced Hearing Loss
Cochlear hair cell injury occurs through mechanical trauma and metabolic injury in response to high-intensity noise exposure. Mechanical destruction of hair cells and

supporting structures has been identifiable in the medical literature for several decades.[35] More recently, animal studies have identified three metabolic pathways that contribute to noise-induced hearing loss (NIHL), including calcium overload, reactive oxidative species, and mitochondrial pathways.[35]

Excessive recreational and/or occupational noise is recognized as a key contributor to permanent hearing loss with nearly 500 million individuals at risk of developing NIHL.[36,37] Hazardous occupational noise exposure affects an estimated 22 million US workers.[36,37] Despite being the mainstay of hearing loss prevention, hearing protection devices compliance is estimated to be only 34.3% in individuals exposed to hazardous noise volumes.[36] Moreover, an estimated 1.1 billion young adults are at risk of hearing loss secondary to noise exposure from nightclubs, sporting events, and personal audio devices.[38] When comparing the prevalence of the incidence of hearing loss from ages 12 to 19 years, the National Health and Nutrition Examination Survey identified an increase in hearing loss prevalence from 3.5% to 5.3% from 1994 to 2006, respectively.[39]

Ototoxicity

The continued use of ototoxic medications relates to the low clinical risk or the lack of treatment alternatives.[40] Platinum-based chemotherapeutic agents and aminoglycosides are two drug classes that show irreversible inner ear damage to both the stria vascularis and the outer hair cells.[40,41] Contrastingly, the ototoxic effects of macrolide antibiotics, loop diuretics, and quinine are reversed with cessation.[41]

Early recognition and close audiologic monitoring are often the standard of care for patients receiving cisplatin and aminoglycosides.[41] Dose modifications, alternative therapies, and trial of otoprotective substances should be explored if hearing loss develops.[40,41] Although preclinical studies for antioxidants have been promising, the potential impairment of antitumor activity of cisplatin deems it a more challenging use.[41]

Trauma

Temporal bone fractures involving the otic capsule may result in permanent SNHL, vertigo, and facial nerve injury. Inner ear barotrauma from scuba diving or sudden and violent pressure changes to the external and middle ear causing damage to the oval or round windows may result in perilymph fistulization and subsequent hearing loss, tinnitus, and vertigo. Injury rates from head and neck radiation for nasopharyngeal carcinoma range from 46% to 67% from intensity-modulated and conventional radiation therapy, respectively.[42]

Vascular

Although vestibular signs are more common in stroke, hearing disturbances have also been described. The auditory pathway possesses both vascular and neural redundancy in comparison with the vestibular pathway, which often require psychoacoustic and electrophysiologic testing to elicit hearing dysfunction.[43] Häusler et al. outlined the auditory symptoms and associated ischemic location from the cochlea to the temporal lobes.[43] In addition, patients with stroke are at an increased risk of SSNHL in comparison with nonstroke patients, with an adjusted hazard ratio of 1.71 (1.24–2.36).[20]

EVIDENCE-BASED CLINICAL ASSESSMENT

A thorough clinical assessment provides a high diagnostic yield and ensures proper management. Beginning with a comprehensive history, a patient's description of their hearing dysfunction and presence of otologic symptoms, including tinnitus, vertigo, otalgia, aural fullness, and otorrhea, should be identified. The patient's past medical history, family history, medication profile, occupational history, and social history should be obtained. Physical examination should include external ear inspection and otoscopy to assess external auditory canal and middle ear integrity. Tuning fork tests and special tests should be performed to help identify and characterize hearing loss.

Audiometric Testing

Standard pure-tone audiometry provides diagnostic information regarding the degree, type, and configuration of hearing loss. Hearing thresholds are obtained to air conduction (0.25–8 kHz) and bone conduction (0.5–4 kHz) stimuli. In addition, an initial audiogram should include speech reception thresholds and word recognition scores. Serial audiometric evaluations document changes in threshold and treatment response, while guiding aural rehabilitation.

With suspected SSNHL, hearing loss should be documented, allowing for prompt intervention.[21] If ASNHL is identified, then further diagnostic steps may be warranted, including MRI. Although definitions of ASNHL vary slightly, studies have shown that an asymmetry of 15 dB or more at 3000 Hz had the highest odds ratio association with a positive VS finding on MRI in the retrospective study population.[44]

Auditory Brainstem Response

Retrocochlear pathology suspicion warrants further investigation beyond standard audiometric testing, which may include ABR audiometry. Sufficient residual hearing thresholds (<75 dB HL) must be present for a response to be observed, however. Waveform morphology and interaural latency of wave V are two parameters used to identify VSs larger than 2.0 cm.[45] Stacked ABR allows for small tumor detection (<1 cm) but with lower specificity than MRI.[46,47]

Vestibular Assessment

Objective vestibular assessment with electronystagmography (ENG), videonystagmography, and/or vestibular evoked myogenic potentials (VEMP) may be useful in predicting the prognosis for hearing recovery. Korres et al. identified a significantly higher number of abnormal ENG and VEMP results in patients with profound hearing loss, as well as a negative correlation between the severity of hearing loss and the likelihood of hearing recovery.[48] In addition, patients with SSNHL and vertigo with normal caloric testing are more likely to have a higher chance of hearing recovery.[49]

Video head impulse testing (vHIT) has been shown to detect vestibuloocular reflex deficits in patients with SSNHL. For example, a posterior canal deficit on vHIT testing associated with SSNHL may be suggestive of common cochlear artery ischemia.[50]

Magnetic Resonance Imaging

MRI is a more sensitive diagnostic test for the detection of VS than ABR.[51] MRI with gadolinium is a preferable method for assessing the cerebellopontine angle and internal auditory canal for identification of potentially treatable causes. Contrast-enhanced MRI is able to detect a variety of abnormalities of patients with SSNHL, including neoplasm, stroke, hemorrhage, or demyelination.[52] The sensitivity and specificity of MRI with gadolinium in the diagnosis of a VS larger than 3 mm approach nearly 100%.[51,53] High-resolution MRI with constructive interference steady state sequence may be performed as an alternative to gadolinium when concerns of nephrotoxicity arise.[53]

A meta-analysis of studies assessing ASNHL with MRI scans demonstrated an overall diagnostic yield of 5.1%.[54] To combat MRI's low accuracy, expensive nature, and limited availability, multiple standardized protocols have been proposed to increase the diagnostic accuracy through unique findings on audiograms.[33,54] A widely popularized and simplistic "rule 3000" was shown to have the highest positive likelihood ratio of 2.91 compared with eight other testing protocols.[55] "Rule 3000" was defined as ASNHL of 15 dB or greater at 3000 Hz.[55,56] Additional clinical factors such as patient age, word recognition score, and character and laterality of tinnitus were other predictors of VS.[54] Further

analysis did not reveal a positive correlation between the severity of ASNHL and MR diagnosis of VS.

Computed Tomography

An MRI scan may be contraindicated in some patients (implanted ferromagnetic materials), or patients may refuse to consent because of claustrophobia or other reasons. Temporal bone computed tomography (CT) scan with intravenous contrast of the head and temporal bones has reasonable sensitivity for lesions greater than 1.5 cm in diameter.[43] When compared with MRI, CT scans remain suboptimal in their diagnostic capabilities for retrocochlear lesions. Exposure to ionizing radiation also makes CT scan less than optimal when compared with MRI.

Laboratory Tests

The use of laboratory tests in the evaluation of patients with SSNHL is variable. There is no evidence to support a "shotgun approach" to serologic testing for patients with SSNHL because of low diagnostic yield.[57] Laboratory tests, including complete blood count, electrolytes, basic metabolic panels, and erythrocyte sedimentation rate (ESR), can be considered on an individual basis.

Serologic markers for metabolic disorders are commonly investigated in patients with SSNHL. Hypercholesterolemia has been identified in 35%–40% of patients with idiopathic SSNHL and hyperglycemia in 18%–37%.[58,59] Hypothyroidism is also common, with a prevalence of up to 15% in patients with SSNHL.[57,60] Most of these conditions have been identified on previous testing performed by the primary care physician before presentation to an otolaryngologist. Information obtained on history and physical examination may indicate specific exposures and risk factors for various health conditions, which should guide further serologic workup if a specific cause is suspected.

Hemostatic parameters such as thrombophilic genetic polymorphisms and coagulation studies have been investigated in patients with SSNHL. A higher rate of polymorphisms in factor V Leiden, prothrombin, methylenetetrahydrofolate reductase, and platelet glycoprotein IIIa has been shown in patients with SSNHL, but our clinical ability to identify these polymorphisms in the general population to reduce the risk of an SSNHL event before it occurs is not feasible.[61-63] Investigations have shown no clear distinction between the coagulation profiles of patients with and without SSNHL. Therefore, coagulation studies, such as prothrombin time, activated partial thromboplastin time, and coagulation factors, are of little diagnostic value in the clinical evaluation of SSNHL.[61]

Laboratory investigations for potential infectious etiologies of SSNHL have been proposed. Influenza B and enterovirus have been shown to have higher rates of seroconversion in patients with SSNHL in some studies.[64,65] Other studies have failed to show an association between SSNHL and human herpes simplex virus, varicella zoster, cytomegalovirus, influenza A1/A3, parainfluenza viruses 1, 2, and 3, enterovirus, Epstein-Barr virus, hepatitis C, adenovirus, rubella, and respiratory syncytial virus.[65–69] Investigations including routine polymerase chain reaction or immunoglobulin titers for these aforementioned viruses have not been shown to influence treatment or improve patient outcomes.

Other nonviral infectious diseases are considered if a patient's history and physical examination are suggestive.[67] Hearing loss caused by Lyme disease rarely presents without other clinical symptoms; thus patients with a history of exposure and positive clinical findings should be considered for serologic testing.[67] If congenital or latent syphilis is suspected, serum fluorescent treponemal antibody absorption or microhemagglutination assay for *Treponema pallidum* may be performed.[69]

Multiple studies have examined the relationship between SSNHL and various systemic autoimmune markers, including ESR, antinuclear antibodies, rheumatoid factor, and anticardiolipin antibodies, all of which have been shown to be increased in patients with SSNHL.[57,70] These tests lack specificity for the diagnosis of autoimmune-mediated SNHL, and there is no evidence to support a positive association between the increase of a nonspecific inflammatory marker and a positive response to corticosteroid treatment of SSNHL.

The diagnostic value of specific inner ear proteins, such as heat shock protein 70 (hsp 70), and their relationship to AIED is limited, as expression in healthy individuals is common.[70] Routine testing for other proteins, including cochlin, b-hector choline transporter like protein 2, and myelin protein Po, is not currently recommended.[71,72]

EVIDENCED-BASED MANAGEMENT

Depending on the degree of hearing loss, word recognition capabilities, and ability to tolerate sound amplification, a patient's unilateral hearing loss may be adequately addressed with traditional hearing amplification devices. In the setting of profound hearing loss, poor word recognition, and intolerance for amplified sounds, contralateral routing of signals CROS systems have been employed. By rerouting sound to the contralateral ear the challenges of monaural hearing stemming

from sound localization, speech discrimination, and hearing in noisy environments are mitigated.[73,74]

In a similar fashion, popularization of the use of bone conduction devices (BCD) to reroute sound to the operational cochlea via bone conduction has expanded candidacy of BCD to include unilateral SNHL.[74] When comparing BCD with CROS strategies for patients with single-sided hearing loss, speech perception in noise, sound localization, and quality-of-life measurements were not statistically significantly different in both modalities.[74,75] Given the lack of objective differences between bone-conducting devices and CROS systems and the avoidance of surgical risks and postoperative complications, CROS devices have been advocated as a first-line treatment in single-sided deafness.[76]

CI is a consideration for treating unilateral SNHL, which transmits electrical impulses directly to the cochlear nerve by circumventing damaged hair cells.[77,78] High-level evidence is lacking given the large degree of heterogeneity arising from the classification, duration, and onset of hearing loss between studies.[78] However, unilateral CIs have demonstrated a statistically significant improvement in speech perception, specifically in open-set sentence or multisyallable word testing.[77] With respect to severe to profound bilateral SNHL, bilateral CIs have been demonstrated to be beneficial for speech perception in noise under certain conditions and several self-reported measures have demonstrated improvement.[79]

Additionally, auditory brainstem implants have employed for patients where CI is not a rehabilitative option such as neurofibromatosis 2, bilateral complete cochlear aplasia, and inner ear aplasia.[79a]

Autoimmune Inner Ear Disease

AIED treatment has been predicated around immunosuppressive therapy given the initial benefit of combined steroid and cyclophosphamide treatment in McCabe's 1979 article.[80] However, in the more current literature cyclophosphamide has not demonstrated clinical efficacy in prospective trials and given its potential adverse effects its use for fluctuating SNHL is not recommended.[81] A multidisciplinary approach for the management of AIED has been advocated, consisting of an otolaryngologist, rheumatologist, and audiologist while monitoring treatment.[10]

Idiopathic Sudden Sensorineural Hearing Loss
Corticosteroids

Purported to address cochlear inflammation and edema, corticosteroids have become the most widely employed treatment despite definitive positive outcomes and

TABLE 2.1
Oral Corticosteroid for Idiopathic Sudden Sensorineural Hearing Loss

Corticosteroid	Dosing (mg/kg/d)	Maximum Dose (mg/d)	Duration
Prednisone	1	60	Full dose for 7–14 days, with taper over similar time period
Methylprednisone	0.8[a]	48	
Dexamethasone	0.17[a]	10	

Adapted from the AAO-HNSF Clinical Practice Guideline: Sudden Hearing Loss.
[a]Based on prednisone daily dosing equivalence.

potential side effects.[21,82] The most recent Cochrane review of steroid management for idiopathic sudden sensorineural hearing loss (ISSNHL) identified just three randomized control trials (RCTs) that met strict inclusion criteria.[82] As a result of small study populations, inconsistent therapies, and variable outcome measurements, the review was unable to provide definitive support for steroid therapy.

Despite the lack of convincing evidence, the small rate of adverse effects and the potential for improved hearing have resulted in the American Academy of Otolaryngology–Head and Neck Surgery Foundation (AAO-HNSF) guidelines recommending steroid therapy consideration.[21] Multiple treatment recommendations exist for ISSNHL, with variability in the type, dosing, and duration of steroid treatment, although the AAO-HNSF guidelines have outlined a straightforward treatment recommendation (Table 2.1).[21] Patients with active infection, poorly controlled diabetes, and prior psychiatric disease are among the numerous contraindications that should be evaluated for before initiation of treatment.[21,83]

Extreme variability exists with therapy initiation, as patients may not present immediately after hearing loss onset. Current consensus favors prompt initiation of therapy for maximum efficacy and potential benefit sustained up until 6 weeks.[21]

Intratympanic steroids
The adverse effects of systemic steroid therapy (SST) have been widely described in the literature with concerning effects such as avascular necrosis, hyperglycemia, and weight alteration.[83] Intratympanic injections provide a higher concentration in the perilymph than intravenous administration, and this has contributed to the popularization of intratympanic steroid (ITS) application as both first-line and salvage therapy.[84–87]

Dexamethasone is most commonly used because it has major antiinflammatory and minor mineralocorticoid activity in comparison with other corticosteroids.[85]

Currently, no consensus exists on the efficacy of ITS over SST, although a meta-analysis of six RCTs favored ITS administration with a slight 3.42 dB (0.17–6.67) improvement in pure-tone audiometry.[86] When comparing ITS and SST combined with ITS alone, a meta-analysis of 14 RCTs favored the combination therapy.[87] Mean differences between both modalities favored the combination therapy with both pure-tone averages and speech discrimination scores of 13.0 dB (9.24–16.77) and 15.7% (5.1–26.3), respectively.[87] The majority of published ITS side effects include otalgia, aural fullness, headache, and brief vertigo, which affected 13% of the pooled study population.[85] The more serious side effects, severe dizziness and self-resolved tympanic membrane perforation, affected 1.2% of the same population.[85]

Antivirals
Hypothesized as a potential etiology of ISSNHL, potential viral infection or reactivation of a latent virus of the cochlea, vestibulocochlear nerve, or the spiral ganglion has prompted the popular use of antivirals to mitigate or potentially reverse resultant hearing loss.[21,27,88]

A Cochrane review of the role of antivirals in SSNHL did not identify any statistically significant advantage of antiviral addition to systemic steroids in all four included RCTs.[89] Although significant adverse effects were not identified, the use of antivirals lacks any definitive evidence to justify its continued use.[21,89]

Hyperbaric oxygen
Hyperbaric oxygen therapy (HBO) was proposed as a therapy to address ISSNHL and the accompanying tinnitus as early as the 1960s.[90] Patients were subjected to 100% oxygen pressured at 1.5–3.0 atm absolute (ATA) within a sealed chamber, and the aim of therapy is to reverse a suspected hypoxic injury sustained by the cochlea.[90] Nearly 5–40 treatments are required, each lasting 1–2 h in duration.[21,90]

A Cochrane review of supplementary HBO therapy for ISSNHL indicated a statistically significant improvement of 15.6 dB (1.5–29.8) in four included RCTs, which comprised 187 patients.[90] Two separate RCTs (104 patients) with different outcome measurements identified more than 25% improvement in pure-tone averages with a risk ratio of 1.39 (1.05–1.84), translating into a number needed to treat of five.[90] Despite these positive findings, various shortcomings of these investigations exist, with moderate variable in methodology, lack of adequate blinding especially with investigators, and variability in outcome timing. In addition, HBO is not without adverse effects, including but not limited to barotrauma of the sinuses, middle ear, and respiratory tract.[91,92]

Rheopheresis

Rheopheresis aims to reduce acute microcirculatory impairment via plasmapheresis, which is used to eliminate a defined spectrum of high-molecular-weight plasma proteins and result in reduced plasma and whole blood viscosity. Two large RCTs demonstrated equivalent efficacy to standard therapy with systemic corticosteroids and hemodilution.[93] These findings have been recognized by the German SSNHL guidelines, which propose similar treatments as part of a multimodality approach.

BOTTOM LINE

SNHL continues to be a realm in which genetic predisposition and various risk factors influence auditory function. SNHL presents in various time frames as a result of equally diverse causes. Despite advances in the diagnosis of SNHL and its etiology, treatment is limited. Nonetheless, SNHL may be a manifestation of other serious disease processes, prompting thorough consideration when faced by clinicians.

CRITICAL POINTS WITH EVIDENCE

- Standard pure-tone audiometry and speech discrimination testing are essential for diagnosing patients with hearing loss (level 1).
- Suspected SSNHL cases should undergo hearing loss evaluation to allow for prompt intervention (level 1).
- For cases of SSNHL, MRI with gadolinium is a more sensitive diagnostic test in detecting VS than ABR (level 2).
- Multiple algorithms utilizing audiometry findings have been developed to improve MRI diagnostic accuracy of VS (level 3).

- Patients with SSNHL and vertigo with normal caloric testing are more likely to experience hearing recovery.
- Common metabolic disturbances associated with hearing loss, such as hypercholesterolemia, hyperglycemia, and hypothyroidism, should be investigated in previously unscreened patients (level 4).
- Routine evaluation of coagulation studies provides little diagnostic value during management of SSNHL (level 3).
- Convincing evidence of a causal relationship between a viral infection and SSNHL is lacking, and routine workup for a viral etiology in SSNHL is not recommended (level 3).
- Studies have not been able to identify specific markers for AIED, and ordering affiliated tests will not provide information for definitive management (level 4).
- There is no clear advantage between the CROS system and BAHA strategies for unilateral SNHL (level 2).
- CI for unilateral SNHL has demonstrated a statistically significant improvement in speech perception, specifically open-set sentence or multisyllable word testing (level 4).
- Extreme variability exists with SSNHL therapy initiation, and current consensus favors prompt initiation of corticosteroid therapy for maximum efficacy and potential benefit sustained up until 6 weeks (level 1).
- ITS can be employed in both first-line and salvage SSNHL therapy, and when combined with systemic steroids, improved outcomes in pure-tone averages and speech discrimination scores have been identified (level 1).
- There is insufficient evidence to recommend antiviral therapy as the primary or steroid adjunctive therapy in patients with SSNHL (level 2).
- Supplementary HBO therapy in combination with SST may further improve hearing (level 2).
- A limited literature exists regarding the benefit of rheopheresis in SSNHL treatment (level 3).

REFERENCES

1. Howick J, Chalmers I, Glasziou P, et al. *The 2011 Oxford CEBM Levels of Evidence (Introductory Document)*; 2011.
2. Gates GA, Mills JH. Presbycusis. *Lancet.* 2005;366: 1111–1120.
3. Yamasoba T, Lin FR, Someya S, Kashio A, Sakamoto T, Kondo K. Current concepts in age-related hearing loss: epidemiology and mechanistic pathways. *Hear Res.* 2013;303:30–38.

4. Zheng Y, Fan S, Liao W, Fang W, Xiao S, Liu J. Hearing impairment and risk of Alzheimer's disease: a meta-analysis of prospective cohort studies. *Neurol Sci.* 2017;38(2):233–239.
5. Cherko M, Hickson L, Bhutta M. Auditory deprivation and health in the elderly. *Maturitas.* 2016;88:52–57.
6. Kujawa SG, Liberman MC. Adding insult to injury: cochlear nerve degeneration after "temporary" noise-induced hearing loss. *J Neurosci.* 2009;29(45):14077–14085.
7. Buniel MC, Geelan-Hansen K, Weber PC, Tuohy VK. Immunosuppressive therapy for autoimmune inner ear disease. *Immunotherapy.* 2009;1(3):425–434.
8. Kishimoto I, Yamazaki H, Naito Y, et al. Clinical features of rapidly progressive bilateral sensorineural hearing loss. *Acta Otolaryngol.* 2014;134(1):58–65.
9. Vambutas A, Pathak S. AAO: autoimmune and autoinflammatory (disease) in otology: what is new in immune-mediated hearing loss. *Laryngoscope Investig Otolaryngol.* 2016. http://dx.doi.org/10.1002/lio2.28.
10. Mijovic T, Zeitouni A, Colmegna I. Autoimmune sensorineural hearing loss: the otology-rheumatology interface. *Rheumatology.* 2013;52(5):780–789.
11. Salt AN, Plontke SK. Endolymphatic hydrops: pathophysiology and experimental models. *Otolaryngol Clin North Am.* 2010;43.
12. Liston SL, Paparella MM, Mancini F, Anderson JH. Otosclerosis and endolymphatic hydrops. *Laryngoscope.* 1984;94.
13. Poulsen MLM, Gimsing S, Kosteljanetz M, et al. von Hippel-Lindau disease: surveillance strategy for endolymphatic sac tumors. *Genet Med.* 2011;13.
14. Clark SK, Rees TS. Posttraumatic endolymphatic hydrops. *Arch Otolaryngol.* 1977;103.
15. Flint PW, Haughey BH, Lund VJ, et al. *Cummings Otolaryngology;* 2015.
16. Fernández-Menéndez S, Redondo-Robles L, García-Santiago R, García-González MÁ, Arés-Luque A. Isolated deafness in multiple sclerosis patients. *Am J Otolaryngol.* 2014;35(6):810–813.
17. Hellmann MA, Steiner I, Mosberg-Galili R. Sudden sensorineural hearing loss in multiple sclerosis: clinical course and possible pathogenesis. *Acta Neurol Scand.* 2011;124.
18. Usami SI, Abe S, Weston MD, Shinkawa H, Van Camp G, Kimberling WJ. Non-syndromic hearing loss associated with enlarged vestibular aqueduct is caused by PDS mutations. *Hum Genet.* 1999;104(2):188–192.
19. Prezant TR, Agapian JV, Bohlman MC, et al. Mitochondrial ribosomal RNA mutation associated with both antibiotic-induced and non-syndromic deafness. *Nat Genet.* 1993;4(3):289–294.
20. Kuo C-L, Shiao A-S, Wang S-J, Chang W-P, Lin Y-Y. Risk of sudden sensorineural hearing loss in stroke patients : a 5-year nationwide investigation of 44,460 patients. *Medicine (Baltimore).* 2016;95.
21. Stachler RJ, Chandrasekhar SS, Archer SM, et al. Clinical practice guideline: sudden hearing loss. *Otolaryngol Head Neck Surg.* 2012;146(3 suppl):S1–S35.
22. Institute on Deafness N, Communication Disorders O. Sudden Deafness.
23. Byl FM. Sudden hearing loss: eight years' experience and suggested prognostic table. *Laryngoscope.* 1984;94(5 Pt 1):647–661.
24. Nosrati-Zarenoe R, Hansson M, Hultcrantz E. Assessment of diagnostic approaches to idiopathic sudden sensorineural hearing loss and their influence on treatment and outcome. *Acta Otolaryngol.* 2009;130(3):1–8.
25. Fetterman BL, Saunders JE, Luxford WM. Prognosis and treatment of sudden sensorineural hearing loss. *Am J Otol.* 1996;17(4):529–536.
26. Xenellis J, Karapatsas I, Papadimitriou N, et al. Idiopathic sudden sensorineural hearing loss: prognostic factors. *J Laryngol Otol.* 2006;120(9):718–724.
27. Cohen BE, Durstenfeld A, Roehm PC. Viral causes of hearing loss: a review for hearing health professionals. *Trends Hear.* 2014;18.
28. Shin JJ, Keamy DG, Steinberg EA. Medical and surgical interventions for hearing loss associated with congenital cytomegalovirus: a systematic review. *Otolaryngol Head Neck Surg.* 2011;144(5):662–675.
29. Acquired hearing loss in children. *Otolaryngol Clin North Am.* 2015;48(6):933–953.
30. Hartnick CJ, Kim HY, Chute PM, Parisier SC. Preventing labyrinthitis ossificans. *Arch Otolaryngol Neck Surg.* 2001;127(2):180.
31. Coelho DH, Tang Y, Suddarth B, Mamdani M. MRI surveillance of vestibular schwannomas without contrast enhancement: clinical and economic evaluation. *Laryngoscope.* 2017. http://dx.doi.org/10.1002/lary.26589.
32. Stangerup S-E, Tos M, Thomsen J, Caye-Thomasen P. True incidence of vestibular schwannoma? *Neurosurgery.* 2010;67(5):1335–1340.
33. Saliba I, Martineau G, Chagnon M. Asymmetric hearing loss: rule 3,000 for screening vestibular schwannoma. *Otol Neurotol.* 2009;30(4):515–521.
34. Obholzer RJ, Rea PA, Harcourt JP. Magnetic resonance imaging screening for vestibular schwannoma: analysis of published protocols. *J Laryngol Otol.* 2004;118(5):329–332.
35. Le Prell CG, Yamashita D, Minami SB, Yamasoba T, Miller JM. Mechanisms of noise-induced hearing loss indicate multiple methods of prevention. *Hear Res.* 2007;226(1–2):22–43.
36. Tak SW, Davis RR, Calvert GM. Exposure to hazardous workplace noise and use of hearing protection devices among us workers-NHANES, 1999-2004. *Am J Ind Med.* 2009;52(5):358–371.
37. Sliwinska-Kowalska M, Davis A. Noise-induced hearing loss. *Noise Health.* 2012;14(61):274–280.
38. Organization WH. *Hearing Loss Due to Recreational Exposure to Loud Sounds: A Review;* 2015.
39. Shargorodsky J, Curhan SG, Curhan GC, Eavey R. Change in prevalence of hearing loss in US adolescents. *JAMA.* 2010;304(7):772–778.

40. Schacht J, Talaska AE, Rybak LP. Cisplatin and aminoglycoside antibiotics: hearing loss and its prevention. *Anat Rec (Hoboken)*. 2012;295(11):1837–1850.

41. Lanvers-Kaminsky C, Zehnhoff-Dinnesen AA, Parfitt R, Ciarimboli G. Drug-induced ototoxicity: mechanisms, pharmacogenetics, and protective strategies. *Clin Pharmacol Ther*. 2017;101(4):491–500.

42. Hsin CH, Chen TH, Young YH, Liu WS. Comparison of otologic complications between intensity-modulated and two-dimensional radiotherapies in nasopharyngeal carcinoma patients. *Otolaryngol Head Neck Surg*. 2010;143(5):662–668.

43. Häusler R, Levine RA. Auditory dysfunction in stroke. *Acta Otolaryngol*. 2000;120(6):689–703.

44. Gimsing S. Vestibular schwannoma: when to look for it? *J Laryngol Otol*. 2010;124.

45. Chandrasekhar SS, Brackmann DE, Devgan KK. Utility of auditory brainstem response audiometry in diagnosis of acoustic neuromas. *Am J Otol*. 1995;16.

46. Kochanek KM, Śliwa L, Gołębiowski M, Piłka A, Skarżyński H. Comparison of 3 ABR methods for diagnosis of retrocochlear hearing impairment. *Med Sci Monit*. 2015;21.

47. Don M, Kwong B, Tanaka C, Brackmann D, Nelson R. The stacked ABR: a sensitive and specific screening tool for detecting small acoustic tumors. *Audiol Neurootol*. 2005;10(5):274–290.

48. Korres S, Stamatiou G, Gkoritsa E, Riga M, Xenelis J. Prognosis of patients with idiopathic sudden hearing loss: role of vestibular assessment. *J Laryngol Otol*. 2011;125(3):251–257.

49. Wilson WR, Laird N, Kavesh DA. Electronystagmographic findings in idiopathic sudden hearing loss. *Am J Otolaryngol*. 1982;3(4):279–285.

50. Pogson JM, Taylor RL, Young AS, et al. Vertigo with sudden hearing loss: audio-vestibular characteristics. *J Neurol*. 2016;263.

51. Cueva RA. Auditory brainstem response versus magnetic resonance imaging for the evaluation of asymmetric sensorineural hearing loss. *Laryngoscope*. 2004;114(10):1686–1692.

52. Jeong K-H, Choi JW, Shin JE, Kim C-H. Abnormal magnetic resonance imaging findings in patients with sudden sensorineural hearing loss: vestibular schwannoma as the most common cause of MRI abnormality. *Medicine (Baltimore)*. 2016;95(17):e3557.

53. Fortnum H, O'Neill C, Taylor R, et al. The role of magnetic resonance imaging in the identification of suspected acoustic neuroma: a systematic review of clinical and cost effectiveness and natural history. *Health Technol Assess*. 2009;13(18):1–176.

54. Egan C. *Asymmetric Hearing Loss Stratification and Vestibular Schwannoma Risk: A Meta-analysis* Bost Univ Theses Diss; 2015.

55. Saliba I, Bergeron M, Martineau G, Chagnon M. Rule 3,000: a more reliable precursor to perceive vestibular schwannoma on MRI in screened asymmetric sensorineural hearing loss. *Eur Arch Otorhinolaryngol*. 2011;268(2):207–212.

56. Ahshan S, Standring R, Osborn D, Peterson E, Seidman M, Jain R. Clinical predictors of abnormal magnetic resonance imaging findings in patients with asymmetric sensorineural hearing loss. *JAMA Otolaryngol Head Neck Surg*. 2015;141(5):451–456.

57. Heman-Ackah SE, Jabbour N, Huang TC. Asymmetric sudden sensorineural hearing loss: is all this testing necessary? *J Otolaryngol Head Neck Surg*. 2010;39(5):486–490.

58. Cadoni G, Agostino S, Scipione S, et al. Sudden sensorineural hearing loss: our experience in diagnosis, treatment, and outcome. *J Otolaryngol*. 2005;34(6):395–401.

59. Aimoni C, Bianchini C, Borin M, et al. Diabetes, cardiovascular risk factors and idiopathic sudden sensorineural hearing loss: a case-control study. *Audiol Neurootol*. 2010;15(2):111–115.

60. Oiticica J, Bittar RSM. Metabolic disorders prevalence in sudden deafness. *Clinics (Sao Paulo)*. 2010;65(11):1149–1553.

61. Ballesteros F, Alobid I, Tassies D, et al. Is there an overlap between sudden neurosensorial hearing loss and cardiovascular risk factors? *Audiol Neurootol*. 2009;14(3):139–145.

62. Capaccio P, Ottaviani F, Cuccarini V, et al. Genetic and acquired prothrombotic risk factors and sudden hearing loss. *Laryngoscope*. 2007;117(3):547–551.

63. Capaccio P, Cuccarini V, Ottaviani F, Fracchiolla NS, Bossi A, Pignataro L. Prothrombotic gene mutations in patients with sudden sensorineural hearing loss and cardiovascular thrombotic disease. *Ann Otol Rhinol Laryngol*. 2009;118(3):205–210.

64. Chau JK, Lin JRJ, Atashband S, Irvine RA, Westerberg BD. Systematic review of the evidence for the etiology of adult sudden sensorineural hearing loss. *Laryngoscope*. 2010;120(5):1011–1021.

65. Wilson WR, Veltri RW, Laird N, Sprinkle PM. Viral and epidemiologic studies of idiopathic sudden hearing loss. *Otolaryngol Head Neck Surg*. 1983;91(6):653–658.

66. Gross M, Wolf DG, Elidan J, Eliashar R. Enterovirus, cytomegalovirus, and Epstein-Barr virus infection screening in idiopathic sudden sensorineural hearing loss. *Audiol Neurootol*. 2007;12(3):179–182.

67. Gagnebin J, Maire R. Infection screening in sudden and progressive idiopathic sensorineural hearing loss: a retrospective study of 182 cases. *Otol Neurotol*. 2002;23(2):160–162.

68. Bakker R, Aarts MCJ, van der Heijden GJMG, Rovers MM. No evidence for the diagnostic value of Borrelia serology in patients with sudden hearing loss. *Otolaryngol Head Neck Surg*. 2012;146.

69. Yimtae K, Srirompotong S, Lertsukprasert K. Otosyphilis: a review of 85 cases. *Otolaryngol Head Neck Surg*. 2007;136(1):67–71.

70. Süslü N, Yilmaz T, Gürsel B. Utility of anti-HSP 70, TNF-alpha, ESR, antinuclear antibody, and antiphospholipid antibodies in the diagnosis and treatment of sudden sensorineural hearing loss. *Laryngoscope*. 2009;119(2):341–346.

71. Tebo AE, Szankasi P, Hillman TA, Litwin CM, Hill HR. Antibody reactivity to heat shock protein 70 and inner ear-specific proteins in patients with idiopathic sensorineural hearing loss. *Clin Exp Immunol*. 2006;146(3): 427–432.

72. Cao MY, Dupriez VJ, Rider MH, et al. Myelin protein Po as a potential autoantigen in autoimmune inner ear disease. *FASEB J*. 1996;10(14):1635–1640.

73. Valente M. Fitting options for adults with unilateral hearing loss. *Hear J*. 2007;60(8):10.

74. Kitterick PT, Smith SN, Lucas L. Hearing instruments for unilateral severe-to-profound sensorineural hearing loss in adults. *Ear Hear*. 2016;37(5):495–507.

75. Baguley DM, Bird J, Humphriss RL, Prevost AT. The evidence base for the application of contralateral bone anchored hearing aids in acquired unilateral sensorineural hearing loss in adults. *Clin Otolaryngol*. 2006;31(1):6–14.

76. Finbow J, Bance M, Aiken S, Gulliver M, Verge J, Caissie RA. Comparison between wireless CROS and bone-anchored hearing devices for single-sided deafness. *Otol Neurotol*. 2015;36(5):819–825.

77. Gaylor JM, Raman G, Chung M, et al. Cochlear implantation in adults. *JAMA Otolaryngol Head Neck Surg*. 2013;139(3):265.

78. van Zon A, Peters JPM, Stegeman I, Smit AL, Grolman W. Cochlear implantation for patients with single-sided deafness or asymmetrical hearing loss. *Otol Neurotol*. 2015;36(2):209–219.

79. van Schoonhoven J, Sparreboom M, van Zanten BGA, et al. The effectiveness of bilateral cochlear implants for severe-to-profound deafness in adults: a systematic review. *Otol Neurotol*. 2013;34(2):190–198.

79a. Merkus P, Di lella F, Di trapani G, et al. Indications and contraindications of auditory brainstem implants: systematic review and illustrative cases. *Eur Arch Otorhinolaryngol*. 2014;271(1):3–13.

80. McCabe BF. Autoimmune sensorineural hearing loss. *Ann Otol Rhinol Laryngol*. 1979;88:585–589.

81. Brant JA, Eliades SJ, Ruckenstein MJ. Systematic review of treatments for autoimmune inner ear disease. *Otol Neurotol*. 2015;36:1585–1592.

82. Wei BPC, Stathopoulos D, O'Leary S. Steroids for idiopathic sudden sensorineural hearing loss. *Cochrane Database Syst Rev*. 2013;(7):CD003998.

83. Rauch S, Halpin C, Antonelli P, et al. Oral vs intratympanic corticosteroid therapy for idiopathic sudden sensorineural hearing loss: a randomized trial. *JAMA*. 2011;305(20):2071–2079.

84. Rauch SD, Halpin CF, Antonelli PJ, et al. Oral vs intratympanic corticosteroid therapy for idiopathic sudden sensorineural hearing loss. *JAMA*. 2011;305(20):2071.

85. El Sabbagh NG, Sewitch MJ, Bezdjian A, Daniel SJ. Intratympanic dexamethasone in sudden sensorineural hearing loss: a systematic review and meta-analysis. *Laryngoscope*. 2017;127(8):1897–1908.

86. Qiang Q, Wu X, Yang T, Yang C, Sun H. A comparison between systemic and intratympanic steroid therapies as initial therapy for idiopathic sudden sensorineural hearing loss: a meta-analysis. *Acta Otolaryngol*. 2016:1–8.

87. Han X, Yin X, Du X, Sun C. Combined intratympanic and systemic use of steroids as a first-line treatment for sudden sensorineural hearing loss. *Otol Neurotol*. 2017;38(4): 487–495.

88. Fasano T, Pertinhez TA, Tribi L, et al. Laboratory assessment of sudden sensorineural hearing loss: a case-control study. *Laryngoscope*. 2017;127(10):2375–2381.

89. Awad Z, Huins C, Pothier DD. Antivirals for idiopathic sudden sensorineural hearing loss. In: Awad Z, ed. *Cochrane Database of Systematic Reviews*. Chichester, UK: John Wiley & Sons, Ltd; 2012:CD006987.

90. Bennett MH, Kertesz T, Perleth M, Yeung P, Lehm JP. Hyperbaric oxygen for idiopathic sudden sensorineural hearing loss and tinnitus. In: Bennett MH, ed. *Cochrane Database of Systematic Reviews*. Chichester, UK: John Wiley & Sons, Ltd; 2012.

91. Plafki C, Peters P, Almeling M, Welslau W, Busch R. Complications and side effects of hyperbaric oxygen therapy. *Aviat Space Environ Med*. 2000;71(2):119–124.

92. Korpinar S, Alkan Z, Yigit O, et al. Factors influencing the outcome of idiopathic sudden sensorineural hearing loss treated with hyperbaric oxygen therapy. *Eur Arch Otorhinolaryngol*. 2011;268(1):41–47.

93. Klingel R, Heibges A, Uygun-Kiehne S, Fassbender C, Mösges R. Rheopheresis for sudden sensorineural hearing loss. *Atheroscler Suppl*. 2009;10(5):102–106.

Laryngopharyngeal Reflux in Chronic Rhinosinusitis: Evidence-Based Practice

LAUREN J. LUK, MD • JOHN M. DELGAUDIO, MD

INTRODUCTION

Gastroesophageal reflux (GER) is a physiologic phenomenon occurring up to 50 times a day (pH < 4) in asymptomatic individuals according to pH studies.[1] The esophagus is equipped with mucosal barriers to protect against brief exposure to gastric contents. However, with prolonged exposure, breakdown in the mucosal barrier can lead to mucosal damage and gastroesophageal reflux disease (GERD). GERD affects up to 30%–40% of the population in Western society and typically presents with symptoms of heartburn and regurgitation.[2]

Advances in multichannel pH-impedance monitoring have demonstrated that gastric refluxate can travel beyond the esophagus, resulting in extraesophageal reflux (EER) or laryngopharyngeal reflux (LPR). Patients with LPR may experience chronic cough, dysphagia, hoarseness, globus pharyngeus, frequent throat clearing, postnasal drip (PND), and sore throat.[2] The addition of intraluminal impedance monitoring to traditional pH testing allows detection of weakly acidic or nonacidic reflux via changes of resistance to current across electrodes positioned along the aerodigestive tract.

In contrast to GER, LPR can cause chronic laryngeal damage with as few as three reflux episodes per week.[3,4] Laryngeal mucosal barriers to reflux are significantly weaker than gastroesophageal barriers. Carbonic anhydrase III (CA-III) is an important physiologic acid–base buffer expressed by gastroesophageal tissue in response to reflux exposure. Interestingly, CA-III expression is decreased in laryngeal tissue in response to reflux.[5] This study highlights important differences between extraesophageal and esophageal mucosal barriers against reflux.

Studies implicate both acid and pepsin exposure in the damage of laryngeal tissues.[4,5] Pepsin has maximal activity at pH 2 and is inactive at a pH of 6.5 or higher but remains stable up to a pH of 8.[5] Pepsin can accumulate in laryngeal tissue after exposure via receptor-mediated endocytosis.[6] It is postulated that pepsin is activated in the acidic intravesicular environment after endocytosis.[5] In addition, pepsin causes intracellular damage to mitochondria in cultured hypopharyngeal and nasal epithelial cells and changes the expression of genes expressed in stress and toxicity that may correlate to the mechanism of nonacidic reflux injury in LPR.[7–9]

Increasingly, EER or LPR has been implicated in several other otolaryngologic disease processes, including chronic rhinosinusitis (CRS), otitis media, cough, sleep-disordered breathing, laryngitis, laryngospasm, and airway stenosis. It has been demonstrated that positive pH probe studies correlated with extraesophageal symptoms and/or evidence of refluxate in extraesophageal subsites.[1] This chapter examines the relationship in adults between CRS and reflux in terms of epidemiology, pathogenesis, and the effect of medical therapy.

EPIDEMIOLOGIC ASSOCIATION BETWEEN REFLUX AND CHRONIC RHINOSINUSITIS

Several case-control studies have examined the epidemiologic association between GERD and CRS (Table 3.1). A large case-control study of 101,366 veteran patients demonstrated that erosive esophagitis or esophageal stricture was associated with sinusitis (odds ratio [OR] 1.6, 95% confidence interval [CI], [1.51–1.7]).[10] Leason and colleagues performed a meta-analysis of six case-control studies and demonstrated reflux was

TABLE 3.1
Epidemiologic Association Between Reflux and CRS

References	Type	Population Studied	Measurement	Result
el-Serag et al.[10]	Cohort	GERD (101,366) Without GERD (101,366)	CRS prevalence by medical record	Erosive esophagitis/esophageal stricture associated with comorbid CRS
Leason et al.[11]	Systematic review of case-control and cohort studies	CRS (143) Without CRS (207)	GERD prevalence by medical record; Prevalence of *Helicobacter pylori* in CRS	Reflux more prevalent in CRS than in control; *H. pylori* more prevalent in CRS than in control
Tan et al.[12]	Cohort	CRSwNP (595) CRSsNP (7523) Without CRS (8118)	GERD prevalence by medical record	Reflux more common in patients with CRS with or without polyps than in those without CRS
Ruhl et al.[13]	Cohort	Hospitalized patients With GERD (537) Without GERD (6391)	CRS incidence by medical record	Development of sinusitis not predicted with presence of reflux
Ruigomez et al.[14]	Cohort	GERD (7159) Without GERD (10,000)	CRS incidence by medical record	Increase in CRS diagnosis 1 year after GERD diagnosis
Lin et al.[15]	Cohort	GERD (15,807) Without GERD (47,421)	CRS incidence by chart review with endoscopy	Patients with GERD at 2.36 times greater risk of developing CRS
Katle et al.[16]	Cohort	GERD (77) Without GERD (480)	CRS prevalence, SNOT-20	Patients with GERD report reduced nose- and sinus-related QOL
Theodoropoulos et al.[17]	Cohort	GERD (36) Without GERD (74)	CRS prevalence, symptom questionnaire	Patients with GERD report increase in general nasal symptoms but not sinus-specific symptoms

CRS, Chronic rhinosinusitis; *CRSwNP*, CRS patients with nasal polyposis; *GERD*, gastroesophageal reflux disease; *QOL*, quality of life; *SNOT-20*, sinonasal outcome test 20.

more common in patients with CRS (75/143) than in those without CRS (40/207) (OR 4.03 [2.37–6.86]).[11] Overall, 52.4% of patients with CRS had comorbid reflux.[11] Similarly, Tan and colleagues found significantly increased GERD prevalence in patients with CRS with nasal polyps (176/595, 29.6%, OR 1.5 [1.2–1.8] vs. control) and CRS without nasal polyps (2220/7523, 29.0%, OR 1.7 [1.6–1.8]) versus controls without CRS (1666/8118, 20.5%).[12]

Among patients initially hospitalized with reflux esophagitis or hiatal hernia, the development of sinusitis could not be predicted with the presence of reflux (relative risk = 1.8, CI 0.8–4).[13] However, this study is unlikely to represent the general population with GERD or CRS, as inclusion criteria required two hospitalizations to follow the development of respiratory

disease on the second hospitalization. In contrast, patients accrued from a general practice in the United Kingdom were more likely to develop sinusitis in the subsequent year after GERD diagnosis (n = 7159) than age/sex-matched controls (n = 10,000) (OR 1.6 [1.2–2.0]).[14] Another prospective population cohort study from Taiwan demonstrated that patients newly diagnosed with GERD were at 2.36 times greater risk of developing CRS ($P < .001$).[15] The risk of developing CRS without nasal polyposis (CRSsNP) was higher than that of CRS with nasal polyposis (CRSwNP) (adjusted hazard ratio 2.48 vs. 1.85).[15]

In addition, patients with GERD diagnosed by gastroscopy report a significantly reduced nose- and sinus-related quality of life (QOL) (average sinonasal outcome test 20, [SNOT-20] of 22.1) compared with a control group without GERD (average SNOT-20 of 9.4).[16] This study highlights the significant overlap in symptoms of reflux and CRS. Similarly, Theodoropoulos and colleagues examined 74 patients with and 74 patients without heartburn with an upper respiratory symptom (URS) questionnaire before 24-h esophageal pH monitoring.[17] Mean URS was 8.31 in patients with GERD and 4.57 in patients without GERD by pH monitoring ($P = .02$).[17] Subjects with negative pH probe studies scored similarly to normal controls on URS.[17] In addition, reflux episodes per 24 h positively correlated with URS scores ($r = 0.47$, $P = .0001$).[17] When the URS was broken down into component questions, there was no statistical significance between sinus symptoms of any duration.[17] However, there was a statistically significant increase in nasal symptoms lasting longer than 4 days in patients with reflux ($P < .02$).[17] Nasal symptoms included congestion, PND, clear rhinorrhea, sneezing, or nasal itching.[17] Sinus symptoms included headache, facial pressure, mucopurulent nasal discharge, or abnormal sinus imaging.[17] This study highlights the distinction between nasal symptoms possibly associated with reflux alone and typical CRS symptoms.

PATHOGENIC ROLE OF REFLUX IN CHRONIC RHINOSINUSITIS

Pathogenesis of CRS involves a complex interaction between host factors, environmental exposure, epigenetics, and microbiota that creates chronic mucosal inflammation and impaired mucociliary clearance. There are several theories of how reflux contributes to CRS supported by the literature, although the true mechanism may involve a combination of these factors (Table 3.2).[37]

Direct acid or pepsin exposure to sinonasal tissue may initiate or worsen inflammation in CRS. Delehaye and colleagues demonstrated impaired sinonasal mucociliary clearance by saccharin test in 74% of patients (37/50) with GERD by symptoms and endoscopic findings.[18] This subgroup primarily reported heartburn and regurgitation without LPR symptoms, such as globus, dysphonia, or coughing. However, their

TABLE 3.2				
Pathogenic Role of Reflux in CRS				
References	**Type**	**Population Studied**	**Measurement**	**Result**
Delehaye et al.[18]	Cohort	GERD (37) LPR (13)	Mucociliary clearance by saccharin test, SNOT-20	Patients with GERD have impaired mucociliary clearance and higher SNOT scores than those with LPR
Katle et al.[19]	Prospective case-control	CRS (46) Control without CRS (45)	Presence of NPR with multichannel impedance-pH probe (measured events >=5 and <4)	Patients with CRS by EPOS criteria have increased median upright, nonacid NPR events versus control
DelGaudio[20]	Prospective case-control	Refractory CRS s/p ESS (38) Controlled CRS s/p ESS (10) Without CRS (20)	Presence of NPR, reflux at UES, or GERD by 3-channel pH probe	Significantly more reflux events (pH < 4 and pH < 5) in the CRS group compared with other two groups
Dinis et al.[21]	Prospective case-control	CRS (15) CB (5)	*Helicobacter pylori* using PCR, pepsin in blood and mucosa	*H. pylori* and pepsin present in both CRS and controls
Loehrl et al.[22]	Case-control	CRS (5) No CRS or GERD (5)	Nasal pepsin lavage	
Ozmen et al.[23]	Prospective case-control	Medically refractory CRS (33) CB (20)	Presence of LPR by dual-channel pH probe and presence of pepsin in middle meatus aspirate	More pharyngeal acid events and pepsin in nasal lavage in CRS group than in control

Continued

TABLE 3.2
Pathogenic Role of Reflux in CRS—cont'd

References	Type	Population Studied	Measurement	Result
Wong et al.[24]	Cohort	Adults without CRS or GERD Given saline (10) Given HCl (10)	Response to saline and HCl administration at GEJ	No significant increase in nasal symptom scores, mucus production, or nasal inspiratory peak flow
Loehrl et al.[25]	Prospective case-control	30 Vasomotor rhinitis with and without EER	Multichannel pH probe, composite autonomic scoring scale	Significantly increased autonomic dysfunction in VR patients with EER compared with those without EER
Morinaka et al.[26]	Case series	CRS (11)	*H. pylori* using IHC, CLO, PCR	Only 1/11 CRS patients with *H. pylori* infection
Koc et al.[27]	Prospective case-control	CRSwNP (30) CB (20)	*H. pylori*	*H. pylori* found in 20% of CRSwNP, none in control
Ozdek et al.[28]	Prospective case-control	CRSwNP (12) CB (13)	*H. pylori* using PCR	*H. pylori* found in 33.3% of CRSwNP, none in control
Cvorovik et al.[29]	Prospective case-control	CRSwNP CB	*H. pylori* using CLO, IHC	*H. pylori* found in 26.1% of CRSwNP, none in control
Kim et al.[30]	Prospective case-control	CRSwNP (48) Septoplasty/pituitary surgery (29)	*H. pylori* using CLO, IHC, CT grade, and symptom scores	*H. pylori* found in 25% of CRSwNP and 3.4% in control; no correlation between *H. pylori* infection and severity of CT or symptoms
Vceva et al.[31]	Prospective case-control	CRSwNP (30) CB (30)	*H. pylori* using PCR	*H. pylori* found in 28.57% of CRSwNP and not in controls
Ozyurt et al.[32]	Prospective case-control	CRSwNP (32) Septoplasty (29)	*H. pylori* using PCR	*H. pylori* found in CRSwNP and controls
Ozcan et al.[33]	Prospective case-control	CRSwNP (25) CB (14)	*H. pylori* by CLO	*H. pylori* found in CRSwNP and controls
Burduk et al.[34]	Prospective case-control	CRSwNP (20) CB (10)	*H. pylori* by PCR	*H. pylori* found in CRSwNP and controls
Nemati et al.[35]	Prospective case-control	CRSwNP (25) CB (25)	*H. pylori* by PCR, culture, rapid urease test	No *H. pylori* in either group
Jelavic et al.[36]	Prospective case-control	CRS s/p ESS With *H. pylori* (28) Without *H. pylori* (12)	*H. pylori* by IHC, pre- and postoperative subjective symptom scores, nasal endoscopy scores	*H. pylori* colonization associated with improved nasal endoscopy scores but not symptom improvement

CB, Concha bullosa; *CRS*, chronic rhinosinusitis; *CRSwNP*, patients with CRS with nasal polyposis; *EER*, extraesophageal reflux; *GEJ*, gastroesophageal junction; *GERD*, gastroesophageal reflux disease; *IHC*, immunohistochemistry; *LPR*, laryngopharyngeal reflux; *NPR*, nasopharyngeal reflux; *PCR*, polymerase chain reaction; *SNOT*, sinonasal outcome test; *s/p*, status post; *EPOS*, European position paper on rhinosinusitis and nasal polyps.

SNOT-20 average was significantly higher than that of patients with normal mucociliary clearance time and LPR symptoms (19.3 vs. 7.4, $P<.005$).[17]

Katle and colleagues used multichannel impedance-pH monitoring and detected an increased median number of total reflux events (supine, upright, acid, and nonacid) in patients with CRS versus control (56.5 vs. 33; $P<.0005$). They also found a specific increase in proximal reflux events (27.3 vs. 3; $P<.0005$), upright reflux events (52.5 vs. 28; $P<.005$), and nonacidic reflux events (pH>4, 19 vs. 8; $P<.005$) in patients with CRS over control.[19] The CRS group also had an increased distal esophageal acid exposure time (pH < 4) as compared with control by traditional pH probe testing ($P = .029$).[19] The groups did not have statistically different supine or acidic reflux episodes.[19]

DelGaudio demonstrated that a significantly higher percentage of patients with surgically refractory CRS had nasopharyngeal reflux (NPR) events (pH < 5) than the control group consisting of patients without CRS and patients without additional CRS symptoms after prior endoscopic sinus surgery (ESS) (76% vs. 24%, $P = .00003$).[20] The reflux area index (RAI) is a measurement that takes into account the number and duration of reflux events at a specific pH cutoff level. In this study, reflux at the upper esophageal sphincter (UES) was considered abnormal if there were more than 6.9 reflux events or if the RAI was greater than 6.3. The UES RAI was abnormal for 58% of the study group versus 21% in the control group ($P = .007$).

A small study by Dinis and colleagues demonstrated the presence of pepsin and pepsinogen I in blood and in biopsied mucosa of both CRS and healthy control patients.[21] However, a study by Loehrl and colleagues demonstrated the presence of pepsin via nasal lavage in patients with CRS and not in healthy controls, whereas pepsin assay from biopsied nasopharyngeal tissue was negative in subjects with CRS.[22]

Ozmen and colleagues correlated pepsin from nasal lavage fluid with results of 24-h dual probe monitoring for LPR with 100% sensitivity and 92.5% specificity.[23] A higher incidence of pharyngeal acid reflux events was found in patients with medically refractory CRS (88%, 29/33) versus concha bullosa (CB) controls (55%, 11/20) ($P = .01$).[23] Similarly, pepsin was identified in the nasal lavage fluid more commonly in patients with CRS (82%), as compared with the control group (50%) ($P = .014$).[23] Notably, a high number of controls also had pepsin identified in nasal lavage, suggesting that nonacid reflux events may be clinically silent. Intranasal pepsin lavage may be a good diagnostic test for LPR. This study did not quantify the amount of pepsin detected.

A second theory postulates that reflux triggers an autonomic response in sinonasal tissues, resulting in the development of CRS or CRS-like symptoms. Wong and colleagues demonstrated an increase in nasal symptom scores, mucus production, and nasal inspiratory peak flow measurements in normal subjects after the administration of both saline and hydrochloric acid at the gastroesophageal junction.[24] Owing to the small sample size, none of these changes were statistically significant. In addition, these subjects did not have a history of GERD and may not exhibit the effect of chronic reflux exposure. Patients with symptoms of both vasomotor rhinitis and extraesophageal reflux by multichannel pH probe have evidence of autonomic dysfunction as measured by the composite autonomic scoring scale as compared with age- and sex-matched controls.[25] In addition, esophageal stimulation by hydrochloric acid in guinea pigs leads to release of tachykinin-like substances that cause plasma extravasation and neurogenic inflammation. The cholinergic and adrenergic nerves were pharmacologically blocked in these guinea pigs. This finding supports the existence of a nonadrenergic noncholinergic excitatory nerve connection between the airways and the esophagus, possibly mediated by the vagus nerve.[38]

Additional studies have attempted to link local sinonasal inflammation directly to the presence of *Helicobacter pylori*. Chronic gastritis as well as development of gastroduodenal ulceration and gastric carcinoma is associated with *H. pylori* infection.[26] Many patients with GERD are infected with *H. pylori*, and the transmission of *H. pylori* from the stomach to the nose and sinuses was investigated. Several techniques for *H. pylori* detection are employed in these studies, including polymerase chain reaction (PCR) to a *H. pylori* ureA gene, (Campylobacter-like organism test)/rapid urease test (CLO test), culture, immunohistochemistry (IHC), and anti-*H. pylori* serum immunoglobulins. Real-time PCR is considered the most sensitive detection method. Many studies compare nasal polyp tissue from patients with CRSwNP and controls with CB. The results of the individual studies are mixed and inconclusive. However, a meta-analysis found an increased OR of *H. pylori* in CRS (OR 2.88 [1.58–5.26]) with an overall prevalence of *H. pylori* in CRS of 31.7% (84/265).[11]

Morinaka and colleagues investigated 11 patients with CRS and found *H. pylori* coinfection of nasal tissues and stomach in one patient using IHC, CLO, and PCR.[26] This study is limited by a small sample size and the lack of a control group. Koc and colleagues found *H. pylori* isolated in nasal polyp tissue in patients with CRSwNP (20%, 6/30) but not in the middle turbinate from control patients with CB (0/20) by IHC.[27] However, they found a high percentage of serum IgG antibodies to *H. pylori* in both patients with CRSwNP (86.7%, 26/30) and controls (85%, 17/20).[27] Ozdek and colleagues used PCR and similarly detected *H. pylori* in nasal polyp tissue from patients with CRSwNP (33.3%, 4/12) and not in the middle turbinate from controls with CB (0/13).[28] Cvorovik used CLO and IHC and found *H. pylori* in nasal polyp tissue from patients with CRSwNP (26.1%, 6/23) and not in the middle turbinate from controls with CB (0/15).[29] Similarly, Kim and colleagues used CLO and IHC and found a higher prevalence of intranasal *H. pylori* in patients with CRSwNP (25%, 12/48) versus controls without CRS undergoing transphenoidal pituitary surgery or septoplasty (3.4%, 1/29) (*P* = .025).[30] However, the severity of sinusitis by computed tomography (CT) grade and symptom scores did not significantly correlate with intranasal *H. pylori* colonization.[30] Vceva and colleagues used PCR and detected *H. pylori* DNA in nasal polyp tissue of patients with CRSwNP (28.57%, 10/30) and not in the middle turbinate from controls with CB (0/30) (*P* < .001).[31] Serum IgG and IgA antibodies were also statistically higher in patients with CRS (85.7%, 30/35) versus control (53.3%, 16/30) (*P* < .006).

However, a number of studies have not found any statistical difference in *H. pylori* infection between patients with CRS and controls using similar techniques. Dinis performed PCR for *H. pylori* and found no statistical difference in patients with CRS (6/15) and controls with CB (1/5).[21] Interestingly, in this study, patients with medically refractory CRS who underwent surgery did not specifically have nasal polyps, unlike other studies. Ozyurt and colleagues found no statistical significance in *H. pylori* DNA by PCR in nasal polyp tissue (59.4%, 19/32) from patients with CRSwNP and nasal mucosa from control patients undergoing septoplasty (70.4%, 19/29).[32] They also performed PCR for cagA (*H. pylori*'s major virulence factor) and did not find statistical significance between groups. Ozcan and colleagues used CLO to detect *H. pylori* and found no statistical difference between patients with CRSwNP (4%, 1/25) and controls with CB (14%, 2/14).[33] Burduk and colleagues found intranasal *H. pylori* by PCR for *ureA* gene in all patients with CRSwNP (20/20) and controls with CB (10/10).[34] The authors discuss that the high incidence of *H. pylori* may be related to the Polish study population that is estimated to have about 100% infection rate.[34] Conversely, Nemati performed PCR, culture, and rapid urease test on 25 patients with CRSwNP and 25 controls with CB and found no intranasal *H. pylori* in either group by all three tests.[35]

Jelavik and colleagues found that *H. pylori* colonization by IHC correlates with greater improvement in nasal endoscopic scores but not symptom scores in patients with CRS after undergoing ESS.[36] It is well established that nasal endoscopic scores correlate poorly with symptoms. Therefore, the clinical significance of *H. pylori* colonization is unclear. Overall, the pathogenic role of *H. pylori* remains unclear, and no studies to date have examined a mechanism in patients with CRS. Preexisting sinonasal inflammation may permit *H. pylori* colonization without additional potentiation of inflammation in patients with CRS.

PROGNOSTIC IMPACT OF REFLUX ON CHRONIC RHINOSINUSITIS SYMPTOMS

Several studies have implicated reflux as an independent predictor of surgically refractory CRS (Table 3.3). Chambers and colleagues performed a retrospective review of 182 patients with CRS and showed that a history of GERD was a predictor of poor symptom outcome after ESS.[39] Patients self-reported whether they had a significant improvement after ESS (Group A) or minimal or no benefit after ESS (Group B). Forty-one percent from Group B (17/42) had a history of GERD, whereas only 20% from Group A (27/140) had a history of GERD (*P* = .006).[39] However, the retrospective nature of the study is limited by recall bias from patients as well as reliance on self-reporting of comorbid GERD.

Ulaulp and colleagues performed a case-control study using a three-channel pH probe to document reflux at the hypopharynx, proximal esophagus, and distal esophagus.[40] Study subjects included patients with posterior laryngitis (PL) (28), surgically refractory CRS (12), patients with both processes (6), and healthy controls (34).[40] Pharyngeal acid reflux events were more prevalent in patients with PL than in patients with CRS and controls.[40] There was no statistical significance in reflux events between patients with isolated CRS and normal controls.[40] It is difficult to interpret the results of patients with PL and CRS, as this group was included with PL and vocal cord nodules or laryngotracheal stenosis. As a whole, this combined group also had a statistically significant increased number of reflux events as compared with CRS and controls. In another study, Ulualp found a significantly increased number of patients with medically refractory CRS with reflux (7/11) as compared with normal controls (2/11) (*P* < .05).[41]

DelGaudio examined patients with refractory CRS after ESS and found an increased number of NPR events by 24-h three-channel pH probe study as compared with the control groups consisting of patients with well-controlled CRS after ESS and patients without CRS.[20] As previously discussed, a significantly higher number of patients from the study group were found to have NPR (pH < 5) as compared with the control group. This finding was maintained with more stringent criteria for reflux events (pH < 4). When patients with refractory isolated frontal disease were

TABLE 3.3
Prognostic Impact of Reflux on CRS Symptoms

References	Type	Size	Measurement	Result
Chambers et al.[39]	Retrospective case-control	CRS s/p ESS Successful (140) Refractory (42)	History of GERD by medical chart, symptom scores	History of a GERD-independent predictor of failure after ESS
Ulualp et al.[40]	Case-control	Posterior laryngitis (28) Surgically refractory CRS (12) PL and CRS (6) Control (34)	Presence of proximal reflux by 3-channel pH probe in patients who failed sinus surgery	No difference in reflux events between isolated CRS and normal controls. Posterior laryngitis with or without CRS associated with increased reflux events
Ulualp et al.[41]	Case-control	Medically refractory CRS (11) Control (11)	Presence of proximal reflux by 3-channel pH probe in patients with medically refractory CRS	Higher percentage of reflux in CRS patients compared with controls
Jecker et al.[42]	Case-control	Surgically refractory CRS (20) Control (20)	Presence of LPR or GERD by dual-channel pH probe (pH < 4)	Significantly more GER events in the CRS patients than in controls, but not in hypopharynx
Wong et al.[43]	Case series	Medically refractory CRS (37)	Presence of acid reflux into the nasopharynx by 4-channel pH probe (pH < 4)	Found nasopharyngeal reflux in only 2 of 37 patients (5%); GER was found in 12 of 37 patients (32.4%)
Zelenik et al.[44]	Case-control	CRSsNP (30) CRSwNP (30) CRSwNP and asthma (30)	EER by RYAN score from Rescher oropharyngeal probe; amount of time exposed to refluxate pH < 5.5	Patients with CRSwNP with asthma have a high incidence of reflux and revision surgery
Wise et al.[45]	Prospective case-control	Refractory CRS s/p ESS (38) Controlled CRS s/p ESS (10) Without CRS (20)	SNOT-20, MRSI, NPR via 3-channel pH probe	Significantly more PND symptoms in patients with NPR events with pH < 5
DeConde et al.[46]	Cohort	CRS s/p ESS With GERD (72) Without GERD (157)	Response to ESS via SNOT-22, GERD history and treatment by medical record	All patients improved after ESS; no significant impact with history of treated or untreated GERD

CRS, Chronic rhinosinusitis; *CRSwNP*, patients with CRS with nasal polyposis; *EER*, extraesophageal reflux; *GER*, gastroesophageal reflux; *GERD*, gastroesophageal reflux disease; *LPR*, laryngopharyngeal reflux; *MRSI*, modified reflux severity index; *NPR*, nasopharyngeal reflux; *PL*, posterior laryngitis; *PND*, postnasal drip; *SNOT*, sinonasal outcome test; s/p, status post.

removed from the dataset, 45% (15/33) of the study group demonstrates NPR events (pH < 4) versus 10% of control groups (1/10, 2/20) (*P* = .002).[20] Patients with CRS also had significantly increased acidic reflux events (pH < 4) in the esophagus than controls (66 vs. 31%, *P* = .007).

Jecker and colleagues similarly evaluated patients with CRS with continuing symptoms after ESS versus healthy controls using dual channel pH monitoring.[42] They also found that patients with CRS had significantly more reflux events in the esophagus with pH < 4 (fourfold increase) than the control cohort.[14] However, they did not find any differences in reflux events at the hypopharynx. They did not examine reflux at the nasopharyngeal level and also did not report data for pH < 5, excluding weakly acidic reflux events. They concluded that recurrent CRS is associated with GERD but not EER.

Wong and colleagues examined patients with medically refractory CRS and tested them with four-channel pH probe for NPR.[43] Only 5.4% (2/37) of patients were diagnosed with NPR, whereas 32% (12/37) were diagnosed with GER.[47] This study group is similar to DelGaudio's control group with CRS that had improved symptoms after ESS. In addition, the threshold in this study was lower with pH less than 4 instead of a pH less than 5, possibly missing a substantial number of NPR events.[43]

Zelenik and colleagues examined three groups of patients for reflux: CRSsNP, CRSwNP, and CRSwNP and comorbid bronchial asthma, with 90 patients in total.[44] In this study, they performed pharyngeal pH-monitoring (ResTech Corp), calculated a RYAN score that represents composite pharyngeal pH score based on normal volunteers without reflux, and calculated the time exposed to contents with pH < 5.5. In addition, patients with comorbid CRS and bronchial asthma had a higher incidence of revision endoscopic sinus surgery (ESS) and pathologic EER.[44] However, this group was statistically significantly older than the other two groups. Therefore, it is unclear whether the increased pathologic EER and surgeries are attributable to age. This study is limited by the case-series design without an appropriate control group. The ResTech device, which lacks a distal sensor, was used to measure oropharyngeal reflux in these studies. This device does not confirm the presence of distal reflux and may overestimate the number of proximal reflux events with confounding events, such as meals. However, previous studies have shown concordance of ResTech measurements with multichannel pH probe testing when patients accurately report meals and activity.[44]

Wise and colleagues demonstrated that increased PND correlates with NPR regardless of the status of sinus disease.[45] Patients with surgically refractory CRS, patients with surgically controlled CRS, and healthy controls completed sinonasal outcomes test 20 (SNOT-20) and modified reflux severity index (MRSI) questionnaires, as well as underwent the 24-h three-channel pH probe study. For NPR events with pH less than 5, reflux-positive patients reported significantly more PND symptoms on SNOT-20 ($P = .030$) and MRSI as compared with patients without PND symptoms. Interestingly, there was no difference in PND reporting with NPR events with pH less than 4 between groups. This finding may support the importance of nonacid reflux events in the development of PND.

DeConde and colleagues found a similar improvement in QOL by SNOT-22 in patients with CRS after ESS with (n = 72) and without (n = 157) self-reported comorbid GERD.[46] Patients with GERD on medical therapy did not experience a significant difference in QOL improvement after ESS as compared with patients not on therapy.[46] All patients in this study experienced a significant QOL improvement after ESS (=<0.021). In addition, no pH studies were performed in these patients and it unclear if the self-reported diagnosis of GERD is reliable. This study group included patients with medically refractory CRS and not surgically refractory CRS and is therefore different from the patient populations in the studies by DelGaudio and Wise.

EFFECT OF MEDICAL TREATMENT OF REFLUX ON CHRONIC RHINOSINUSITIS SYMPTOMS

Many patients with CRS report PND as a bothersome symptom. Whether this symptom is secondary to CRS or a by-product of comorbid LPR is unknown. Vaezi and colleagues performed a double-blinded randomized controlled trial (RCT) in 75 patients and found that PND significantly improved with twice-daily lansoprazole versus placebo.[48] Patients given lansoprazole had 50% median improvement at 16 weeks of therapy as compared with 5% in the placebo arm.[48] The presence of heartburn, regurgitation, and abnormal esophageal acid or nonacid reflux by impedance-pH probe studies did not predict response to therapy.[48] Patients with chronic sinusitis or allergy were excluded from this study, and therefore results may not be generalizable to this population. However, treatment of patients with proton pump inhibitor (PPI) for PND seems to be effective.

DiBaise treated a small prospective cohort of patients with surgically refractory CRS (n = 11) with twice-daily omeprazole 20 mg for 3 months and found a modest sustained improvement by 8 weeks of therapy.[49] Nine patients had an abnormal pH probe study, and eight patients reported heartburn at least once a week. The greatest improvement was seen in sinus pressure and facial pain.[49] Endoscopic scores did not parallel symptomatic improvement.

Pincus identified 25 patients with positive pH probe studies (NPR, LPR, or GERD) and CRS recalcitrant to medical and surgical therapy and treated them with a PPI once daily for 1 month.[50] Pre- and posttreatment symptom scores were obtained. Only 15 patients completed the PPI course, and 93.3% (14/15) demonstrated a reduction in their symptom score by one or more, whereas 46.7% (7/15) experienced nearcomplete improvement.[50] Again, this study is limited by the lack of a placebo group, small sample size, lack of objective data, and also attrition of patients.

TABLE 3.4
Effect of Medical Treatment of Reflux on CRS Symptoms

References	Type	Size	Measurement	Result
Vaezi et al.[48]	Randomized controlled trial	75 (11 patients excluded) PPI (30) Placebo (34)	Improvement in PND symptoms following treatment with BID lansoprazole versus placebo	Significantly greater percentage improvement in the treatment arm versus control
DiBaise et al.[49]	Case series	CRS (11)	Response to twice-daily PPI therapy in patients with CRS	Modest symptom improvement
Pincus et al.[50]	Case series	Surgically refractory CRS and GERD by pH testing (25)	Response to daily PPI therapy in patients with medically and surgically refractory CRS	Modest symptom improvement
Dagli et al.[51]	Case series Controls not treated with PPI	LPR (29) Control (27)	Total nasal resistance, NOSE score before and after PPI therapy as compared with control (no therapy)	Treatment of patients with LPR with PPI decreases TNR and NOSE score to control levels

BID, Twice a day; *CRS,* chronic rhinosinusitis; *GERD,* gastroesophageal reflux disease; *LPR,* laryngopharyngeal reflux; *PND,* postnasal drip; *PPI,* proton pump inhibitor; *NOSE,* nasal obstruction symptom evaluation scale.

CRS is more often associated with symptoms of nasal obstruction or congestion than PND. However, a recent study demonstrates that patients with LPR alone also experience these symptoms, which are reported to be treatable with PPI. Interestingly, Dagli and colleagues demonstrated significant improvement in total nasal resistance and NOSE score symptoms in patients with LPR after 12 weeks of PPI therapy.[51] The NOSE score in the study group normalized to control levels after PPI therapy. The study participants all had objective evidence of GERD with gastritis or esophagitis on endoscopy and were diagnosed with LPR using the reflux finding score questionnaire (RFS > 7). Patients with CRS and other nasal allergies were excluded. Patients in this study received a maximal PPI therapy of pantoprazole 40 mg twice daily.

The mechanism by which PPIs improve PND and decrease nasal resistance is not clear. PPIs have been shown to reduce both esophageal acid and nonacid reflux, likely by reducing gastric contents, and therefore reduce overall nasal inflammation by direct contact or via autonomic reflex pathway.[43,48] PPIs may also dry nasal secretions and improve nasal airflow secondary to their antihistaminergic and antiinflammatory properties (Table 3.4).[47]

Recommendation of medical treatment of comorbid reflux for patients with CRS:
1. Aggregative quality of evidence: B (mainly cohort and case-control studies with one RCT)
2. Benefit: significant improvement of PND and nasal congestion in patients with reflux with PPI with or without comorbid CRS

3. Harm: Overall incidence of adverse effects to PPI is similar to placebo and <5% (headache, diarrhea, abdominal pain, nausea). PPIs contraindicated in patients with known hypersensitivity to PPIs, and used in caution in patients with severe liver disease. Not recommended in breast-feeding mothers
4. Cost: Over-the-counter PPI cost around $0.5 per pill; 40 mg taken twice daily leads to a cost of $60/month
5. Benefits-harm assessment: benefit over harm
6. Value judgments: The strongest evidence for use of PPI is for the treatment of PND in patients with reflux (Vaezi, RCT, evidence-based medicine grade 1b) and not specifically for CRS; however, given the high incidence of comorbid GERD/CRS and high safety profile of PPI, PPI would be recommended for empiric treatment of surgically refractory nasal obstruction and PND in patients with CRS
7. Recommendation level: Recommendation for patients with CRS with comorbid reflux with symptoms of PND and nasal congestion

REFERENCES

1. Johnston N, et al. Airway reflux. *Ann N Y Acad Sci.* 2016; 1381(1):5–13.
2. Wright MR, Sharda R, Vaezi MF. Unmet needs in treating laryngo-pharyngeal reflux disease: where do we go from here? *Expert Rev Gastroenterol Hepatol.* 2016;10(9):995–1004.

3. Johnston N, et al. Effect of pepsin on laryngeal stress protein (Sep70, Sep53, and Hsp70) response: role in laryngopharyngeal reflux disease. *Ann Otol Rhinol Laryngol.* 2006;115(1):47–58.

4. Koufman JA. The otolaryngologic manifestations of gastroesophageal reflux disease (GERD): a clinical investigation of 225 patients using ambulatory 24-hour pH monitoring and an experimental investigation of the role of acid and pepsin in the development of laryngeal injury. *Laryngoscope.* 1991;101(4 Pt 2 suppl 53):1–78.

5. Johnston N, et al. Activity/stability of human pepsin: implications for reflux attributed laryngeal disease. *Laryngoscope.* 2007;117(6):1036–1039.

6. Johnston N, et al. Receptor-mediated uptake of pepsin by laryngeal epithelial cells. *Ann Otol Rhinol Laryngol.* 2007;116(12):934–938.

7. Johnston N, et al. Pepsin in nonacidic refluxate can damage hypopharyngeal epithelial cells. *Ann Otol Rhinol Laryngol.* 2009;118(9):677–685.

8. Johnston N, et al. Rationale for targeting pepsin in the treatment of reflux disease. *Ann Otol Rhinol Laryngol.* 2010;119(8):547–558.

9. Southwood JE, et al. The impact of pepsin on human nasal epithelial cells in vitro: a potential mechanism for extraesophageal reflux induced chronic rhinosinusitis. *Ann Otol Rhinol Laryngol.* 2015;124(12):957–964.

10. el-Serag HB, Sonnenberg A. Comorbid occurrence of laryngeal or pulmonary disease with esophagitis in United States military veterans. *Gastroenterology.* 1997;113(3):755–760.

11. Leason SR, et al. Association of gastro-oesophageal reflux and chronic rhinosinusitis: systematic review and meta-analysis. *Rhinology.* 2017;55(1):3–16.

12. Tan BK, et al. Incidence and associated premorbid diagnoses of patients with chronic rhinosinusitis. *J Allergy Clin Immunol.* 2013;131(5):1350–1360.

13. Ruhl CE, Sonnenberg A, Everhart JE. Hospitalization with respiratory disease following hiatal hernia and reflux esophagitis in a prospective, population-based study. *Ann Epidemiol.* 2001;11(7):477–483.

14. Ruigomez A, et al. Natural history of gastro-oesophageal reflux disease diagnosed in general practice. *Aliment Pharmacol Ther.* 2004;20(7):751–760.

15. Lin YH, et al. Increased risk of chronic sinusitis in adults with gastroesophgeal reflux disease: a nationwide population-based cohort study. *Medicine (Baltimore).* 2015;94(39):e1642.

16. Katle EJ, et al. Nose- and sinus-related quality of life and GERD. *Eur Arch Otorhinolaryngol.* 2012;269(1):121–125.

17. Theodoropoulos DS, et al. Prevalence of upper respiratory symptoms in patients with symptomatic gastroesophageal reflux disease. *Am J Respir Crit Care Med.* 2001;164(1):72–76.

18. Delehaye E, et al. Correlation between nasal mucociliary clearance time and gastroesophageal reflux disease: our experience on 50 patients. *Auris Nasus Larynx.* 2009;36(2):157–161.

19. Katle EJ, et al. Gastro-oesophageal reflux in patients with chronic rhino-sinusitis investigated with multichannel impedance – pH monitoring. *Rhinology.* 2017;55(1):27–33.

20. DelGaudio JM. Direct nasopharyngeal reflux of gastric acid is a contributing factor in refractory chronic rhinosinusitis. *Laryngoscope.* 2005;115(6):946–957.

21. Dinis PB, Subtil J. *Helicobacter pylori* and laryngopharyngeal reflux in chronic rhinosinusitis. *Otolaryngol Head Neck Surg.* 2006;134(1):67–72.

22. Loehrl TA, et al. The role of extraesophageal reflux in medically and surgically refractory rhinosinusitis. *Laryngoscope.* 2012;122(7):1425–1430.

23. Ozmen S, et al. Nasal pepsin assay and pH monitoring in chronic rhinosinusitis. *Laryngoscope.* 2008;118(5):890–894.

24. Wong IW, et al. Gastroesophageal reflux disease and chronic sinusitis: in search of an esophageal-nasal reflex. *Am J Rhinol Allergy.* 2010;24(4):255–259.

25. Loehrl TA, et al. Autonomic dysfunction, vasomotor rhinitis, and extraesophageal manifestations of gastroesophageal reflux. *Otolaryngol Head Neck Surg.* 2002;126(4):382–387.

26. Morinaka S, Ichimiya M, Nakamura H. Detection of *Helicobacter pylori* in nasal and maxillary sinus specimens from patients with chronic sinusitis. *Laryngoscope.* 2003;113(9):1557–1563.

27. Koc C, et al. Prevalence of *Helicobacter pylori* in patients with nasal polyps: a preliminary report. *Laryngoscope.* 2004;114(11):1941–1944.

28. Ozdek A, et al. A possible role of *Helicobacter pylori* in chronic rhinosinusitis: a preliminary report. *Laryngoscope.* 2003;113(4):679–682.

29. Cvorovic L, et al. Detection of *Helicobacter pylori* in nasal polyps: preliminary report. *J Otolaryngol Head Neck Surg.* 2008;37(2):192–195.

30. Kim HY, et al. Intranasal *Helicobacter pylori* colonization does not correlate with the severity of chronic rhinosinusitis. *Otolaryngol Head Neck Surg.* 2007;136(3):390–395.

31. Vceva A, et al. The significance of *Helicobacter pylori* in patients with nasal polyposis. *Med Glas (Zenica).* 2012;9(2):281–286.

32. Ozyurt M, et al. Real-time PCR detection of *Helicobacter pylori* and virulence-associated cagA in nasal polyps and laryngeal disorders. *Otolaryngol Head Neck Surg.* 2009;141(1):131–135.

33. Ozcan C, et al. Does *Helicobacter pylori* play a role in etiology of nasal polyposis? *Auris Nasus Larynx.* 2009;36(4):427–430.

34. Burduk PK, et al. Detection of *Helicobacter pylori* and cagA gene in nasal polyps and benign laryngeal diseases. *Arch Med Res.* 2011;42(8):686–689.

35. Nemati S, et al. Investigating *Helicobacter pylori* in nasal polyposis using polymerase chain reaction, urease test and culture. *Eur Arch Otorhinolaryngol.* 2012;269(5):1457–1461.

36. Jelavic B, et al. Prognostic value of *Helicobacter pylori* sinonasal colonization for efficacy of endoscopic sinus surgery. *Eur Arch Otorhinolaryngol.* 2012;269(10):2197–2202.
37. Lupa M, DelGaudio JM. Evidence-based practice: reflux in sinusitis. *Otolaryngol Clin North Am.* 2012;45(5):983–992.
38. Hamamoto J, et al. Esophageal stimulation by hydrochloric acid causes neurogenic inflammation in the airways in guinea pigs. *J Appl Physiol (1985).* 1997;82(3):738–745.
39. Chambers DW, et al. Long-term outcome analysis of functional endoscopic sinus surgery: correlation of symptoms with endoscopic examination findings and potential prognostic variables. *Laryngoscope.* 1997;107(4):504–510.
40. Ulualp SO, Toohill RJ, Shaker R. Pharyngeal acid reflux in patients with single and multiple otolaryngologic disorders. *Otolaryngol Head Neck Surg.* 1999;121(6):725–730.
41. Ulualp SO, et al. Possible relationship of gastroesophagopharyngeal acid reflux with pathogenesis of chronic sinusitis. *Am J Rhinol.* 1999;13(3):197–202.
42. Jecker P, et al. Gastroesophageal reflux disease (GERD), extraesophageal reflux (EER) and recurrent chronic rhinosinusitis. *Eur Arch Otorhinolaryngol.* 2006;263(7):664–667.
43. Wong IW, et al. Nasopharyngeal pH monitoring in chronic sinusitis patients using a novel four channel probe. *Laryngoscope.* 2004;114(9):1582–1585.
44. Zelenik K, et al. Patients with chronic rhinosinusitis and simultaneous bronchial asthma suffer from significant extraesophageal reflux. *Int Forum Allergy Rhinol.* 2015;5(10):944–949.
45. Wise SK, Wise JC, DelGaudio JM. Association of nasopharyngeal and laryngopharyngeal reflux with postnasal drip symptomatology in patients with and without rhinosinusitis. *Am J Rhinol.* 2006;20(3):283–289.
46. DeConde AS, Mace JC, Smith TL. The impact of comorbid gastroesophageal reflux disease on endoscopic sinus surgery quality-of-life outcomes. *Int Forum Allergy Rhinol.* 2014;4(8):663–669.
47. Kedika RR, Souza RF, Spechler SJ. Potential anti-inflammatory effects of proton pump inhibitors: a review and discussion of the clinical implications. *Dig Dis Sci.* 2009;54(11):2312–2317.
48. Vaezi MF, et al. Proton pump inhibitor therapy improves symptoms in postnasal drainage. *Gastroenterology.* 2010;139(6):1887–1893. e1; quiz e11.
49. DiBaise JK, et al. Role of GERD in chronic resistant sinusitis: a prospective, open label, pilot trial. *Am J Gastroenterol.* 2002;97(4):843–850.
50. Pincus RL, et al. A study of the link between gastric reflux and chronic sinusitis in adults. *Ear Nose Throat J.* 2006;85(3):174–178.
51. Dagli E, et al. Association of Oral Antireflux Medication with laryngopharyngeal reflux and nasal resistance. *JAMA Otolaryngol Head Neck Surg.* 2017;143.

CHAPTER 4

Evidence-Based Practice: Balloon Catheter Dilation in Rhinology

PETE S. BATRA, MD, FACS • BOBBY A. TAJUDEEN, MD • DANNY JANDALI, MD

KEY POINTS

- Numerous studies have evaluated the utility of balloon dilatation for surgical management of adult chronic rhinosinusitis; however, existing data include extensive exclusionary criteria thus narrowing the evaluable literature to a subgroup of patients with chronic rhinosinusitis (CRS) with more limited disease.

- One study provides sufficiently powered level 1 evidence that balloon catheter dilation (BCD) may be a potential treatment option for patients with limited sinus disease involving the maxillary sinus only or maxillary with anterior ethmoid disease.

- Four studies that assess BCD for pediatric chronic rhinosinusitis are graded level 4 and 2b; they are confounded by concurrent adenoidectomy in significant number of the children, precluding the ability to discern the impact of each intervention.

- Most studies that report the use of BCD for frontal sinus disease are level 4, although recent prospective studies suggest possible utility of the technology for select cases.

- The overall recommendation is grade C for the use of BCD for paranasal sinus inflammatory disease, with a higher level grade being reserved until well-controlled randomized trials are available in representative populations with CRS.

BACKGROUND ON CHRONIC RHINOSINUSITIS

Chronic rhinosinusitis (CRS) represents a clinical disorder characterized by inflammation of the mucosa of the nose and paranasal sinuses of 12 weeks duration.[1] The International Consensus Statement on Allergy and Rhinology clinically defines CRS by two or more of the following symptoms: mucopurulent discharge, nasal obstruction/congestion, decreased or absent smell, and facial pressure/pain.[2] Symptomatology is supported by endoscopic evidence of mucopurulence, edema, or polyps and/or computed tomography (CT) presence of mucosal thickening or air-fluid levels in the sinuses. Indeed, CRS is one of the most common chronic medical conditions in the United States, afflicting approximately 31 million Americans.[3] The illness accounts for 18–22 million office visits annually, resulting in an estimated $6 billion in direct and indirect healthcare expenditures.[4] CRS not only causes physical symptoms but also results in significant functional and emotional impairment, and the quality of life (QOL) scores measured are similar to those of patients with other chronic debilitating illnesses, including congestive heart failure,

angina, and back pain.[5] The exact pathophysiologic mechanisms resulting in CRS remain elusive to date. A variety of host and environmental factors have been implicated, including derangements in innate and adaptive immunity, ciliary dysfunction, inhalant allergies, infectious agents (viral, bacterial, and/or fungal), superantigens, biofilms, and osteitis.

Medical therapy remains the cornerstone in the overall management schema of patients with CRS. This typically entails various oral and topical agents, such as antibiotics, steroids, antihistamines, leukotriene receptor antagonists, saline irrigations, and mucolytics. Functional endoscopic sinus surgery (FESS) represents the main surgical strategy for the management of medically recalcitrant CRS. FESS is a minimally invasive, mucosal-sparing surgical technique that hopes to achieve one or more of the following goals: (1) to open the sinuses to facilitate ventilation and drainage, (2) to remove polyps and/or osteitic bone fragments to reduce the inflammatory load, (3) to enlarge the sinus ostia to achieve optimal instillation of topical therapies, and (4) to obtain bacterial and fungal cultures and tissue for histopathology. FESS has been demonstrated to be effective in improving symptoms and QOL in adult patients with CRS.[6] A multiinstitutional prospective trial has illustrated improvement in QOL in both medically and surgically treated patients with CRS; however, the FESS group experienced significantly more improvement in disease-specific QOL, reduction in the need for systemic antibiotics and steroids, and decrease in missed work/school days.[7]

OVERVIEW OF BALLOON CATHETER TECHNOLOGIES
Balloon Sinuplasty
The use of balloon catheters for frontal sinus dilation was initially described by Lanza in 1993.[8] He utilized Fogarty balloon catheters under endoscopic guidance in post-FESS patients to achieve temporary ventilation and drainage of the frontal recess. In 2002, California-based engineers started the process of adapting cardiac catheters to perform paranasal sinus balloon dilation.[9] The balloon catheter technology cleared the US Food and Drug Administration (FDA) 510(k) pathway in April 2005 and was launched as Balloon Sinuplasty (Acclarent, Inc., Menlo Park, CA).[10] In contrast to traditional balloons that are compliant with and conform to regional anatomy, the new device is semirigid and non-compliant, with the ability to displace adjacent bone and tissue on inflation. The basic premise of balloon catheter dilation (BCD) is the Seldinger technique, with initial access being gained by endoscopic placement of a guide catheter. A flexible guide is introduced through the guide catheter and its position in the targeted sinus confirmed by fluoroscopy, transillumination, or image guidance. The balloon catheter is then advanced over the guidewire and gradually inflated to dilate the obstructed sinus ostium.[10]

The initial cadaver study on BCD was presented at the annual American Rhinologic Society meeting in 2005.[11] Technical feasibility and safety were evaluated by dilation of 31 sinus ostia (9 maxillary, 11 sphenoid, and 11 frontal) in six cadaver heads. BCT successfully dilated all 31 sinuses and did not result in adjacent skull base or orbital injury in any case. The authors posited that balloon technology also appeared to impart less mucosal trauma than standard endoscopic instruments, although no comparative analysis was performed in the study. This was followed by the first patient trial on BCD in 10 patients with persistent CRS after failed medical therapy.[12] A total of 18 sinuses were dilated, with 8 of 10 patients undergoing concurrent ethmoidectomy. All sinuses were successfully dilated without adverse events, although the authors noted

that the maxillary sinus was the most difficult to cannulate given the relative position of the natural ostium to the uncinate process. This study served to provide proof of concept in limited number of patients without any follow-up period. The impact on the underlying disease process was unclear.

LacriCATH
The LacriCATH system (Quest Medical, Inc., Allen, TX) is an established balloon device utilized for dilation of the lacrimal outflow system for chronic epiphora.[13] Citardi and Kanowitz performed endoscopic paranasal sinus dissection in three cadaver heads using conventional FESS instrumentation concurrently with the lacrimal balloon for BCD.[14] Frontal recess dissection was successfully performed in all six sinuses with FESS instruments and BCD, while all six sphenoid sinuses were also successfully dilated. They noted that it was not feasible to reliably pass the balloon through the maxillary natural ostium, with only three of six being successfully dilated with this technique. This study provided proof of concept in a cadaver model, precluding extrapolation of the intervention in patients with CRS. The study highlighted the potential technical limitation of BCD of the maxillary sinus in patients with an intact uncinate process.

FinESS
FinESS or Functional Infundibular Endoscopic Sinus System (Entellus Medical, Inc., Maple Grove, MN) obtained FDA clearance in April 2008 and was launched at the annual American Academy of Otolaryngology meeting later that year.[10] The transantral dilation system uses a flexible 0.5-mm endoscope and dual-channel cannula to localize the maxillary sinus ostia via the canine fossa approach. BCD of the maxillary ostium and ethmoid infundibulum is then performed under endoscopic visualization. The initial data on this device were reported in a multicenter Balloon Remodeling Antrostomy Therapy study (BREATHE I) that assessed outcomes and safety in patients with CRS.[15] Of 58 maxillary ostia, 55 (94.8%) were successfully treated, with 97% being performed under local anesthesia with or without minimal sedation. Mean Sinonasal Outcome Test (SNOT-20) scores had statistically significant improvement at 6 months, with patency in 95.8% by CT imaging. Follow-up data demonstrated sustained improvement in all four domains on SNOT-20 at 1 year.[16] These two studies serve to provide a proof of clinical concept of this technology. The technology may be applicable to patients with limited disease focused at the maxillary infundibulum; however, broader application to the larger subset of CRS is not afforded by the data.

EVIDENCE-BASED CLINICAL ASSESSMENT

Given the paucity of randomized, controlled studies, the exact role of the various balloon catheter devices in the management of CRS and its subtypes remains to be elucidated to date. Thus definitive recommendations on how to evaluate patients thought suitable for BCD are limited at the present juncture. Nonetheless, the available database has reported on a multitude of potential applications in patients with paranasal sinus inflammatory disease. Studies have reported on both adult and pediatric CRS refractory to maximal medical therapy.[17–24] Several studies have explored the utility of BCD in frontal sinus disease.[25–31] The surgical technique section evaluates the evidence base available for the various applications.

EVIDENCE-BASED SURGICAL TECHNIQUE

Adult Medically Refractory Chronic Rhinosinusitis

Multiple retrospective and prospective case series have reported on the utility of BCD on medically refractory adult CRS. The present analysis does not purport to analyze every available study on this topic. Instead, it focuses on the salient studies to highlight the current state of the evidence. The initial large-scale investigation, dubbed the CLEAR study, reported on 109 patients with nonpolypoid CRS unresponsive to medical management who underwent planned FESS.[17] Follow-up evaluations were performed at 1, 2, 12, and 24 weeks, with the main outcomes measures being ostial patency, SNOT-20 scores, and global rating of improvement. Overall, 52% of patients underwent concomitant FESS, or so-called hybrid procedures. The mean Lund-Mackay scores for the balloon-only and hybrid groups were 6.1 and 10.4, respectively.

Most procedures were performed uneventfully without any cases of cerebrospinal fluid (CSF) leaks, orbital injury, or epistaxis requiring packing. BCD appeared to be technically feasible, although there were 12 device malfunctions. Endoscopic sinus ostial patency rates at 24 weeks were 91% for maxillary sinus, 82% at frontal sinus, and 60% for sphenoid sinus. A significant number of frontal (17%) and sphenoid (39%) sinuses were not evaluable because of inadequate postoperative endoscopic visualization. A statistically significant decrease in SNOT-20 scores was noted for both the balloon and hybrid groups. Specifically, the scores of the balloon group patients decreased from 2.14 to 1.27, whereas the hybrid group scores improved from 2.42 to 1.02.

One-year follow-up data were reported on 66 patients from the original cohort.[18] The remainder were excluded from the analysis because of attrition, loss to follow-up, and loss of study sites. Postoperative ostial patency by endoscopy and CT was 93.5% for maxillary sinus, 91.9% for frontal sinus, and 86.1% for sphenoid sinus. Mean SNOT-20 scores for balloon-only and hybrid subsets improved to 0.95 and 0.87, respectively. Additional 2-year follow-up data were published on 65 of the above-mentioned patients.[19] The SNOT-20 scores for the balloon-only and hybrid groups dropped to 1.09 and 0.66, respectively. The Lund-Mackay scores improved from 5.7 to 1.8 and from 12.1 to 3.3 for patients of the balloon-only and hybrid groups, respectively. Overall, 85% of patients reported symptom improvement, with 15% same and 0% worse.

Many important observations can be gleaned from the aforementioned series. They attest to the technical feasibility and safety of the balloon to achieve sinus ostia dilation. Furthermore, 1- and 2-year follow-up studies demonstrated the potential for reasonable ostial patency over this time period. Yet many questions remain unanswered. The patient cohort for these studies was not clearly defined; moreover, a uniform management algorithm was not applied to tailor the medical and surgical therapy. Thus it is unclear if the data can be generalized to all patients with CRS.

The CLEAR study represents a single-arm, uncontrolled, observational study. However, the lack of a comparison group greatly limits meaningful interpretation of the results; importantly, it precludes any efficacy claims relative to FESS. Comparison of the mean SNOT-20 scores for the balloon-only and hybrid groups offers an insightful analysis.[32] The balloon-only group improved from a baseline of 2.14 to 0.99 and 1.09 at 1 and 2 years, respectively. On the other hand, the hybrid group started at a higher mean SNOT-20 score of 2.42 and improved to 0.68 and 0.64 at 1 and 2 years, respectively. This would suggest that patients undergoing concurrent ethmoidectomy not only have higher baseline SNOT-20 scores but also derive greater benefit from surgery. Although the data were intended to be interpreted exactly in this manner, it does serve to highlight the potential usefulness of direct comparative trials to better understand the role of BCD compared with FESS.

In one of the largest retrospective studies to date, Levine et al. reported outcomes of BCD on 1036 patients from a multicenter registry.[20] BCD was used in 3276 sinuses, with a mean of 3.2 sinuses per patient. Sinonasal symptoms improved in 95.2%, were unchanged in 3.8%, and became worse in 1.0% of patients.

Postoperative infections were significantly less frequent and less severe compared with preoperatively. No major adverse events were attributable to balloons, although two CSF leaks were documented in patients who underwent concurrent ethmoidectomy. Six cases had minor bleeding, requiring use of packing or cautery. Perhaps the most important observation that stems from the data is the safety profile of BCD. However, the study does not afford the ability to reliably assess the impact of BCD on CRS. The data are pooled across 27 sites with no standardization of medical treatment or indications for surgery. The starting burden of disease by endoscopy and/or CT was not defined. The use of subjective symptom improvement as the primary end point and lack of validated outcome measures prevent robust assessment of BCD on the underlying disease process.

Friedman et al. performed a comparative retrospective analysis of prospectively collected data in 70 patients who underwent BCD versus FESS.[21] Inclusion criteria included recurrent rhinosinusitis in patients with either a persistently abnormal CT after 4 weeks of continuous therapy or an abnormal CT during treatment, with posttreatment normalization and three or more recurrences per year. Exclusion criteria included Lund-McKay scores >12, significant polyposis, osteoneogenesis, or systemic disease. Thirty-five patients in each treatment arm were assessed by SNOT-20 scores, global patient assessment, postoperative narcotic usage, and cost at a minimum of 3-month follow-up. The SNOT-20 scores improved from 2.8 to 0.78 for the balloon group and from 2.7 to 1.29 for the FESS group,

demonstrating clinically and statistically significant improvement in both groups. Patient satisfaction was higher and narcotic usage was lower in the BCD group. The average cost of BCD ($12,657) was less than that of FESS ($14,471); the lower charges were attributed to shorter operative and recovery times and the reduced need for general anesthesia with BCD.

On the surface, the results may suggest superiority of BCD over FESS in this comparative study. However, delving deeper into the data, it becomes apparent the study represents a highly selective patient sample that did not undergo matching or randomization. The patients decided on their surgical intervention, thus likely influencing the symptom and satisfaction scores. Furthermore, the study did not report on ostial patency for this patient group, acknowledging the inherent limitations in adequate endoscopic visualization in patients with an intact uncinate process. The relatively short follow-up time period in a chronic inflammatory process that often spans years is an additional drawback that precludes meaningful interpretation of the data. In addition, the operative charges are estimation at best.

Since 2012, there have been numerous additional studies that reported the evaluation of postoperative outcomes among patients who underwent BCD for CRS both in the office and operating room setting (Table 4.1). The largest studies to date include the Optimization and Refinement of Technique in In-Office Sinus Dilation 2 (ORIOS) and Randomized Evaluation of Maxillary Antrostomy Versus Ostial Dilation Efficacy Through Long-Term Follow-up (REMODEL) groups. The ORIOS

TABLE 4.1
Evidence-Based Prospective Studies of Balloon Catheter Dilation of Adult CRS Since 2012

Study	Study Design	Outcome Measure	Level of Evidence	Findings	Polyp Disease
Abreu[33]	Prospective	SNOT-20, LM scores	2b	Positive	Excluded
Achar[34]	Prospective	SNOT-20, CT sinus	2b	Positive	Excluded
Albritton[35]	Prospective	SNOT-20, LM scores	2b	Positive	Included
Bikhazi[36] Cutler[37]	Prospective	SNOT-20	1b	Positive	Excluded
Brodner[38]	Prospective	Safety, patency, SNOT-20	2b	Positive	Included
Gould[39]	Prospective	SNOT-20/RSI	2b	Positive	Excluded
Karanfilov[40] Sikand[41]	Prospective	SNOT-20, LM scores	2b	Positive	Limited
Payne[42]	Prospective	CSS score, SNOT-20, RSDI	2b	Positive	Limited
Raghunandhan[43]	Prospective	SNOT-20, endoscopy, LM	2b	Positive	Excluded

CSS, Chronic Sinusitis Survey; *CRS*, chronic rhinosinusitis; *LM*, Lund-Mackay; *RSI*, Rhinosinusitis Symptom Inventory; *RSDI*, Rhinosinusitis Disability Index; *SNOT-20*, Sinonasal Outcome Test.

study began as an initial prospective, single-arm, nonrandomized, multicenter evaluation of in-office BCD in 38 patients with CRS.[35] The goal of the study was to assess technical success of BCD in the office setting. The ORIOS investigators reported in-office technical success as 89% with no adverse complications. As a secondary outcome, patients were assessed at 1, 4, 24, and 52 weeks with point-of-care CT scans obtained at 24 weeks. The authors note a statistically significant reduction of mean SNOT-20 from baseline of −0.98, −1.32, −1.25, and −1.43 at 1, 4, 24, and 52 weeks, respectively ($P < .0001$). An improvement in the mean Lund-Mackay score of 6.62 at baseline to 2.79 was noted at 24 weeks ($P < .001$). The study demonstrated safety and technical feasibility of BCD in the in-office setting. The secondary outcomes, however, suffer from several limitations. As with single-arm studies, the lack of a control group limits the evaluation of BCD for therapy of CRS. Furthermore, 24% of subjects (9/37) underwent adjunctive in-office procedures such as turbinoplasty, further limiting the assessment of BCD in patient outcomes. In addition, there was significant loss to follow-up, with only 57% of patients reaching the 52-week time point. Lastly, medical therapy after BCD was not standardized and was determined by the treating physician, adding additional confounding variables.

Following the results of the ORIOS study, the ORIOS2 study was initiated to compile a larger cohort with 203 patients from 14 centers.[40] The study group included patients with medically refractory CRS as defined by failure of >3 weeks of antibiotics and >3 weeks of intranasal and/or oral steroids. Patients with grade 3 nasal polyposis were excluded. Unlike the previous ORIOS study, patients needing adjunctive procedures were excluded. All patients underwent in-office BCD and were followed up to 24 weeks. Primary end points included change in SNOT-20 and Lund-Mackay scores from baseline and 24 weeks. Secondary outcome measures included safety, technical success, patient tolerability, satisfaction, return to normal activity, need for postoperative debridements, and need for revision surgery. Balloon dilation was successful in 552 of 592 sinuses (93.2%). No device-related or procedure-related serious adverse events occurred. One patient developed periorbital swelling that resolved spontaneously after the procedure. Overall, 113 of the original 203 patients completed follow-up to 24 weeks. The mean SNOT-20 change from a baseline SNOT-20 of 2.1 was −1, −1.2, and −1.1 at 2, 8 and 24 weeks, respectively. Statistical significance was present to <0.0001 at all time points. The baseline Lund-Mackay score was 6.9 (±3.6), with reduction to 2.5 (±3) at 24 weeks ($P < .0001$). Patients rated the procedure as "highly tolerable" in 82.3%, with 3% reporting the procedure as intolerable. The average number of debridements was 0.15 per patient.

As an extension of the ORIOS2 study, a follow-up study was conducted in which the original cohort of patients was invited for 52-week follow-up.[41] This extended study included 122 patients of the original 203 patients, all of whom completed the 52-week follow-up. Baseline SNOT-20 reduced from 2.1 (±0.9) to 1.0 (±0.9) at 52 weeks ($P < .001$).

Many positive conclusions can be gathered from the results of the ORIOS2 studies. Most importantly, the studies demonstrate in a large cohort of patients that in-office BCD is technically feasible with good patient tolerability and low complication rate. The authors also purport that QOL improvements are seen as early as 2 weeks, with maintenance to 52 weeks. Although the results appear promising, the ORIOS2 study suffers from the same weaknesses of the original ORIOS study. Again, owing to the lack of a control group, the effect of BCD is difficult to determine. Postprocedure management significantly varied depending on physician preference. Therefore, it is unclear to what degree close follow-up and medical management played in improving outcomes. In addition, reenrollment in the 52-week extension study was on a voluntary basis, in which only 122 of the original 203 patients elected to participate. This introduces additional potential for bias, as patients who were not satisfied with their outcome may have opted to not reenroll. Nonetheless, the study provides level 2b evidence in a large cohort that in-office BCD is safe and patients who undergo the procedure in conjunction with close follow-up and medical therapy may derive QOL improvement.

To date, two randomized control trials have been performed to assess the efficacy of BCD to FESS.[34,36,37] The REMODEL trial is the largest of these trials including 92 patients; it is the only randomized control trial of sufficient power to draw conclusions.[37] Eligible patients were at least 18 years of age and were diagnosed with either chronic or recurrent sinusitis. Importantly, patients with posterior ethmoid, sphenoid, frontal, fungal disease and polypoid disease were excluded. This yielded a study cohort of patients with maxillary disease only (62%) or maxillary and anterior ethmoid disease (38%). Patients were randomized to obtain either in-office balloon dilation of the maxillary sinus or operative FESS including uncinectomy and maxillary antrostomy with or without anterior ethmoidectomy. Postoperative follow-up assessments were conducted at 1 week and 1, 3, and 6 months. The primary end point included improvement in sinus symptoms as measured by mean SNOT-20 scores and number of postoperative debridements. The six-month follow-up was excellent at 98.9%. Important findings noted by the authors included equivalent mean SNOT-20 score change between groups (1.67 ± 1.10 in the balloon arm and 1.60 ± 0.96 in the FESS arm). On the other hand, FESS had a higher requirement for debridement (0.1 ± 0.6 in the balloon arm and 1.2 ± 1.0 in the FESS arm, P < .0001). Secondary findings included a 0% complication rate in both arms, faster return to normal daily activity (1.6 vs. 4.8 days, P = .001) in the balloon arm, and less pain medication requirement in the balloon arm (0.9 vs. 2.8 days, P < .001).

A follow-up study of the REMODEL trial included the same cohort of patients with follow-up to 12 months.[36] Overall, 89 of the original 92 patients completed follow-up to 1 year. Again, improvement in the baseline SNOT-20 score in both arms was nearly equivalent (−1.64 ± 1.06 in the balloon arm and −1.65 ± 0.94 in the FESS arm). A 0% complication rate was maintained.

The REMODEL trial was the first and only prospective RCT with sufficient power. Although the results of the REMODEL trial support noninferiority of balloon dilation to FESS, significant caution should be exercised when interpreting the results. Most importantly, the external validity of the analysis is limited, as patients in the participating head-to-head trial had limited disease severity. The study did not include patients with nasal polyposis, posterior ethmoid, sphenoid, or frontal disease. In addition, the average Lund-Mackay score was 3.2 at baseline. A mean "normal" Lund-Mackay score of 4.26 (confidence interval: 3.43–5.0) has been reported in the literature of patients undergoing CT of the paranasal sinus region for reasons unrelated to sinusitis.[44] Although it has been established that the Lund-Mackay score does not correlate with the SNOT score, the low opacification score combined with exclusion criteria of patients with advanced CRS limits the evaluated population to a select subset of patients with CRS with very limited disease. Additional study of patients with more advanced CRS is necessary to further support the use of BCD among all patients with CRS. This point was also supported by a recent meta-analysis by Levy et al. in which collective review of the literature failed to support BCD as an indication for CRS.[45] This conclusion stemmed primarily from extensive exclusion criteria noted in the literature. In addition, the authors note a high prevalence of industry support introducing significant potential conflict of interest and inherent bias. Aside from these highlighted issues, the REMODEL study provides level 1 evidence that BCD may be a potential treatment option for patients with limited maxillary only or maxillary with anterior ethmoid disease.

Pediatric Medically Refractory Chronic Rhinosinusitis

Ramadan reported initial data on technical feasibility and safety of BCD in children.[22] Thirty children with medically recalcitrant CRS underwent BCD; concurrent adenoidectomy was performed in 13 patients (43%). The procedures were technically feasible in 51 of 56 sinuses (91%), with no complications attributable to BCD. The feasibility rate was 98% in normal sinuses, decreasing to 60% in hypoplastic sinuses. The average fluoroscopy time was 18 s per sinus, with a mean fluoroscopy exposure of 0.18 mGy. The preliminary data again attest to the safety of BCD. It does suggest that, although the procedure is technically feasible in children, the inherent limitations posed by the smaller, especially hypoplastic, sinuses result in a lower cannulation rate in children. The study provides proof of concept in pediatric patients with CRS. The short- or long-term impact on the underlying disease process was unclear.

In a follow-up study, Ramadan and Terrell presented experience on 49 pediatric patients with CRS who underwent BCD and/or adenoidectomy with a postoperative follow-up of 1 year.[24] The groups were matched except for age, with the adenoidectomy alone group being statistically younger (4.8 years) than the balloon group (7.7 years). The comparative groups included adenoidectomy alone (19) or BCD (30); 17 in the latter group also underwent adenoidectomy. Symptom improvement, defined as a decrease of 0.5 or more on the sinonasal-5 (SN-5) questionnaire, was seen in 24 (80%) and 10 (52.6%) in the balloon and adenoidectomy alone groups, respectively. These data suggest the potential utility of BCD in the pediatric patients. However, similar to the study by Friedman et al.,[21] the two groups represent highly selective samples without any attempt at randomization. Moreover, given that 17 of the 30 in the balloon group underwent concomitant adenoidectomy, the exact impact of BCD on the underlying disease process and SN-5 scores is unclear. In fact, the intervention of adenoidectomy in both groups greatly confounds the ability to interpret the findings.

A subsequent prospective, multicenter, nonrandomized study evaluated the efficacy of BCD in 32 children with CRS.[23] Concurrent adenoidectomy was performed in 15 patients. Twenty-four patients (75%) completed the 52-week follow-up. BCD was successful in 56 of 63 (89%) sinuses. The seven failed sinuses comprised three hypoplastic maxillary sinuses, three sphenoid sinuses, and one frontal sinus. The SN-5 score improved from 4.9 at baseline to 2.95 at 52 weeks. Overall, improvement was deemed significant in 50%, moderate in 29%, and mild in 8%. One had no improvement, whereas two worsened in the postoperative period. Although this study makes a compelling case for BCD in pediatric patients, the impact of BCD is difficult to discern, given that 15 (46.9%) had simultaneous adenoidectomy and 6 (18.9%) had concurrent ethmoidectomy.

The largest and most recent study of pediatric BCD was performed by Soler et al.[46] In this prospective, multicenter, single-arm investigation, 50 children (age 2–21 years) with medically refractory CRS were treated with BCD and followed up for 6 months post procedure. Multiple concurrent procedures were performed, including concurrent adenoidectomy in 42%, inferior turbinate reduction in 26%, ethmoidectomy in 12%, and concha bullosa resection in 6%. Visit compliance for follow-ups was 99%, with all participants completing the 6-month follow-up. A total of 157 sinus dilations were attempted (98 maxillary, 30 frontal, and 29 sphenoid sinuses) with 100% technical success rate. No adverse events were reported through the 6-month follow-up for all participants. Across the entire cohort, there was mean improvement in overall SN-5 scores from baseline to 6 months (4.6 vs. 1.7, $P < .0001$). Overall, 82% of participants had achieved large improvement, 10% moderate improvement, 2% slight improvement, and 6% no clinical change. In participants greater than 12 years of age, SNOT-22 scores showed significant improvement from baseline (from 42.4 to 10.4, $P < .0001$). Multivariate regression analysis noted no difference in SN-5 outcomes when comparing those with and without concurrent sinonasal procedures.

Data from this study provide additional feasibility of BCD in children with a success rate of 100% with no serious adverse events reported. Review and oversight by the FDA was provided for this study, and the data were used to obtain FDA clearance for the expanded indication for treating maxillary sinuses in children 2 years and older and frontal and sphenoid sinuses in children 12 years and older. Clinical efficacy was a secondary outcome of the study, and although the results were reassuring, the study has similar shortcomings to the previous investigations. First, the study is a single-arm study with no control group, leaving uncertainty to conclude that BCD itself provided the entirety of the QOL improvement. In addition, 60% of patients had concurrent procedures, most commonly adenoidectomy (40%), and therefore the relative contribution of each procedure is not discernible. The authors in this study performed multivariate analysis and supported that improvements in SN-5 were obtained controlling for concomitant procedures. In addition, a subgroup analysis of the patients who underwent BCD alone (40%) showed significant improvement in QOL with shorter recovery times (3.1 vs. 1.1 days, $P = .0002$).

The potential beneficial effect of adenoidectomy in pediatric patients with CRS cannot be understated. The adenoid may serve as a reservoir of potentially pathogenic bacteria; the overall adenoid bacterial isolation rate has been noted to be as high as 79%, with the isolate rate increasing with sinusitis grade.[47] A meta-analysis of adenoidectomy in medically refractory CRS demonstrated improvement of sinusitis symptoms or outcomes in 69.3% of the patients.[48] Given its simplicity, effectiveness, and low risk profile, adenoidectomy likely represents a first-line therapy for uncomplicated pediatric CRS. Direct comparative trials of adenoidectomy, BCD, and FESS would be required to better understand the role of balloons in the management algorithm of pediatric CRS.

Frontal Sinus Disease

BCD has been touted as a potential minimally invasive alternative to endoscopic frontal sinusotomy (EFS) for frontal sinus disease. Several studies to date have evaluated the utility of balloons in this regard (Table 4.2).[25-31,49] Khalid et al. performed frontal recess BCD in eight cadaver heads to evaluate the patterns of fracture of bony lamellae and change in frontal recess dimensions using pre- and postintervention endoscopy and CT.[26] This in turn was compared with the degree of change seen with EFS. BCD resulted in statistically less change in mean coronal (0.9 mm vs. 2.6 mm) and sagittal (1.0 mm vs. 4.0 mm) dimensions compared with EFS. The most commonly fractured lamella after BCD was the anterior face of the ethmoid bulla (56%). The clinical significance of these two interventions on frontal sinus disease is not afforded by the cadaveric data; from a technical perspective, it does suggest that BCD results in smaller frontal sinus outflow tract (FSOT) dimensions and may not produce consistent fracture patterns of the bony lamellae of the frontal recess cells.

Catalano and Payne performed BCD in 20 patients with medically refractory chronic frontal sinusitis.[25] A total of 29 frontal sinuses were accrued with either complete opacification or partial opacification with a total Lund-McKay score of ≥10. The disease was categorized grade I (<5 mm of mucosal thickening), II (≥5 mm of mucosal thickening, partial opacification, air-fluid level), and III (total opacification) in 10, 5, and 14 frontal sinuses, respectively. Overall, improvement was noted in 14 of 29 frontal sinuses (48.3%) using CT as the primary outcome measure. Success rate by disease subtype for Samter triad, CRS with polyposis, and CRS without polyposis was 36.4%, 40%, and 61.5%, respectively. The authors felt that "…50% of the frontal sinuses in this study group were spared aggressive

TABLE 4.2
Evidence-Based Studies on Balloon Catheter Dilation for Frontal Sinus Disease

Author	Indication	N	Study Design	Evidence Based Medicine (EBM) Level	Outcome
Catalano[25]	Chronic frontal sinusitis +/- polyps	20	Retrospective	4	Mixed
Khalid[26]	Anatomic dimensions in normal sinuses	8	Cadavers	5	Mixed
Heimgartner[27]	Chronic frontal sinusitis	64	Retrospective	4	Mixed
Hopkins[28]	Acute frontal sinusitis	1	Case report	5	Positive
Wycherly[29]	Revision frontal sinus surgery	13	Retrospective	4	Positive
Plaza[30]	Chronic rhinosinusitis with polyposis	32	Prospective	2b	Positive
Andrews[31]	Recurrent sinus barotrauma	1	Case report	5	Negative
Luong[49]	Postop frontal stenosis	6	Retrospective	4	Positive
Bowles[50]	Recurrent and chronic and frontal sinusitis without nasal polyps	60	Prospective	2b	Positive

endoscopic intervention and its associated morbidity…."[25] Viewed differently, one could also argue that the failure rate of BCD in patients with chronic frontal sinusitis approximates 50%, approaching 60%–65% in patients with hyperplastic sinus disease. It is possible that the reported failure rate was high given that many of the frontal mucosal changes seen on CT may be potentially irreversible in patients with severe polyp disease and, thus, not respond favorably to BCD. Furthermore, the study did not consider patient symptomatology or endoscopic patency for outcome measures.

Heimgartner et al. retrospectively evaluated the limitation of BCD in frontal sinus surgery, specifically to determine the technical failure rate and to assess the potential reasons for failed access to the frontal sinus.[27] BCD was unsuccessful in 12 of 104 frontal sinuses (12%). The CT anatomy of the failed cases revealed that complex frontal recess pneumatization pattern, such as agger nasi cell, frontoethmoidal cell, and/or frontal bullar cell, or the presence of significant osteoneogenesis, may result in BCD being "challenging or impossible." This study underscores the potential limitation of BCD in difficult anatomic configurations; it also emphasizes the ability of the surgeon to perform EFS or other endoscopic frontal sinus procedures if BCD is unable to achieve the desired result.

Plaza et al. have performed the only randomized clinical trial of BCD and Draf I for frontal sinus disease to date.[30] A total of 40 patients with CRS with polyposis were enrolled, with 32 successfully concluding the study. All patients had failed an 8-week course

of antibiotics, oral steroids, and saline irrigations. Exclusionary criteria included previous sinus surgery, advanced CRS, defined as Samter triad or symptomatic asthma, severe systemic disease (i.e., diabetes), and smoking >20 cigarettes daily. All patients underwent "hybrid procedures," which included a minimum of maxillary antrostomy and anterior ethmoidectomy, with posterior ethmoidectomy and sphenoidotomy performed in select cases. Preoperative and 12-month postoperative measures were obtained, including visual analog scores (VAS), Rhinosinusitis Disability Index (RSDI), olfactory threshold, Lund-McKay scores, and frontal recess patency.

The VAS, RSDI, olfactory thresholds, and polyp scores were statistically improved in both groups. Furthermore, the frontal sinus Lund-McKay scores improved from 1.9 to 0.5 and 2.0 to 0.4 in the BCD and Draf I groups, respectively, with both being statistically significant. Resolution of frontal sinus disease was more common after BCD compared with Draf I or Draf IIa procedures (80.8% vs. 75%), although neither was statistically significant. Frontal patency was statistically more common after BCD (73.1% vs. 62.5%), whereas synechiae formation was more common in BCD, although it was not statistically significant.

This is the first prospective comparative analysis of BCD and FESS. The strengths of the study include independence from commercial conflicts, use of several validated outcome tools, low attrition rate, and long follow-up. However, the study does not provide sufficient data to suggest equivalency of BCD and Draf

I procedures. As noted by Ahmed et al., the study did not perform a pretrial power analysis; thus the group sizes may have not been large enough to discern a true difference in the frontal radiologic scores.[51] The study also suffers from a selective reporting bias, as it failed to conduct a between-group analysis for CT, VAS, RSDI, and polyp scores, which would have facilitated direct comparison. Often statistical significance was reported, although confidence intervals and exact P-values were omitted. Given the "hybrid" nature of the surgical procedures, the ability to differentiate the direct impact of the frontal intervention from concurrent ethmoidectomy is limited.

Luong et al. reported a multiinstitutional case series on BCD for frontal sinus ostial stenosis in the office setting.[49] Six adult patients underwent a total of seven BCD with change of ostia size from 1–2 to 5–7 mm immediately after treatment. All procedures were performed using topical anesthesia without any complications. One frontal sinus ostia contracted >50%, requiring revision BCD in the office. All frontal ostia were patent with follow-up ranging from 4 to 9 months, with no patients requiring formal surgical revision in the operating room. Similarly, Eloy et al. performed in-office BCD in five patients who developed frontal stenosis after Draf I and II surgery.[52] All procedures were well tolerated with the use of topical and injection local anesthesia. All procedures were deemed successful, with improvement of frontal headaches and establishment of patent drainage pathway at mean follow-up of 5 months. Both studies provide proof of concept of potential utility of balloon technology in the office setting. Importantly, it may provide the ability to temporize sinus ostia stenosis in a subset of patients without the need for formal surgical revision in the operative suite. This potential application merits further investigation with accrual of additional patients and longer term follow-up.

WHAT DOES THE EVIDENCE TELL US?

The accrued evidence to date has reported on the utility of BCD on a variety of indications, including adult and pediatric CRS, limited CRS, and frontal sinusitis. Studies have also explored the use of the technology in alternate practice settings, including the office. The current database suggests that balloon technology is relatively safe; BCD provides the ability to reliably dilate frontal, sphenoid, and maxillary sinuses and to achieve patency in a large number of these cases for up to 2 years. However, limitations to the current state of evidence preclude meaningful recommendations on how

TABLE 4.3

Grade of Recommendation for Potential Indications of Balloon Catheter Technology for Paranasal Sinus Inflammatory Disease

Indication	Recommendation Grade
DISEASE SPECIFIC	
Adult medically refractory CRS	C
Pediatric medically refractory CRS	C
SPECIFIC SINUS	
Frontal sinus disease	C
Limited maxillary with or without anterior ethmoid disease	B

CRS, chronic rhinosinusitis.

to apply BCD in the treatment schema of CRS. In fact, the majority of the data comprises uncontrolled, retrospective, and prospective studies with poorly characterized patient cohorts lacking a matched control group. In addition, exclusion criteria in more well-designed studies limit patient selection to limited disease and thus is not a representative population with CRS. This seriously hinders the ability make any comparative efficacy claims relative to FESS. Table 4.3 highlights the grade of evidence available of these several applications of BCD. The overall grade of the data is C given that most available higher level studies do not comprise a representative population of patients with CRS. Given the widespread adoption of BCD, this underscores the importance of timely randomized clinical trials, preferably with inclusion of appropriately matched controls and validated outcome measures that offer the ability to discern impact of BCD, relative to FESS, on the underlying disease process.

REFERENCES

1. Benninger MS, Ferguson BJ, Hadley JA. Adult chronic rhinosinusitis: definitions, diagnosis, epidemiology, and pathophysiology. *Otolaryngol Head Neck Surg.* 2003;129 (3 suppl):S1–S32.
2. Orlandi RR, Kingdom TT, Hwang PH. International consensus statement on allergy and rhinology: rhinosinusitis executive summary. *Int Forum Allergy Rhinol.* 2016;6(suppl 1):S3–S21.
3. Slavin RG. Management of sinusitis. *J Am Geriatr Soc.* 1991;39(2):212–217.

4. Cohen M, Kofonow J, Nayak JV. Biofilms in chronic rhinosinusitis: a review. *Am J Rhinol Allergy.* 2009;23(3): 255–260.

5. Senior BA, Glaze C, Benninger MS. Use of the rhinosinusitis disability index (RSDI) in rhinologic disease. *Am J Rhinol.* 2001;15(1):15–20.

6. Smith TL, Batra PS, Seiden AM, Hannley M. Evidence supporting endoscopic sinus surgery in the management of adult chronic rhinosinusitis: a systematic review. *Am J Rhinol.* 2005;19(6):537–543.

7. Smith TL, Kern RC, Palmer JN. Medical therapy vs surgery for chronic rhinosinusitis: a prospective, multi-institutional study. *Int Forum Allergy Rhinol.* 2011;1(4):235–241.

8. Lanza DC. Postoperative care and avoiding frontal recess stenosis. In: *Abstracts of the International Advanced Sinus Symposium Philadelphia.* 1993.

9. Vaughan WC. Review of balloon sinuplasty. *Curr Opin Otolaryngol Head Neck Surg.* 2008;16(1):2–9.

10. Batra PS, Ryan MW, Sindwani R, Marple BF. Balloon catheter technology in rhinology: reviewing the evidence. *Laryngoscope.* 2011;121(1):226–232.

11. Bolger WE, Vaughan WC. Catheter-based dilation of the sinus ostia: initial safety and feasibility analysis in a cadaver model. *Am J Rhinol.* 2006;20(3):290–294.

12. Brown CL, Bolger WE. Safety and feasibility of balloon catheter dilation of paranasal sinus ostia: a preliminary investigation. *Ann Otol Rhinol Laryngol.* 2006;115(4): 293–299.

13. Tao S, Meyer DR, Simon JW. Success of balloon catheter dilatation as a primary or secondary procedure for congenital nasolacrimal duct obstruction. *Ophthalmology.* 2002;109(11):2108–2111.

14. Citardi MJ, Kanowitz SJ. A cadaveric model for balloon-assisted endoscopic paranasal sinus dissection without fluoroscopy. *Am J Rhinol.* 2007;21(5):579–583.

15. Stankiewicz J, Tami T, Truitt T. Transantral, endoscopically guided balloon dilatation of the ostiomeatal complex for chronic rhinosinusitis under local anesthesia. *Am J Rhinol Allergy.* 2009;23(3):321–327.

16. Stankiewicz J, Truitt T, Atkins J. One-year results: transantral balloon dilation of the ethmoid infundibulum. *Ear Nose Throat J.* 2010;89(2):72–77.

17. Bolger WE, Brown CL, Church CA. Safety and outcomes of balloon catheter technology: a multicenter 24-week analysis of 115 patients. *Otolaryngol Head Neck Surg.* 2007;37(1):10–20.

18. Kuhn FA, Church CA, Goldberg AN. Balloon catheter sinusotomy: one-year follow-up – outcomes and role of in functional endoscopic sinus surgery. *Otolaryngol Head Neck Surg.* 2008;139(3S3):S27–S37.

19. Weiss RL, Church CA, Kuhn FA. Long-term outcome analysis of balloon catheter sinusotomy: two-year follow-up. *Otolaryngol Head Neck Surg.* 2008;139(3S3):S38–S46.

20. Levine HL, Sertich AP, Hoisington II DR. Multicenter registry of balloon catheter sinusotomy. Outcomes for 1036 patients. *Ann Otol Rhinol Laryngol.* 2008;117(4): 263–270.

21. Friedman M, Schalch P, Lin HC. Functional endoscopic dilatation of the sinuses: patient satisfaction, postoperative pain, and cost. *Am J Rhinol.* 2008;22(2):204–209.

22. Ramadan HH. Safety and feasibility of balloon sinuplasty for treatment of chronic rhinosinusitis in children. *Ann Otol Rhinol Laryngol.* 2009;118(3):161–165.

23. Ramadan HH, McLaughlin K, Josephson G. Balloon catheter sinuplasty in young children. *Am J Rhinol Allergy.* 2010;24(1):e54–e56.

24. Ramadan HH, Terrell AM. Balloon catheter sinuplasty and adenoidectomy in children with chronic rhinosinusitis. *Ann Otol Rhinol Laryngol.* 2010;119(9):578–582.

25. Catalano PJ, Payne SC. Balloon dilation of the frontal recess in patients with chronic frontal sinusitis and advanced sinus disease: an initial report. *Ann Otol Rhinol Laryngol.* 2009;118(2):107–112.

26. Khalid AN, Smith TL, Anderson JC. Fracture of bony lamellae within the frontal recess after balloon catheter dilatation. *Am J Rhinol Allergy.* 2010;24(1):55–59.

27. Heimgartner S, Eckardt J, Simmen D. Limitations of balloon sinuplasty in frontal sinus surgery. *Eur Arch Otorhinolaryngol.* 2011;268(10):1463–1467.

28. Hopkins C, Noon E, Roberts D. Balloon sinuplasty in acute frontal sinusitis. *Rhinology.* 2009;47(4):375–378.

29. Wycherly BJ, Manes RP, Mikula SK. Initial clinical experience with balloon dilation in revision frontal sinus surgery. *Ann Otol Rhinol Laryngol.* 2010;119(7):468–471.

30. Plaza G, Eisenberg G, Montojo J. Balloon dilation of the frontal recess: a randomized clinical trial. *Ann Otol Rhinol Laryngol.* 2011;120(8):511–518.

31. Andrews JN, Weitzel EK, Eller R. Unsuccessful frontal balloon sinuplasty for recurrent sinus barotrauma. *Aviat Space Environ Med.* 2010;81(5):514–516.

32. Marple BF, Stringer SP, Batra PS. Going to the next level: health care's evolving expectations for evidence. *Otolaryngol Head Neck Surg.* 2009;141:551–554.

33. Abreu CB, Balsalobre L, Pascoto GR, Pozzobon M, Fuchs SC, Stamm AC. Effectiveness of balloon sinuplasty in patients with chronic rhinosinusitis without polyposis. *Braz J Otorhinolaryngol.* 2014;80(6):470–475.

34. Achar P, Duvvi S, Kumar BN. Endoscopic dilatation sinus surgery (FEDS) versus functional endoscopic sinus surgery (FESS) for treatment of chronic rhinosinusitis: a pilot study. *Acta Otorhinolaryngol Ital.* 2012;32(5):314–319.

35. Albritton FD, Casiano RR, Sillers MJ. Feasibility of in-office endoscopic sinus surgery with balloon sinus dilation. *Am J Rhinol Allergy.* 2012;26(3):243–248.

36. Bikhazi N, Light J, Truitt T, Schwartz M, Cutler J, Investigators RS. Standalone balloon dilation versus sinus surgery for chronic rhinosinusitis: a prospective, multicenter, randomized, controlled trial with 1-year follow-up. *Am J Rhinol Allergy.* 2014;28(4):323–329.

37. Cutler J, Bikhazi N, Light J, Truitt T, Schwartz M, Investigators RS. Standalone balloon dilation versus sinus surgery for chronic rhinosinusitis: a prospective, multicenter, randomized, controlled trial. *Am J Rhinol Allergy.* 2013;27(5):416–422.

38. Brodner D, Nachlas N, Mock P, et al. Safety and outcomes following hybrid balloon and balloon-only procedures using a multifunction, multisinus balloon dilation tool. *Int Forum Allergy Rhinol.* 2013;3(8):652–658.
39. Gould J, Alexander I, Tomkin E, Brodner D. In-office, multisinus balloon dilation: 1-Year outcomes from a prospective, multicenter, open label trial. *Am J Rhinol Allergy.* 2014;28(2):156–163.
40. Karanfilov B, Silvers S, Pasha R, et al. Office-based balloon sinus dilation: a prospective, multicenter study of 203 patients. *Int Forum Allergy Rhinol.* 2013;3(5):404–411.
41. Sikand A, Silvers SL, Pasha R, et al. Office-based balloon sinus dilation: 1-year follow-up of a prospective, multicenter study. *Ann Otol Rhinol Laryngol.* 2015;124(8): 630–637.
42. Payne SC, Stolovitzky P, Mehendale N, et al. Medical therapy versus sinus surgery by using balloon sinus dilation technology: a prospective multicenter study. *Am J Rhinol Allergy.* 2016;30(4):279–286.
43. Raghunandhan S, Bansal T, Natarajan K, Kameswaran M. Efficacy & outcomes of balloon sinuplasty in chronic rhinosinusitis: a prospective study. *Indian J Otolaryngol Head Neck Surg.* 2013;65(suppl 2):314–319.
44. Ashraf N, Bhattacharyya N. Determination of the "incidental" Lund score for the staging of chronic rhinosinusitis. *Otolaryngol Head Neck Surg.* 2001;125(5):483–486.
45. Levy JM, Marino MJ, McCoul ED. Paranasal sinus balloon catheter dilation for treatment of chronic rhinosinusitis: a systematic review and meta-analysis. *Otolaryngol Head Neck Surg.* 2016;154(1):33–40.
46. Soler ZM, Rosenbloom JS, Skarada D, Gutman M, Hoy MJ, Nguyen SA. Prospective, multicenter evaluation of balloon sinus dilation for treatment of pediatric chronic rhinosinusitis. *Int Forum Allergy Rhinol.* 2017;7(3):221–229.
47. Shin KS, Cho SH, Kim KR. The role of adenoids in pediatric rhinosinusitis. *Int J Pediatr Otorhinolaryngol.* 2008;72:1643–1650.
48. Brietzke SE, Brigger MT. Adenoidectomy outcomes in pediatric rhinosinusitis: a meta-analysis. *Int J Pediatr Otorhinolaryngol.* 2008;72:1541–1545.
49. Luong A, Batra PS, Fakhri S. Balloon catheter dilatation for frontal sinus ostium stenosis in the office setting. *Am J Rhinol.* 2008;22(6):621–624.
50. Bowles PF, Agrawal S, Salam MA. Efficacy of balloon sinuplasty in treatment of frontal rhinosinusitis: a prospective study in sixty patients. *Clin Otolaryngol.* 2016;42.
51. Ahmed J, Pal S, Hopkins C. Functional endoscopic balloon dilation of sinus ostia for chronic rhinosinusitis. *Cochrane Database Syst Rev.* 2011;(7):CD008515.
52. Eloy JA, Friedel ME, Eloy JD. In-office balloon dilation of the failed frontal sinusotomy. *Otolaryngol Head Neck Surg.* 2012;146. Epub ahead of print. October 13, 2011.

CHAPTER 5

Epistaxis: An Update on Contemporary Evidence-Based Approach

A. SHAO, FRACS-ORLHNS • M.L. BARNES, FRCS-ORL(ED), MD •
P.M. SPIELMANN, FRCS-ORL(ED) • P.S. WHITE, FRACS, FRCS(ED), MBCHB

INTRODUCTION

Epistaxis is the second most common cause for emergency admission to ear, nose, and throat (ENT) services (following sore throat). In 2009/2010, there were more than 21,000 emergency admissions in England, with a mean inpatient stay of 1.9 days. The majority of patients admitted are aged 60–70 years,[1] but there is a bimodal age incidence, with an earlier peak in childhood.[2]

Death caused by epistaxis is rare. In 2005 in the United States, seven epistaxis-related deaths were recorded, all from the 75-year or older population,[3] an approximate incidence in that age group of 1:2,500,000 and an overall incidence of 2:100 million. The epidemiology of epistaxis in Scotland has been well reviewed,[4] and readers are referred here for more details.

Despite the heavy caseload, there are no national or consensus guidelines to inform management decisions and the most junior members of staff are often the main caregivers.[5] Across different centers investigation profiles and treatment preferences vary. There are areas of controversy and nonstandardized practice exists, which need to be addressed in an evidence-based fashion. The purpose of this article, therefore, is to review the literature concerning the management of epistaxis and to make recommendations (evidence based where available) for treatment.

This article provides a contemporary management protocol for adult epistaxis admissions, evidence based where possible, otherwise based on our own experience.

METHODS

A literature review was performed in March 2017, Pubmed was searched using the term "Epistaxis"[Majr], limited to reviews within the last 10 years. Relevant papers were identified and obtained, as well as important ancestor references. Further specific searches were conducted without limits, to address each theme within the review, e.g., "Epistaxis"[Majr] AND "Blood Coagulation Disorders"[Mesh]. More than 200 articles were reviewed, although few provided primary evidence beyond expert opinion to guide the development of an overall management protocol.

RESULTS–A MANAGEMENT PATHWAY
Management

A stepwise approach to epistaxis management is advocated. In order, this should be "Initial Management, Direct Therapy, Tamponade, and Vascular Intervention." Where control of bleeding is not achieved, timely progression through the management steps is essential (see Fig. 5.1).

Pathway progression—uncontrolled epistaxis
Direct therapy or tamponade will almost invariably reduce bleeding, but sometimes control is not absolute and intermittent or minor ongoing bleeding may occur. In such cases, a clinical decision must be made whether to progress with further management as per uncontrolled epistaxis or to observe the patient. This is not uncommon in cases of coagulopathy, where bleeding times may be significantly prolonged. The decision must be based on the ongoing rate of bleeding and the patient's risks. In some cases, a little further air in a tamponade balloon (often required within the hour after initial insertion), application of Haemostatic matrix (Floseal), or a procoagulant dressing to an oozing cautery site (e.g., Surgicel) may be helpful. Patients must not, however, sit for prolonged periods with poor control, multiple nasal packs, and no further intervention—these patients must receive a pack or vascular intervention if required.

Protocol completion—treated epistaxis
Where possible, epistaxis should only be considered adequately treated when a topical therapy or vascular intervention has been used, although where a thorough

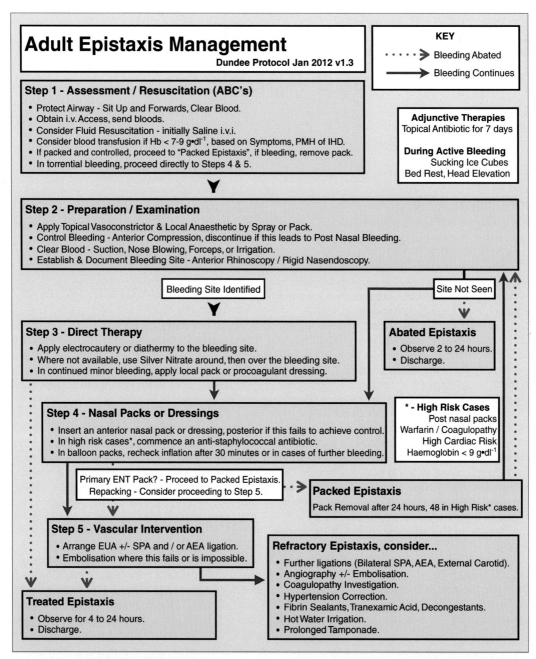

FIG. 5.1 **Adult Epistaxis Management Pathway.** *AEA*, anterior ethmoid artery; *SPA*, sphenopalatine artery; *PMH*, past medical history; *IHD*, ischaemic heart disease; *EUA*, examination under anaesthesia.

examination has not identified a bleeding site, and simple vasoconstriction or tamponade has led to initial control, longer-term resolution may be achieved through normal haemostatic and tissue repair mechanisms in some cases.

Step 1. Initial management. Immediate management includes an Adult Life Support-type Airway, Breathing, Circulaion assessment and resuscitation. Epistaxis is not usually an immediate airway concern, but the patient should be made to sit upright and encouraged to lean forward and clear any clots from the pharynx. An assessment of blood loss (e.g., volume, time, number of tissues, towels, or bowls) and the degree of any hypovolemic shock should be made, while establishing venous access and fluid resuscitation where indicated. Gloves, gowns, and goggles are essential to protect both yourself and the patient from contamination. A medical and drug history, including complementary and alternative medicine, may elucidate precipitants.[6] The side of bleeding as well as whether it is predominantly anterior or posterior should be determined.

In exceptional circumstances, postnasal bleeding may be so heavy as to warrant an immediate balloon pack (e.g., Foley catheter and anterior pack) to prevent further blood loss, with arrangements for transfer to theater. In general, however, the first priority is to visualize the bleeding area through initial hemostatic measures and examination. Depending on the bleeding site, local skills, and facilities, this may be best achieved with a nasal thudicum or speculum in conjunction with a headlight or mirror, an auroscope, a microscope, or an endoscope, noting that each approach has its limitations. Nasendoscopy are essential for identifying 80% of bleeding sites not otherwise seen.[7]

Blood will likely obstruct the view to the bleeding site. In anterior nasal bleeding, this can be controlled through anterior nasal compression for 10–60 min in conjunction with topical vasoconstrictors.[8,9] If hemostasis is not achieved, or nasal compression only leads to postnasal bleeding, it should be discontinued and an attempt made to clear blood and visualize the site with suction, forceps, irrigation,[10] or nose blowing. These methods may achieve initial hemostasis, and/or allow bleeding site visualization necessary for direct therapies such as cautery.

Topical vasoconstrictor preparations recommended include 1:1000 adrenalin (epinephrine),[11] 0.5% phenylephrine hydrochloride,[9] 4% cocaine, or 0.05% oxymetazoline solution,[8] but few comparisons have been conducted. One study suggested that oxymetazoline may be more effective than 1:100,000 (dilute) adrenalin and equally effective with less propensity to induce hypertension when compared with 4% cocaine.[12] Topical vasoconstrictors can be applied in conjunction with topical anesthetics, such as 4% lignocaine, to improve patient comfort.

Investigations. A full blood count will facilitate assessment of blood loss and shock. A biochemistry profile may indicate circulatory effects on renal function or the breakdown products of a large volume of ingested blood. A sample should be sent to establish blood group and match of transfusion products (e.g., red cells, plasma, or platelets). Routine coagulation profiles are not recommended[13-15] unless the patient takes warfarin or the patient is a child.[16] Angiography has an essential but infrequent role in trauma and cases of heavy postsurgical bleeding to exclude potentially fatal carotid aneurisms.

Step 2. Direct therapy

Silver nitrate cautery. Cautery using topical anesthetic is advocated by most authors as the optimal management in adult epistaxis. Nonetheless, in 1993, only 24% of UK cases referred to specialist otolaryngology units were managed in this way, whereas 76% underwent nasal packing.[5]

Silver nitrate cautery is common but difficult in the context of active bleeding, in which case electrocautery or electrocoagulation (diathermy) may be more effective. A local cauterizing solution is achieved by touching a dry salt silver nitrate-tipped applicator against moist mucosa. The objective is direct cautery of the bleeding site by application with gentle pressure to the bleeding point for a few seconds. Initial circumferential contact may facilitate control of bleeding and more definitive results.[10]

Silver nitrate is available in 75% and 95% preparations. A histopathologic study comparing the two found that 95% silver nitrate caused twice the depth of burn, and it was thought to increase the risk of complications including septal perforation.[17] It is thought that bilateral cautery may increase the risk of septal perforation,[18] with a 4- to 6-week interval being advocated between sides,[19] although Link et al.[20] found this not to be the case using silver nitrate (n = 46).

Silver nitrate ($AgNO_3$) can cause dark staining on the vestibular skin. This may be addressed by application of saline (NaCl) to form silver chloride (AgCl) and sodium nitrate ($NaNO_3$)[21]; both are white crystals, and the latter is readily soluble in water. Stains usually resolve over a period of weeks,[22] but permanent mucosal tattooing has been reported.[23-25]

Electrocautery and electrocoagulation (diathermy). Toner et al.[26] compared routine use of hot wire electrocautery with silver nitrate and found no difference in the rates of recurrent bleeding at 2 months, although the confidence interval (CI) was broad, with some trend toward greater benefit with electrocautery (95% CI 11%–24%). Although specialist equipment is required, electrocautery or diathermy may have advantages over silver nitrate, which can be difficult to apply to the site in cases of uncontrolled bleeding. No further electrocautery or electrocoagulation studies were identified.

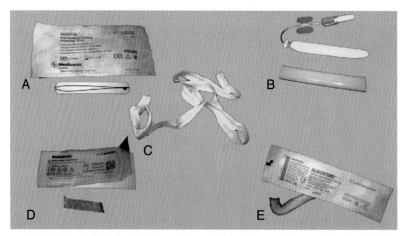

FIG. 5.2 **Common Forms of Nasal Pack.** Common nasal packs and dressings. **(A)** Merocel (polyvinyl acetal polymer sponge pack); **(B)** Rapid Rhino (self-lubricating hydrocolloid covered balloon pack); **(C)** a traditional ribbon pack, in this case BIPP (Bismuth Iodoform Paraffin Paste); **(D)** Surgicel (oxidized regenerated cellulose absorbable hemostat); **(E)** Algosteril (alginate fiber absorbable hemostat).

After direct therapy, in some cases of minor ongoing bleeding, the addition of a hemostatic dressing, such as Surgicel (Ethicon Inc. Somerville, NJ) or Kaltostat (ConvaTec Ltd. Skillman, NJ), or the use of a very localized pack over the bleeding site may help to prevent further pathway progression.

Step 3. Nasal packs or dressings. Where local therapy fails, control of bleeding can be achieved by tamponade, by using a variety of nasal packs, or by promotion of hemostasis through nasal dressings. Modern nasal packs are easily and relatively comfortably inserted by practitioners outwith otorhinolaryngology, e.g., in the emergency department, ambulance, or family practice. As a consequence, many patients now arrive in our department with packs inserted. This does prevent immediate direct therapy, however, which might otherwise allow a treated patient to be sent home. The authors therefore advocate removal of the packing for proper examination if possible. Once a pack is inserted, it is usually recommended to be left for 24 h, necessitating admission, although care at home with packs has been described.[9]

A variety of nasal packing materials are available. Examples include polyvinyl acetal polymer sponges (e.g., Merocel, Medtronic Inc., Minneapolis, MN), nasal balloons (e.g., the Rapid Rhino Balloon pack with a self-lubricating hydrocolloid fabric covering, Arthro-Care Corp., Austin, TX), nasal dressings (e.g., Kaltostat calcium alginate, ConvaTec Ltd., Skillman, NJ), and traditional ribbon packs, e.g., BIPP (Bismuth, Iodoform,

Paraffin Paste) or petroleum jelly-coated ribbon gauze. Each of these packs is illustrated in Fig. 5.2. Some (e.g., Rapid Rhino, Kaltostat) are reported to provide procoagulant surfaces, which may be helpful in coagulopathic patients, most commonly those given warfarin.

FloSeal hemostatic sealant can be considered as an alternative or adjunct to nasal packing for both anterior and posterior epistaxis. The current literature supports the use of FloSeal as an alternative method for anterior epistaxis. A recent study has demonstrated a success rate of 90% in controlling epistaxis with improved patient tolerance.[27,28]

A nasopharyngeal pack may be placed in posterior epistaxis (approximately 5% of cases[29]), especially when initial anterior packs fail. Traditional postnasal packs were rolled gauze attached to tapes passed out through the nose and mouth to secure.[29] More recently, Brighton or Foley catheters have been used, inflated with saline and secured transnasally with an anterior clamp, e.g., umbilical clip.

Postnasal packs are extremely uncomfortable and prone to cause significant hypoxia.[30] Hospitalization, oxygen therapy via face mask, and in some cases sedation are required, a combination that increases the risks of hypoxia and aspiration. Other complications of nasal packs (especially nasopharyngeal) include displacement with airway obstruction; pressure necrosis of the palate, alar, or columellar skin; and sinus infection or toxic shock syndrome. The last condition is caused by staphylococcal exotoxin TSST-1 and presents with fever, diarrhea, hypotension, and rash.[29] *Staphylococcus aureus* can be isolated in one-third of patients, of which 30% produce the exotoxin.[31] Therefore, prolonged packing should be avoided and antistaphylococcal antibiotics prescribed if a pack is to remain in situ for more than 24 h[10]; see notes on high-risk cases.

Balloon packs may deflate over time,[32] so they should be checked after the first hour or if bleeding recommences. Some minor ongoing bleeding is not uncommon immediately following pack insertion and may resolve given careful observation.

Following pack removal it is imperative to examine the nasal cavity to exclude underlying pathology and identify and manage the bleeding source if possible.

Step 4. Ligation/embolization

Surgery. In a 1993 UK national survey of practice, 9.3% of patients with epistaxis referred to an otolaryngologist required a posterior nasal pack (commonly a Foley catheter). A general anesthetic was required in 5.6% to control bleeding, and <1% had a formal arterial ligation (ethmoid, maxillary, or external carotid).[5]

In authors's center, with 593 admissions for acute epistaxis over the last 2 years, 47% had hospital stays of 1 day or less. Of the 317 longer-term cases, 7% were taken to theater and underwent arterial ligation: 21 of the sphenopalatine artery (SPA) and 2 of the anterior ethmoid artery (AEA). In some cases, the theater equipment and anesthetic will facilitate bleeding site visualization, bleeding control, and direct cautery. In cases in which this remains impossible, or uncertainty is present about the control established, arterial ligation is performed.

In the past, ligation was commonly of the maxillary artery, or the external carotid. Although the distribution of these arteries is wider, recent studies suggest that SPA ligation is more successful—possibly because of difficulties completing the other procedures or a failure to address more distal collateral circulation.[33] SPA ligation is associated with minor complications such as nasal crusting, decreased lacrimation, and paresthesia of the palate or nose.[34] Septal perforation and inferior turbinate necrosis have also been reported.[35,36]

In contrast, ligation of the maxillary artery through a canine fossa approach can be complicated by dental or nasolacrimal duct injury, facial and gum numbness, or oroantral fistula.[37] External carotid artery ligation is associated with a small risk of injury to the hypoglossal and vagus nerves and a lower success rate.[33]

When compared with traditional packing techniques, SPA ligation has been shown to enable a reduced inpatient stay, improved patient satisfaction, and cost reductions.[38] Feusi et al.[39] reviewed SPA ligation efficacy studies in 2005: 13 authors reported 264 patients with 1-year success rates between 70% and 100%. More recent studies with longer-term follow-up (15–25 months) reported success rates between 75% and 100%.[40-43] Ligation of all SPA branches is essential.[44,45]

AEA ligation has an essential role in traumatic or postsurgical epistaxis in which nasal or ethmoid bony injury leads to bleeding outwith the SPA distribution. Attempts have been made to avoid the external scar by performing AEA ligation by the endonasal or transcaruncular approach. The endonasal approach, first described by Woolford and Jones,[46] requires either an artery within a mesentery[47] or an approach to the artery through the lamina papyracea.[48] The former was feasible in 20% or less of cases.[47] The latter, performed through the lamina, seems to be safe and feasible in most cases,[48,49] although this is likely an approach best left to expert hands. In both cases, pre- or intraoperative CT scans and image guidance are advised.

A transcaruncular approach is an appealing alternative. Morera et al.[50] report a case series of nine patients in which all cases were successful with no reported complications. For now, however, a pragmatic approach may be to use an endoscope in a conventional external approach, allowing the scar to be minimized.[51]

The choice of surgical ligation type is a clinical decision, which must be based on the history and examination findings. Traditionally, epistaxis has been defined as anterior or posterior, with posterior bleeds considered to relate to Woodruff plexus. The definitions have been inconsistent, however,[52] and the relevance of Woodruff plexus recently questioned.[53]

An understanding of the anatomy is essential for both surgeons and interventional radiologists. To this end, the reader is referred to excellent texts by Wormald, Lee, Biswas, and others.[45,54]

Interventional radiology—embolization. A number of studies have demonstrated that surgical ligation is more cost-effective and safer than embolization[55-57]; however, selective embolization of the maxillary or facial arteries should be considered in cases in which surgical ligation fails or is impossible because of anesthetic concerns. A variety of materials have been used, including metal coils, Gelfoam, and cyanoacrylate glue. Success rates between 79% and 96% are reported,[58] but complications are not uncommon: Cerebral Vascular Accident, arterial dissection, facial skin necrosis, facial numbness, and groin hematoma can occur with historic rates up to 47% but only 6% in larger, more recent series.[59]

Percutaneous angiography is performed to identify the vascular anatomy. Extravasation may suggest the site of epistaxis but is not often seen. Radiopaque nasal packing (such as BIPP) must be removed. Selective embolization of the relevant arterial supply, typically the internal maxillary artery, reduces the hydrostatic pressure of blood to the nasal cavity, allowing hemostasis. This must be balanced against devascularizing the facial soft tissues. Embolization of the ethmoidal arteries is not possible; cannulation of the ophthalmic arteries carries a high risk of blindness.

Refractory Acute Epistaxis

Occasionally bleeding will continue (usually slowly or intermittently) despite all conservative measures, good nasal packs, examination under anesthetic, and even arterial ligations. In such cases, it is important to reconsider the anatomy and physiology.

For anatomy: Which side is it bleeding? Is it passing through a perforation, or around the choana? Has a competent practitioner visualized the area of bleeding directly? In cases with a history of trauma, is there an anterior ethmoid laceration or a carotid aneurysm? Is there a role for further ligations—of the bilateral sphenopalatine, anterior and posterior ethmoid arteries? Will a maxillary artery or external carotid ligation add anything, e.g., minor contributions from the facial and greater palatine branches? Will angiography be informative and potentially therapeutic?

For physiology: Is the patient coagulopathic? Is the patient bleeding diffusely? Have measures been taken to reverse any drug-induced coagulopathy? If the patient has bled extensively, have the clotting factors been replaced? Has hypertension been addressed? Will tranexamic acid,[60] topical hemostatics,[61] or fibrin sealants[27,62,63] help?

Adjunctive Treatments

For the purposes of the current protocol relating to epistaxis requiring admission, topical treatments are considered to be inappropriate as sole therapy. They may have a role as an adjunct, however, and noting their efficacy in minor recurrent epistaxis especially in childhood,[64] we recommend them in all cases. Options include Naseptin cream (0.1% chlorhexidine dihydrochloride with 0.5% neomycin sulfate), petroleum jelly, Bactroban (xx), Triamcinolone 0.025%,[65] and others.[66]

Ice packs are a tradition on many of our wards. When ice cubes are sucked, there is a measurable reduction in nasal blood flow assessed by nasal laser Doppler flowmetry.[67] However, no change is seen when ice is applied to the forehead or neck.[67,68]

Preventing Epistaxis Deaths

In 1961, Quinn[69] wrote of his own experience and reviewed previous cases of fatal epistaxes, recognizing the groups at risk: those with significant comorbidity (e.g., ischemic heart disease, coagulopathy), those with endonasal tumors, or following head and facial trauma or surgery. He advocated angiography following trauma, as well as "adequate blood replacement and an informed attitude toward surgical interruption of the blood supply." He also reported the association of anterior ethmoid bleeding with trauma, the use of ferrous sulfate, and the association of cranial nerve signs with internal carotid laceration or aneurism. His observations seem just as relevant today as then and still address the most important issues, in particular, the recognition of high-risk groups and the need in such cases for early and relatively aggressive fluid resuscitation to prevent complications and deaths, most commonly in elderly patients with ischemic heart disease.

Quinn[69] recognized the difficulty of balancing the need to transfuse anemic patients with epistaxis against risks, noting the possible contribution of a blood transfusion to the death of at least one patient. Prolonged admissions with nasal packs and poorly controlled bleeding will exacerbate this risk, and for these reasons, Kotecha et al.[5] recommended earlier surgical intervention in some elderly patients with compromised respiratory or cardiovascular systems.

In the current protocol, we recommend a transfusion threshold of 7–9 g/dL. This is based primarily on a study in critically unwell patients in which a restrictive policy (transfusion indicated if Hb < 8 g/dL cf. < 10 g/dL) was shown to improve survival outcomes, particularly in the young (<55 years) and those relatively less unwell.[70]

Although rare, death in association with epistaxis has also been reported to occur because of airway obstruction. Again, significant comorbidity (e.g., neurologic impairment caused by preexisting disease or head injury) may be present. Airway obstruction secondary to nasal packing is a risk, caused by either pack or clot dislodgement.[71] In some patients, nasal obstruction itself can lead to significant arterial oxygen desaturation.[30] Again, an awareness of these potential scenarios with appropriate measures to prepare the patient, protect the airway, and monitor oxygenation is important to prevent fatal complications.

The most common case report of death secondary to epistaxis relates to rupture of an internal carotid aneurysm, often of traumatic or surgical origin. In torrential bleeds of this nature, only early suspicion with angiography, coil occlusion, stenting, or surgical ligation of the aneurism or the internal carotid in the neck will prevent death.[72] In the operative context, Valentine et al.[73] compared several measures for initial hemostasis in carotid injury, concluding that crushed muscle hemostasis followed by u-clip repair was the most effective, achieving primary hemostasis, while maintaining vascular patency in all cases.

DISCUSSION

In reviewing the epistaxis literature, one is confronted with a wealth of expert opinion and descriptive articles. Few primary research studies are conducted, and those available focus on management techniques rather than on pathway decisions. Without placing their patients in the context of a management pathway, these studies may lack transferability—our own patients may represent a different population at a different point in the pathway. It is for these reasons that a management pathway must be defined, and as a starting point, we advocate the protocol herein described.

In developing a contemporary protocol, we must recognize the changing emphasis of epistaxis management with a move away from traditional approaches of prolonged admissions and reliance on extensive nasal packing. Refined arterial ligation procedures are increasingly commonly used, offering higher success rates and lesser morbidities. These have facilitated shorter admissions, with happier patients as well as hospital managers.

The current protocol excludes contexts such as coagulopathy, Hereditary Haemorrhage Telangiectasia (HHT), and children, although useful generalizations can be made. Of admitted patients with epistaxis, 62% have an iatrogenic coagulopathy (21% warfarin, 41% antiplatelet). This group requires longer in-patient stays and more aggressive management.[74,75] Although management follows the same principles, the coagulopathy itself must be addressed and care must be taken not to cause further trauma through aggressive cautery, nasal packing, or vascular intervention. Procoagulant dressings may be helpful. We hope to provide further guidance on the management of this group in a later manuscript.

We are aware of a number of different approaches to epistaxis that have not been recommended in this guideline—from simple vasoconstrictor treatments[76] to hot water irrigation[77-79] or cryotherapy.[80] Although efficacy studies are reported, few if any comparisons have been performed against conventional techniques in the context of a defined management protocol. We hope that the current article will facilitate future scientific comparisons to allow us to establish the best timing of such interventions.

As always, further research in the field is needed. Despite the frequency of epistaxis as a presentation, little formal research has been conducted. We recommend (as before) that any interventional studies place themselves in the context of the overall patient management pathway, as well as tightly defining patient flow (stepwise by protocol) and demographics, e.g., age, sex, blood pressure, anticoagulant use, other medications (including herbal), HHT, prior episodes, trauma, or operative history. We are developing an epistaxis admission dataset, which will be optically captured from an admission proforma. We would be happy to hear from any other interested centers.

REFERENCES

1. The Information Centre for Health and Social Care. 2011. Available at: http://www.hesonline.nhs.uk.
2. Epistaxis JH. A clinical study of 1,724 patients. *J Laryngol Otol.* 1974;88:317–327.
3. Centers for Disease Control and Prevention, National Center for Health Statistics. *Vitalstats;* 2005. Available at: http://www.cdc.gov/nchs/vitalstats.htm.
4. Walker TW, Macfarlane TV, McGarry GW. The epidemiology and chronobiology of epistaxis: an investigation of Scottish hospital admissions 1995-2004. *Clin Otolaryngol.* 2007;32:361–365.
5. Kotecha B, Fowler S, Harkness P, et al. Management of epistaxis: a national survey. *Ann R Coll Surg Engl.* 1996;78:444–446.
6. Melia L, McGarry GW. Epistaxis: update on management. *Curr Opin Otolaryngol Head Neck Surg.* 2011;19(1):30–35.
7. McGarry GW. Nasal endoscope in posterior epistaxis: a preliminary evaluation. *J Laryngol Otol.* 1991;105:428–431.
8. Kucik CJ, Clenney T. Management of epistaxis. *Am Fam Physician.* 2005;71:305–311.
9. Upile T, Jerjes W, Sipaul F, et al. A change in UK epistaxis management. *Eur Arch Otorhinolaryngol.* 2008;265:1349–1354.
10. Viehweg TL, Roberson JB, Hudson JW. Epistaxis: diagnosis and treatment. *J Oral Maxillofac Surg.* 2006;64:511–518.
11. Middleton PM. Epistaxis. *Emerg Med Australas.* 2004;16:428–440.
12. Katz RI, Hovagim AR, Finkelstein HS, et al. A comparison of cocaine, lidocaine with epinephrine, and oxymetazoline for prevention of epistaxis on nasotracheal intubation. *J Clin Anesth.* 1990;2:16–20.
13. Supriya M, Shakeel M, Veitch D, et al. Epistaxis: prospective evaluation of bleeding site and its impact on patient outcome. *J Laryngol Otol.* 2010;124:744–749.
14. Thaha MA, Nilssen EL, Holland S, et al. Routine coagulation screening in the management of emergency admission for epistaxis—is it necessary? *J Laryngol Otol.* 2000;114:38–40.

15. Padgham N. Epistaxis: anatomical and clinical correlates. *J Laryngol Otol.* 1990;104:308–311.

16. Sandoval C, Dong S, Visintainer P, et al. Clinical and laboratory features of 178 children with recurrent epistaxis. *J Pediatr Hematol Oncol.* 2002;24:47–49.

17. Amin M, Glynn F, Phelan S, et al. Silver nitrate cauterisation, does concentration matter? *Clin Otolaryngol.* 2007;32:197–199.

18. Lanier B, Kai G, Marple B, et al. Pathophysiology and progression of nasal septal perforation. *Ann Allergy Asthma Immunol.* 2007;99:473–479. [quiz: 480–1, 521].

19. Schlosser RJ. Clinical practice. Epistaxis. *N Engl J Med.* 2009;360:784–789.

20. Link TR, Conley SF, Flanary V, et al. Bilateral epistaxis in children: efficacy of bilateral septal cauterization with silver nitrate. *Int J Pediatr Otorhinolaryngol.* 2006;70: 1439–1442.

21. Maitra S, Gupta D. A simple technique to avoid staining of skin around nasal vestibule following cautery. *Clin Otolaryngol.* 2007;32:74.

22. *Oxford Hands-on Science (H-Sci) Project: Chemical Safety Database.* Chemical safety data: silver nitrate. Available at: http://cartwright.chem.ox.ac.uk/hsci/chemicals/silver_nit rate.html.

23. Kayarkar R, Parker AJ, Goepel JR. The Sheffield nose—an occupational disease? *Rhinology.* 2003;41(2):125–126.

24. Mayall F, Wild D. A silver tattoo of the nasal mucosa after silver nitrate cautery. *J Laryngol Otol.* 1996;110:609–610.

25. Nguyen RC, Leclerc JE, Nantel A, et al. Argyremia in septal cauterization with silver nitrate. *J Otolaryngol.* 1999;28:211–216.

26. Toner JG, Walby AP. Comparison of electro and chemical cautery in the treatment of anterior epistaxis. *J Laryngol Otol.* 1990;104:617–618.

27. Wakelam OC, Dimitriadis PA, Stephens J. The use of Flo-Seal haemostatic sealant in the management of epistaxis: a prospective clinical study and literature review. *Ann R Coll Surg Engl.* 2017;99:28–30.

28. Lau AS, Upile NS, Lazarova L, Swift AC. Evaluating the use of Floseal haemostatic matrix in the treatment of epistaxis: a prospective, control-matched longitudinal study. *Eur Arch Otorhinolaryngol.* 2016;273:2579–2584.

29. Tan LK, Calhoun KH. Epistaxis. *Med Clin North Am.* 1999;83:43–56.

30. Lin YT, Orkin LR. Arterial hypoxemia in patients with anterior and posterior nasal packings. *Laryngoscope.* 1979;89: 140–144.

31. Breda SD, Jacobs JB, Lebowitz AS, et al. Toxic shock syndrome in nasal surgery: a physiochemical and microbiologic evaluation of Merocel and Nugauze nasal packing. *Laryngoscope.* 1987;97:1388–1391.

32. Ong CC, Patel KS. A study comparing rates of deflation of nasal balloons used in epistaxis. *Acta Otorhinolaryngol Belg.* 1996;50:33–35.

33. Srinivasan V, Sherman IW, O'Sullivan G. Surgical management of intractable epistaxis: audit of results. *J Laryngol Otol.* 2000;114:697–700.

34. Snyderman CH, Goldman SA, Carrau RL, et al. Endoscopic sphenopalatine artery ligation is an effective method of treatment for posterior epistaxis. *Am J Rhinol.* 1999;13:137–140.

35. Gifford TO, Orlandi RR. Epistaxis. *Otolaryngol Clin North Am.* 2008;41:525–536. viii.

36. Moorthy R, Anand R, Prior M, et al. Inferior turbinate necrosis following endoscopic sphenopalatine artery ligation. *Otolaryngol Head Neck Surg.* 2003;129:159–160.

37. Schaitkin B, Strauss M, Houck JR. Epistaxis: medical versus surgical therapy: a comparison of efficacy, complications, and economic considerations. *Laryngoscope.* 1987;97:1392–1396.

38. Moshaver A, Harris JR, Liu R, et al. Early operative intervention versus conventional treatment in epistaxis: randomized prospective trial. *J Otolaryngol.* 2004;33:185–188.

39. Feusi B, Holzmann D, Steurer J. Posterior epistaxis: systematic review on the effectiveness of surgical therapies. *Rhinology.* 2005;43:300–304.

40. Harvinder S, Rosalind S, Gurdeep S. Endoscopic cauterization of the sphenopalatine artery in persistent epistaxis. *Med J Malaysia.* 2008;63:377–378.

41. Nouraei SA, Maani T, Hajioff D, et al. Outcome of endoscopic sphenopalatine artery occlusion for intractable epistaxis: a 10-year experience. *Laryngoscope.* 2007;117: 1452–1456.

42. Asanau A, Timoshenko AP, Vercherin P, et al. Sphenopalatine and anterior ethmoidal artery ligation for severe epistaxis. *Ann Otol Rhinol Laryngol.* 2009;118:639–644.

43. Abdelkader M, Leong SC, White PS. Endoscopic control of the sphenopalatine artery for epistaxis: long-term results. *J Laryngol Otol.* 2007;121:759–762.

44. Holzmann D, Kaufmann T, Pedrini P, et al. Posterior epistaxis: endonasal exposure and occlusion of the branches of the sphenopalatine artery. *Eur Arch Otorhinolaryngol.* 2003;260:425–428.

45. Lee HY, Kim HU, Kim SS, et al. Surgical anatomy of the sphenopalatine artery in lateral nasal wall. *Laryngoscope.* 2002;112:1813–1818.

46. Woolford TJ, Jones NS. Endoscopic ligation of anterior ethmoidal artery in treatment of epistaxis. *J Laryngol Otol.* 2000;114:858–860.

47. Solares CA, Luong A, Batra PS. Technical feasibility of transnasal endoscopic anterior ethmoid artery ligation: assessment with intraoperative CT imaging. *Am J Rhinol Allergy.* 2009;23:619–621.

48. Pletcher SD, Metson R. Endoscopic ligation of the anterior ethmoid artery. *Laryngoscope.* 2007;117:378–381.

49. Camp AA, Dutton JM, Caldarelli DD. Endoscopic transnasal transethmoid ligation of the anterior ethmoid artery. *Am J Rhinol Allergy.* 2009;23:200–202.

50. Morera E, Artigas C, Trobat F, et al. Transcaruncular electrocoagulation of anterior ethmoidal artery for the treatment of severe epistaxis. *Laryngoscope.* 2011;121:446–450.

51. Douglas SA, Gupta D. Endoscopic assisted external approach anterior ethmoidal artery ligation for the management of epistaxis. *J Laryngol Otol.* 2003;117:132–133.

52. McGarry GW. Epistaxis. In: Gleeson M, Browning GG, Burton MJ, et al., eds. *Scott-Brown's Otorhinolaryngology, Head and Neck Surgery*. London: Hodder Arnold; 2008:1596–1608.

53. Chiu TW, McGarry GW. Prospective clinical study of bleeding sites in idiopathic adult posterior epistaxis. *Otolaryngol Head Neck Surg*. 2007;137:390–393.

54. Biswas D, Ross SK, Sama A, et al. Non-sphenopalatine dominant arterial supply of the nasal cavity: an unusual anatomical variation. *J Laryngol Otol*. 2009;123:689–691.

55. Sylvester MJ, Chung SY, Guinand LA, Govindan A. Arterial ligation versus embolization in epistaxis management: counterintuitive national trends. *Laryngoscope*. 2017;127(5):1017–1020.

56. Rudmik L, Smith TL. Management of intractable spontaneous epistaxis. *Am J Rhinol*. 2012;26(1):55–60.

57. Rudmik L, Leung R. Cost-effectiveness analysis of endoscopic sphenopalatine artery ligation vs arterial embolization for intractable epistaxis. *JAMA Otolaryngol Head Neck Surg*. 2014;140(9):802–808.

58. Smith TP. Embolization in the external carotid artery. *J Vasc Interv Radiol*. 2006;17:1897–1912. [quiz: 1913].

59. Elahi MM, Parnes LS, Fox AJ, et al. Therapeutic embolization in the treatment of intractable epistaxis. *Arch Otolaryngol Head Neck Surg*. 1995;121:65–69.

60. Sabbà C, Gallitelli M, Palasciano G. Efficacy of unusually high doses of tranexamic acid for the treatment of epistaxis in hereditary hemorrhagic telangiectasia. *N Engl J Med*. 2001;345:926.

61. Shinkwin CA, Beasley N, Simo R, et al. Evaluation of Surgicel Nu-Knit, Merocel and Vaseline gauze nasal packs: a randomized trial. *Rhinology*. 1996;34:41–43.

62. Walshe P, Harkin C, Murphy S, et al. The use of fibrin glue in refractory coagulopathic epistaxis. *Clin Otolaryngol Allied Sci*. 2001;26:284–285.

63. Walshe P. The use of fibrin glue to arrest epistaxis in the presence of a coagulopathy. *Laryngoscope*. 2002;112:1126–1128.

64. Kubba H, MacAndie C, Botma M, et al. A prospective, single-blind, randomized controlled trial of antiseptic cream for recurrent epistaxis in childhood. *Clin Otolaryngol Allied Sci*. 2001;26:465–468.

65. London SD, Lindsey WH. A reliable medical treatment for recurrent mild anterior epistaxis. *Laryngoscope*. 1999;109:1535–1537.

66. Kara N, Spinou C, Gardiner Q. Topical management of anterior epistaxis: a national survey. *J Laryngol Otol*. 2009;123:91–95.

67. Porter MJ. A comparison between the effect of ice packs on the forehead and ice cubes in the mouth on nasal submucosal temperature. *Rhinology*. 1991;29:11–15.

68. Teymoortash A, Sesterhenn A, Kress R, et al. Efficacy of ice packs in the management of epistaxis. *Clin Otolaryngol Allied Sci*. 2003;28:545–547.

69. Quinn FB. Fatal epistaxis. *Calif Med*. 1961;94:88–92.

70. Hébert PC, Wells G, Blajchman MA, et al. A multicenter, randomized, controlled clinical trial of transfusion requirements in critical care. *N Engl J Med*. 1999;340:409–417.

71. Williams M, Onslow J. Airway difficulties associated with severe epistaxis. *Anaesthesia*. 1999;54:812–813.

72. Lehmann P, Saliou G, Page C, et al. Epistaxis revealing the rupture of a carotid aneurysm of the cavernous sinus extending into the sphenoid: treatment using an uncovered stent and coils. Review of literature. *Eur Arch Otorhinolaryngol*. 2009;266:767–772.

73. Valentine R, Boase S, Jervis-Bardy J, et al. The efficacy of hemostatic techniques in the sheep model of carotid artery injury. *Int Forum Allergy Rhinol*. 2011;1:118–122.

74. Smith J, Siddiq S, Dyer C, et al. Epistaxis in patients taking oral anticoagulant and antiplatelet medication: prospective cohort study. *J Laryngol Otol*. 2011;125:38–42.

75. Soyka MB, Rufibach K, Huber A, et al. Is severe epistaxis associated with acetylsalicylic acid intake? *Laryngoscope*. 2010;120:200–207.

76. Doo G, Johnson DS. Oxymetazoline in the treatment of posterior epistaxis. *Hawaii Med J*. 1999;58:210–212.

77. Stangerup SE, Thomsen HK. Histological changes in the nasal mucosa after hotwater irrigation. An animal experimental study. *Rhinology*. 1996;34:14–17.

78. Stangerup SE, Dommerby H, Lau T. Hot-water irrigation as a treatment of posterior epistaxis. *Rhinology*. 1996;34:18–20.

79. Stangerup SE, Dommerby H, Siim C, et al. New modification of hot-water irrigation in the treatment of posterior epistaxis. *Arch Otolaryngol Head Neck Surg*. 1999;125:686–690.

80. Hicks JN, Norris JW. Office treatment by cryotherapy for severe posterior nasal epistaxis–update. *Laryngoscope*. 1983;93:876–879.

CHAPTER 6

Evidence-Based Practice: Functional Rhinoplasty

SEAN T. MASSA, MD • ZACHARY FARHOOD, MD • SCOTT G. WALEN, MD

KEY POINTS

- Functional rhinoplasty consists of a well-established group of techniques to correct nasal obstruction, especially when caused by nasal valve collapse.
- The nasal valve contributes the majority of nasal resistance. It is functionally and anatomically divided into the internal and external nasal valve.
- Nasal obstruction is primarily assessed using validated patient-reported symptom scores. Quantitative tools exist and continue to evolve but have not correlated well with symptoms.
- New techniques and evidence continue to emerge to further improve outcomes and to explore less invasive treatments.

BACKGROUND

Scope of the Problem

Rhinoplasty is defined by the American Academy of Otolaryngology (AAO) as "a surgical procedure that alters the shape or appearance of the nose" with functional rhinoplasty specifically aimed at "enhancing the nasal airway."[1] Traditionally, this procedure was classified dichotomously as aesthetic or functional based on the surgical goal, but the overlap between these categories is increasingly recognized. The functional consequences of cosmetic rhinoplasty became apparent in the 1990s when a high rate of delayed nasal valve collapse developed after the reductive rhinoplasties that were popular in the preceding decades.[2,3] Only recently has the cosmetic impact of functional rhinoplasty been emphasized.[4]

In the United States, more than $5 billion is spent annually on the treatment of nasal obstruction.[5] Functional rhinoplasty seeks to address nasal obstruction primarily through reconstruction of nasal valve collapse, which occurs in 13% of the population.[6] A survey completed by plastic surgeons estimated that 223,000 rhinoplasties were performed in 2016 for all indications.[7]

In 2008, Cannon and Rhee provided a review of the evidence supporting functional rhinoplasty up to that date.[8] In the past decade the facial plastic surgery community strove to improve the evidence base of

treatments,[9] expanding the literature available to guide practice. This has been synthesized by several meta-analyses on specific treatments and outcomes and culminated with a Clinical Practice Guideline produced by the AAO.[1] The present review aims to summarize the most clinically relevant evidence published over the past decade to guide the management of nasal valve obstruction.

Anatomy and Pathophysiology

The nasal valve is the narrowest part of the nasal airway.[10] More than half the resistance in the nasal airway results from the nasal valve.[11] Physiologically this valve is thought to regulate the nasal airflow to allow sufficient time for the nasal cavity to heat, humidify, and filter the inspired air. Given its contribution to nasal resistance, it is logical that augmentation of the nasal vale is the primary focus of functional rhinoplasty.

The nasal valve was first described by Mink in 1903.[12] The definition has evolved and is now divided into internal and external valves (Fig. 6.1). The internal nasal valve (INV) is defined by its borders: the septum, the caudal margin of the upper lateral cartilage (ULC), and the head of the inferior turbinate. The average cross-sectional area of the internal valve is 55–60 mm², with a 15- to 20-degree angle created by the septum and ULC.[13] These data are based on studies of Caucasian noses and may vary in patients of other ethnicities. The

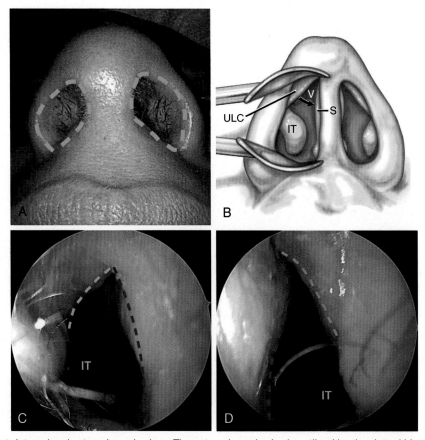

FIG. 6.1 Internal and external nasal valves. The external nasal valve is outlined by the *dotted blue line* **(A)**. The internal nasal valve is shown schematically **(B)** and endoscopically with the caudal upper lateral cartilage (*blue line*) and septum (red) outlined **(C** and **D)**. *IT*, turbinate; *ULC*, upper lateral cartilage. (Panel B from Weaver EM. Nasal valve stabilization. *Op Tech Otolaryngol Head Neck Surg*. 2012;23. Elsevier, with permission.)

external nasal valve (ENV) contributes less to resistance in a normal nasal airway. It is bordered by the nasal sill and caudal margin of the ala. The ENV is supported primarily by the lower lateral cartilage (LLC) and the fibrofatty tissue of the ala.[14]

Compromise of the nasal valves can be categorized as static or dynamic and by etiology. The vast majority of nasal valve narrowing is iatrogenic (79%), followed by traumatic (15%) and congenital (6%).[15] Iatrogenic causes usually occur during rhinoplasty, including disruption of the scroll (the junction of the ULC and LLC), overresection of the LLC, and vestibular scarring.[16] Narrowing may be static, as in the case of a septal deviation, inferior turbinate hypertrophy, scarring, or concave cartilages.[10] Even small changes in airway diameter can have dramatic effects on resistance,

as described by Poiseuille's law. Collapse can also be dynamic because of the negative pressure induced by rapid air flow, as described by Bernoulli's principle.[11] Some dynamic valve collapse is physiologic, and pathologic dynamic collapse is more often related to the ENV.[17] These variations can also coexist and may exacerbate one another.

EVALUATION OF NASAL OBSTRUCTION
History and Physical Examination
Evaluation of the nasal valve starts with a thorough history and physical examination. Other tools may be useful adjuncts but are not required to make the diagnosis and are not necessary for most patients. A patient's general medical condition must be suitable for surgical

treatment, especially if general anesthesia is planned. The details of the nasal symptoms and their impact on quality of life should be assessed. In research, this is often quantified with validated tools such as the Nasal Obstruction Symptom Evaluation (NOSE) scale[18] or Visual Analogue Scale (VAS).[19,20] These tools also have clinical utility to demonstrate changes to the patient after treatment. A history of prior surgery and trauma may explain anatomic anomalies seen on physical examination. The patient's motivation for the current consultation and any prior surgery should be assessed. Prior operative reports should be sought to understand the anatomic alternations before attempting revision surgery. Patients may have mimicked the results of a nasal valve repair by trialing nasal airway modifiers such as Breathe-Right strips (CNS Inc, Minneapolis, MN). Patients who benefit from these tools are considered good candidates for nasal valve surgery if a permanent treatment is desired.

A history of comorbidities whose symptomatology overlaps with mechanical nasal obstruction should also be investigated, including rhinosinusitis, allergies, and obstructive sleep apnea (OSA). Rhinitis can independently cause nasal obstruction or exacerbate existing mechanical obstruction. Empiric medical treatment of rhinitis in patients with mechanical nasal obstruction is not recommended by a clinical consensus statement from 2010, unless the history supports a diagnosis of rhinitis.[21] However, some third-party payers require a trial of medical therapy before approving reimbursement for surgery. The role of nasal obstruction in OSA should be discussed with patients in whom OSA is diagnosed or suspected.[22] Surgical treatment of nasal obstruction improves sleep symptoms, but the impact on the apnea-hypopnea index is modest.[23] Patients with a history suggestive of rhinosinusitis may be candidates for sinus surgery, which can safely be performed concurrently.[24]

Cosmetic concerns should be discussed for all rhinoplasty patients. Specifically, patient expectations for their airway and cosmetic appearance must be addressed. In appropriate patients, concurrent functional and cosmetic rhinoplasty maneuvers can be considered. Psychiatric comorbidities, such as body dysmorphic disorder, are less common among functional rhinoplasty patients compared with cosmetic patients,[25] but screening is reasonable given potential changes to the patient's external appearance.

Physical examination to evaluate nasal obstruction should include internal and external assessment of the nasal valve in repose and with inspiration. The external nose is typically analyzed in thirds. Externally

visible midvault narrowing predisposes to interval valve narrowing, and excessive dynamic lateral wall collapse suggests valve instability. The external nose should be assessed for cosmetic features that nasal valve surgery may affect. Anterior rhinoscopy is used to assess the INV as well as concurrent nasal cavity pathology, such as septal deviation, turbinate hypertrophy, or polyposis. The assessment of symptoms while supporting the ULC with a cerumen curette or similar tool can simulate a patient's response to surgery (Fig. 6.2). This technique is known as the "modified Cottle maneuver" and can predict successful surgery and pinpoint the anatomic region causing the most obstruction.[26] However, it is important to remember that, with aggressive inspiration some dynamic nasal valve collapse is physiologic and all patients will have an improved nasal airway with an overly aggressive Cottle maneuver.[17] Ideally, a proper Cottle maneuver pulls the cheek lateral with enough pressure to make the skin slightly taut. Creating a supraphysiologic nasal airway is not the treatment goal, and patients should be counseled appropriately.

Endoscopy and Imaging

Nasal endoscopy is frequently used by otolaryngologists to assess a variety of nasal pathology, including nasal obstruction. Some authors feel endoscopy is mandatory to rule out concomitant sinus disease or alternative diagnoses. Lanfranchi et al. reported 30% of rhinoplasty patients had additional diagnoses that changed the operative plan, including concha bullosa, posterior septal deviation, adenoid hypertrophy, choanal stenosis, and even one nasal tumor.[13] Others report much lower rates of incidental nasal cavity findings without a suggestive history and emphasize the limited contribution posterior septal deviations have on airway resistance.[27] Guidelines acknowledge these differences and provide leeway for either approach.[1] Similarly, imaging is not routinely needed but should be obtained based on history and examination findings. In most cases, computed tomography without contrast is the imaging modality of choice for the nasal cavity and paranasal sinuses.

Finally, patient photographs should be taken in the preoperative consultation. Photographs should be taken with an appropriate digital camera, and a blue background is preferred. For rhinoplasty, frontal, lateral, left and right oblique, and basal views are recommended. In addition, a photograph looking down to the nasal dorsum, or a "bird's eye view," can be helpful to determine dorsal asymmetries and midvault stenosis.

The author senior also takes pictures and video of the patient breathing gently and deeply through the nose. In addition, some surgeons use 3-D imaging and photo morphology to better communicate the operative plan to the patient and understand their aesthetic goals. Morphologic imaging has been shown to improve patient satisfaction score.[28]

Objective Measures of Nasal Obstruction

To avoid reliance on subjective patient reports, many investigators have sought objective measurements of nasal airflow and resistance. An ideal tool would differentiate normal and abnormal airways, guide treatment, and correlate with subjective changes. Existing tools continue to evolve and new tools are being created, but there is currently no gold standard for the objective assessment of the nasal airway.[29] The main limitation of existing tools is a lack of correlation to patient symptoms,[8,30] which is the motivation for patients to seek treatment and ultimately define success. The following section summarizes the strengths and weaknesses of several methods commonly used in research and occasionally in clinical practice.

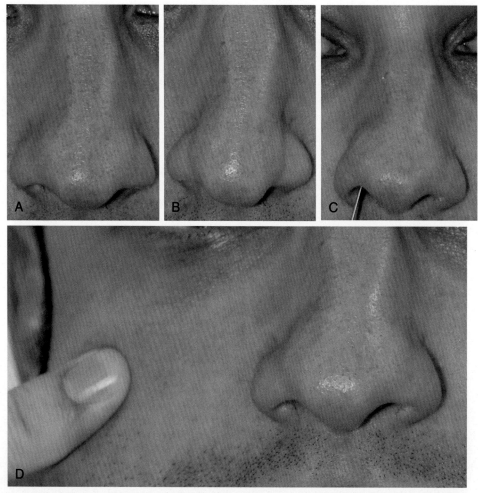

FIG. 6.2 Cottle maneuver. An anterior view of the external nose in repose **(A)** and with inspiration **(B)**, a Modified Cottle maneuver **(C)** and a traditional Cottle maneuver **(D)**. These maneuvers aim to mechanically stent open the nasal valve. Originally it was described by externally tensioning the cheek skin, but the maneuver can be modified by internally supporting the nasal valve with a cerumen curette or similar instrument. Subjective improvement in nasal obstruction is assessed during this maneuver.

1. *Rhinomanometry*—Air is instilled into the nasal cavity through a mask, and airflow is directly measured. Resistance is then computed based on the pressure required to produce various flow rates. This provides an accurate and objective measure but requires specialized equipment and does not localize the site of obstruction.

2. *Acoustic Rhinometry*—Sound waves are produced into the nasal cavity and the reflected waves are used to estimate the cross-sectional area as a function of distance from the nasal aperture.[31,32] The assessment of the nasal valve area correlates well with radiographic measurements.[33] The technique is simple to perform but requires specialized equipment, and its accuracy is dependent on technique and anatomy.[33,34]

3. *Peak Nasal Airflow*—The maximum flow through one or both nostrils is measured during maximal forced nasal inspiration. This does not simulate flows during natural breathing but has proved to be a simple, cheap, reproducible tool to quantify nasal obstruction.[10,35] It does not reliably differentiate symptomatic from asymptomatic patients[35] but does correlate with symptom scores[36] and improves after treatment.[37]

4. *Computational Fluid Dynamics*—A 3-D rendering of the nasal airway is created from cross-sectional imaging. Airflow models can then be created to assess complex fluid dynamics and the resulting airway resistance contributed by each anatomic area.[38] Modifications from treatment can also be simulated.[27] Currently this technology remains investigational, utilizes specialized software and expertise, and requires patient imaging. These factors all contribute to additional costs and clinical burden.

NONSURGICAL MANAGEMENT OF THE NASAL VALVE

Surgical management remains the mainstay of mechanical nasal obstruction, but nonsurgical techniques are often necessary to optimize results. As discussed earlier, sinonasal comorbidities should be assessed and treated. When the history suggests allergic rhinitis, a regimen including nasal saline irrigations and topical nasal steroids is an appropriate first-line treatment. Hypertrophied turbinates and sinus disease can also be treated medically before functional rhinoplasty. Failure of medical management may necessitate concurrent turbinate or sinus surgery.

Nonsurgical options directed at the nasal valve are also available. Intranasal dilators or external taping can support the nasal valve.[39] Patients with primarily nocturnal symptoms may be satisfied with continuing use of these products and prefer to avoid surgery.

SURGICAL MANAGEMENT OF THE NASAL VALVE

The optimal surgical technique to improve the nasal airway varies between patients and depends on the individual surgeon's expertise. This section focuses on the treatment of the nasal valve; however, other causes of nasal obstruction should be evaluated and addressed as needed. The traditional algorithm for nasal valve surgery could be distilled to two options: (1) spreader grafts if the INV is narrowed and (2) alar batten grafts for ENV collapse. A variety of techniques have proliferated to supplement, replace, and improve on these classic techniques.[40] The following section reviews several common and promising techniques, although this list is not exhaustive. Most techniques can be performed either open or endonasally, and both approaches have their advocates. An open approach provides unparalleled visualization of the structural deficiency and the reconstruction, whereas closed approaches result in less edema and avoid a columellar scar. Regardless of the approach, the technique is defined by the anatomic reconstruction rather than the surgical access. Intraoperatively, dynamic nasal valve collapse can be recreated by applying suction tubing directly to the nostril to create negative intranasal pressure.[41] Although the applied suction is supraphysiologic, it can be helpful to identify the area of maximal lateral wall collapse and to confirm improvement after reconstruction.

Perioperative Management

The nuances of operative management often rely upon the surgeon's initial training or anecdotal experience. The evidence supporting these decisions has grown. Patients on antiplatelet therapy are typically instructed to stop these medications 7 days before surgery to minimize intraoperative bleeding and the risk of postoperative hematoma. Prophylactic antibiotics are often given before surgery and may be continued for up to 1 week. However, recent evidence recommends against antibiotics for clean cases of the head and neck.[1,11,42,43] Rhinoplasty-specific guidelines recognize the limitations of the current evidence, so do not recommend against perioperative antibiotics but suggest their use be limited to within 24 h of surgery.[1] Nasal packing, previously standard of care, is also not recommended for routine rhinoplasty.[1] Perioperative corticosteroids may be utilized to help with edema or ecchymosis,

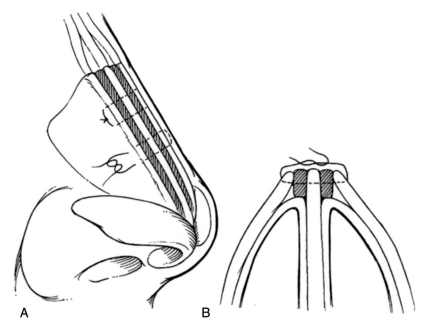

FIG. 6.3 Spreader grafts. Spreader grafts are placed between the dorsal septal cartilage and upper lateral cartilages and then secured with mattress suture. Shown in oblique view **(A)** and cross-section **(B)**. (From Farrior, et al. Special rhinoplasty techniques. In: *Cummings Otolaryngology-Head and Neck Surgery*. 6th ed. Philadelphia, PA: Elsevier Inc; 2015 [chapter 35]; with permission.)

especially in the context of more traumatic procedures such as osteotomy.[44] It is important to emphasize that all guidelines are intended to guide surgeons, not replace clinical judgment based on the unique characteristics of individual patients.

Specific Techniques
Spreader grafts
Spreader grafts were first described by Sheen in 1984 as a means to widened the midvault,[45] but they have evolved into the most common means of addressing INV narrowing.[46] These elongated rectangular cartilage grafts are inserted into a submucosal pocket between the septum and ULC (Fig. 6.3). Grafts should span the length of the ULC and insert cephalad under the nasal bone. Autologous grafts, especially septal cartilage, are typically used, but auricular, rib, and even synthetic grafts are options. Grafts generally must be 20–25 mm long and 2–3 mm thick,[46] but exact dimensions should be tailored to the individual patient. Spreader grafts have two main benefits, the opening of the INV and the ability to correct dorsal midvault asymmetries. Open approaches allow precise placement and suture fixation, although endonasal "pocket spreader" techniques are also described.[47]

Stabilization with a 30-gauge needle placed through the native nasal cartilage and the grafts can be helpful while fixation sutures are placed.[46] In a case series of 53 consecutive patients who presented with nasal valve collapse, Khosh et al. used spreader grafts alone in 79% of patients and reported subjective improvement in 89% of these patients.[15]

Batten grafts
Batten grafts are placed overlying the lateral crura of the LLC and fibrofatty tissue of the ala when the intrinsic mechanical support is deficient (Fig. 6.4). As such, they are primarily used for dynamic ENV collapse or to support the reconstruction of a stenotic ENV. Alternatively, battens can be placed over the scroll to support the INV.[48] These are often amenable to endonasal placement through intercartilagenous or marginal incisions but can also be placed through an open approach. Various donor sites can be used, but the curvature of the ala makes costal or auricular cartilage particularly well suited. Typical dimensions are 8–10 mm wide, 15–20 mm long, and 1 mm thick.[14] The graft is typically beveled at the edges, and some advocate for leaving the perichondrium on one side in an effort to improve vascularity and avoid resorption. The most important

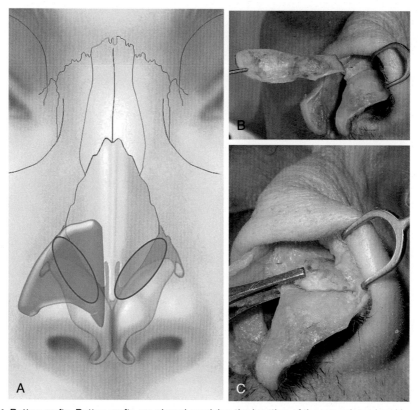

FIG. 6.4 Batten grafts. Batten grafts are placed overlying the junction of the upper lateral and lower lateral cartilage, known as the scroll. This is shown schematically **(A)**, after dissection **(B)** and after graft placement **(C)**. (From Brenner, Hilger. Grafting in rhinoplasty. *Facial Plast Surg Clin North Am*. 2009;17(1):91–113, with permission.)

aspects of the batten graft are placement in the specific point of lateral wall weakness and extension of the graft over the pyriform aperture. In a prospective observational study of 126 patients with ENV collapse, Sufyan et al. reported subjective improvement in 97% after batten grafts without other concurrent nasal surgery.[49]

Alar rim grafts can further support the alar margin but are rarely sufficient independently.[50,51] Rim grafts are smaller and placed along the alar rim. These can be placed through a pocket stab incision or through a marginal incision.

Lateral crural reposition and struts

Malpositioning or insufficiency of the LLC's lateral crura results in a mechanical disadvantage and a susceptibility to ENV collapse, as first noted by Sheen and Sheen in 1987.[52] This anatomy is identifiable in up to 87% of rhinoplasty patients.[53] Aesthetic indications for crural repositioning includes malpositioned (cephalically oriented) crura, retracted ala, and pinched tip. Meanwhile, its popularity has grown for functional repair.[54] Although definitive comparative studies are lacking, this technique is reported to be more powerful than batten grafts for ENV repair. However, it is also more technically challenging—requiring separation of the vestibular skin from the lateral crura–and requires careful consideration of the effects on nasal tip aesthetics. Hydrodissection greatly facilitates vestibular skin elevation. Crural reposition and struts are typically performed via an open approach where the lateral crura is mobilized and separated from the vestibular skin and accessory cartilages.[52] Most often the cartilage is repositioned caudally, overlying the piriform aperture. If the alar rim is deficient, strut grafts further project the lateral crura off the piriform aperture (Fig. 6.5).[55] Alternatively the lateral crura can be supported by other means such as the stair step graft described by Gassner et al.[56]

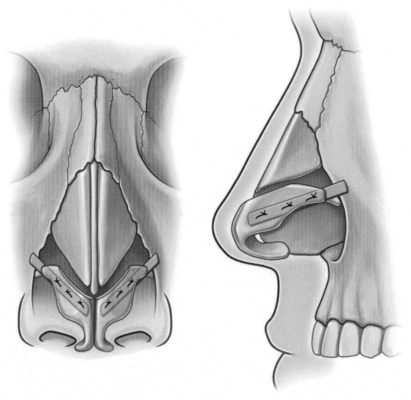

FIG. 6.5 Lateral crural strut grafts. Grafts are seen in place over the lateral crura of the lower lateral cartilages and supported by the bone of the piriform aperture. (From Rohrich, Ahmad, *Open Technique Rhinoplasty. Plastic Surgery*. vol. 2. Philadelphia, PA: Elsevier Inc; 2013 [chapter 18], with permission.)

Barham et al. performed lateral crural strut grafts in 25 patients and compared these with a cohort of lateral crural turn-in flaps in a nonrandomized, prospective cohort study.[57] The strut group showed improvement in NOSE, SNOT-22 (Sino-Nasal Outcome Test), and VAS scores and outperformed the turn-in graft group for objective measures of nasal resistance. Ilhan et al. prospectively identified 80 patients with lateral crural malposition and ultimately selected 71 to undergo lateral crural repositioning based on intraoperative findings.[52] The NOSE score improved from 6.96 preoperatively to 3.18 at 6 months postoperatively and continued to improve to 0.39 at 12 months. Aesthetic scores also improved.

Local cartilage flaps

The benefits of spreader and alar grafts can also be obtained using flaps of local cartilage, thus avoiding the need to harvest donor cartilage.[58] This is particularly useful in revision cases when no septal cartilage is available. Examples of local cartilage flaps include the spreader flap[59,60] and the cephalic crural turn-in[54]

to address the INV and ENV, respectively. Spreader flaps make use of the excess ULC that can be preserved after a dorsal hump reduction. After the dorsal septal cartilage is removed, the excess dorsal ULC is folded into the space between the septum and ULC, performing the same function as a spreader graft. Similarly, the benefit of alar strut grafts can also be obtained using lateral crural turn-in flaps. The cephalic margin of the LLC is scored and then folded into pocket under the vestibular skin, creating a thicker LLC at the expense of reducing the craniocaudal dimension. Compared with lateral crural strut grafts, these turn-in flaps improved patient-reported outcome scores similarly based on a single observation cohort study of 41 patients.[57]

Butterfly grafts

The butterfly graft was first described by Cook in 2002 and uses the mechanical resilience of cartilage placed over the nasal tip and secured to the LLC to outwardly rotate the LLC and widen the INV.[61] Auricular cartilage is typically used because of its natural curvature. Grafts can be placed via open or endonasal approaches and can be used for primary or revision rhinoplasty.[62] Excellent results are reproducible with this technique[61-63]; however, cosmetic effects on the nasal tip and supratip are noticeable to most patients and unacceptable for up to 19%.[64] Thus caution is warranted in thin-skinned or cosmetically sensitive individuals.

Suturing techniques

Park first described flaring sutures for INV augmentation in 1998.[65] A suture is passed through the lateral ULC, over the nasal dorsum and then through the contralateral ULC. Tensioning this suture serves to flair the ULC and widen the INV angle. In observational studies of patients without septal deviation, this technique improves NOSE scores with similar results to spreader grafts.[66,67]

Repair of a deviated or deficient caudal septum is more challenging than addressing the posterior septum because of its role supporting the nasal tip.[68] However, caudal septum repair can significantly widen the nasal valve. Several techniques are available depending on the degree of deformity. These range from cartilage scoring and suture fixation to the nasal spine to caudal extension grafts and anterior septal reconstruction.[69,70] A stable, midline septum is the foundation for further nasal valve repair.

Minimally invasive techniques

Office-based interventions addressing the nasal valve remain in their infancy but will likely expand following the broader trends in facial plastics.[71] For more than a decade, office-based techniques have been used to treat inferior turbinate hypertrophy.[72] More recently, the lateral nasal wall is also being addressed. Saban et al. presented a 45-patient case series that described the elevation of the lateral nasal wall by nonsurgical placement of polylactic acid threads.[73] As these threads absorb they stimulate collagen production and fibrosis, which contracts and elevates the lateral nasal wall. Similarly, Seren used radiofrequency-induced thermotherapy to increase lateral nasal wall support through scar contracture.[74] In a randomized comparison with bone-anchored suspension sutures, radiofrequency techniques produced similar improvements in NOSE and VAS scores, while avoiding the operating room.[75]

Dolan described an in-office excision of the caudal 1–2 mm of ULC through a limited endonasal incision.[76] A related technique, known as a J-flap, involves a J-shaped endonasal incision, excision of excess ULC

and vestibular skin, then closure by advancing vestibular skin.[67,77] Even releasing the INV nasal lining through a Z-plasty can improve the obstructive score.[78] Mean NOSE scores improved among the 29 patients in the study.

Injection of fillers into the submucoperichondrial space of the keystone area can also widen the INV. Nyte used both calcium hydroxylapatite and hyaluronic acid and reported subjective improvement in all 23 subjects using this technique.[79]

The results from these minimally invasive techniques have not yet been reproduced.

Outcomes

Two systematic reviews have analyzed the available data on surgical outcomes after functional rhinoplasty.[29,80] Both recognize the limitations in the available data, including the lack of level I evidence and the convolution of results by multiple techniques and concomitant surgery. Concomitant surgery, especially septoplasty and turbinate reduction, is often indicated, but separating the relative effect of each surgery can be challenging.[29] Outcome studies of individual techniques are detailed in the relevant sections earlier in the discussion.

Despite the inherent subjectivity, patient-reported outcomes are increasingly used as the gold-standard measurement tool in facial plastics[81] and functional rhinoplasty specifically.[80] This may be in response to the lack of correlation between objective measures and patient symptoms[30] or the recognition that symptoms rather than anomalous anatomy are the main motivation for nasal obstruction treatments.

Level 1 evidence for functional rhinoplasty compared with nonsurgical treatment will likely remain elusive because of challenges with randomization and blinding. However, opportunities exist to strengthen the evidence supporting functional rhinoplasty and specific techniques. Based on systematic reviews of level 2b evidence, it is still reasonable to conclude that functional rhinoplasty techniques are highly effective in the management of nasal obstruction.[29,80] Overall, success rates range from 65% to 100%, depending on the patient population and techniques employed.[29] NOSE, VAS, and general quality of life scores improve after functional rhinoplasty.[82-84] Most recently, a meta-analysis of 77 articles analyzed NOSE scores after functional rhinoplasty and found a 50-point improvement, which persisted beyond 12 months.[85] For comparison, an earlier meta-analysis found a 31.1 decrease in NOSE scores at 6 months after septoplasty and a 45.1 decrease after septoplasty with turbinate reduction.[86]

Complications

The most common complications after functional rhinoplasty are acute postoperative concerns and persistent symptoms. Acute complications include infection, delayed or unfavorable wound healing, bruising, and poorly controlled pain. Infection is uncommon, ranging up to 5%[87] but more often reported as less than 1%.[42] Persistent symptoms are more troublesome and suggest a failure to accurately diagnose or correct the underlying cause. Adequate time should be allowed for edema to resolve and wound healing to occur before evaluating the postoperative result. Diligent pre- and postsurgical counseling is helpful to mitigate patient's anxiety during the initial healing phase. Branham et al. established an overall 3.3% rate of revision surgery after rhinoplasty using administrative databases,[88] but reports range up to 15%–20%. Most revisions are due to functional compromise after aesthetic rhinoplasty.[89] Yet, aesthetic revisions after functional rhinoplasty may also be occasionally required because of unintended cosmetic consequences of airway improvements. Minor irregularities may be amenable to nonsurgical options, such as steroid injection, fillers, and laser scar treatments.[90]

BOTTOM LINE

Functional rhinoplasty is an effective treatment for chronic nasal obstruction. It is the first-line treatment when the history and physical examination reveal mechanical nasal valve obstruction in a symptomatic patient without contraindications for surgery. The diagnosis is made based on history and physical examination. Numerous operative and nonoperative techniques are available and more continue to be developed. Traditional techniques, including spreader and batten grafts, provide consistent results. Emerging techniques hold promise to further improve success rates through less invasive means. Outcomes assessment should focus primarily on subjective improvement. Ongoing research is needed to establish high-quality evidence to guide the selection of specific techniques.

REFERENCES

1. Ishii LE, Tollefson TT, Basura GJ, et al. Clinical practice guideline: improving nasal form and function after rhinoplasty executive summary. *Otolaryngol Head Neck Surg.* 2017;156(2):205–219. http://dx.doi.org/10.1177/0194599816683156.
2. Beekhuis GJ. Nasal obstruction after rhinoplasty: etiology, and techniques for correction. *Laryngoscope.* 1976;86(4):540–548. http://dx.doi.org/10.1288/00005537-197604000-00010.
3. Courtiss EH, Goldwyn RM. The effects of nasal surgery on airflow. *Plast Reconstr Surg.* 1983;72(1):9–21.
4. Marcus BC. The nasal valve – not just for functional surgery anymore. *JAMA Facial Plast Surg.* 2016;18(2):135. http://dx.doi.org/10.1001/jamafacial.2015.1967.
5. Shemirani NL, Rhee JS, Chiu AM. Nasal airway obstruction: allergy and otolaryngology perspectives. *Ann Allergy Asthma Immunol.* 2008;101(6):593–598. http://dx.doi.org/10.1016/S1081-1206(10)60221-9.
6. Haight JS, Cole P. The site and function of the nasal valve. *Laryngoscope.* 1983;93(1):49–55.
7. *Plastic Surgery Statistics.* https://d2wirczt3b6wjm.cloudfront.net/News/Statistics/2016/2016-plastic-surgery-statistics-report.pdf.
8. Cannon DE, Rhee JS. Evidence-based practice: functional rhinoplasty. *Otolaryngol Clin North Am.* 2012;45(5):1033–1043. http://dx.doi.org/10.1016/j.otc.2012.06.007.
9. Dedhia R, Hsieh T-Y, Tollefson TT, Ishii LE. Evidence-based medicine in facial plastic surgery: current state and future directions. *Facial Plast Surg Clin North Am.* 2016;24(3):265–274. http://dx.doi.org/10.1016/j.fsc.2016.03.005.
10. Chan D, Shipchandler TZ. Update on the evidence for functional rhinoplasty techniques. *Curr Opin Otolaryngol Head Neck Surg.* 2015;23(4):265–271. http://dx.doi.org/10.1097/MOO.0000000000000172.
11. Rhee JS, Weaver EM, Park SS, et al. Clinical consensus statement: diagnosis and management of nasal valve compromise. *Otolaryngol Head Neck Surg.* 2010;143(1):48–59. http://dx.doi.org/10.1016/j.otohns.2010.04.019.
12. Yarlagadda BB, Dolan RW. Nasal valve dysfunction: diagnosis and treatment. *Curr Opin Otolaryngol Head Neck Surg.* 2011;19(1):25–29. http://dx.doi.org/10.1097/MOO.0b013e3283419507.
13. Lanfranchi PV, Steiger J, Sparano A, et al. Diagnostic and surgical endoscopy in functional septorhinoplasty. *Facial Plast Surg.* 2004;20(3):207–215. http://dx.doi.org/10.1055/s-2004-861776.
14. Hamilton GS. The external nasal valve. *Facial Plast Surg Clin North Am.* 2017;25(2):179–194. http://dx.doi.org/10.1016/j.fsc.2016.12.010.
15. Khosh MM, Jen A, Honrado C, Pearlman SJ. Nasal valve reconstruction: experience in 53 consecutive patients. *Arch Facial Plast Surg.* 2004;6(3):167–171. http://dx.doi.org/10.1001/archfaci.6.3.167.
16. Wittkopf M, Wittkopf J, Ries WR. The diagnosis and treatment of nasal valve collapse. *Curr Opin Otolaryngol Head Neck Surg.* 2008;16(1):10–13. http://dx.doi.org/10.1097/MOO.0b013e3282f396ef.
17. Lee J, White WM, Constantinides M. Surgical and nonsurgical treatments of the nasal valves. *Otolaryngol Clin North Am.* 2009;42(3):495–511. http://dx.doi.org/10.1016/j.otc.2009.03.010.
18. Stewart MG, Witsell DL, Smith TL, Weaver EM, Yueh B, Hannley MT. Development and validation of the nasal obstruction symptom evaluation (NOSE) scale. *Otolaryngol Head Neck Surg.* 2004;130(2):157–163. http://dx.doi.org/10.1016/j.otohns.2003.09.016.

19. Hirschberg A, Rezek O. Correlation between objective and subjective assessments of nasal patency. *ORL J Otorhinolaryngol Relat Spec.* 1998;60(4):206–211.

20. Sipilä J, Suonpää J, Silvoniemi P, Laippala P. Correlations between subjective sensation of nasal patency and rhinomanometry in both unilateral and total nasal assessment. *ORL J Otorhinolaryngol Relat Spec.* 1995;57(5):260–263.

21. Pawar SS, Garcia GJM, Kimbell JS, Rhee JS. Objective measures in aesthetic and functional nasal surgery: perspectives on nasal form and function. *Facial Plast Surg.* 2010;26(4):320–327. http://dx.doi.org/10.1055/s-0030-1262314.

22. Friedman M, Maley A, Kelley K, et al. Impact of nasal obstruction on obstructive sleep apnea. *Otolaryngol Head Neck Surg.* 2011;144(6):1000–1004. http://dx.doi.org/10.1177/0194599811400977.

23. Choi JH, Kim EJ, Kim YS, et al. Effectiveness of nasal surgery alone on sleep quality, architecture, position, and sleep-disordered breathing in obstructive sleep apnea syndrome with nasal obstruction. *Am J Rhinol Allergy.* 2011;25(5):338–341. http://dx.doi.org/10.2500/ajra.2011.25.3654.

24. Inanli S, Sari M, Yazici MZ. The results of concurrent functional endoscopic sinus surgery and rhinoplasty. *J Craniofac Surg.* 2008;19(3):701–704. http://dx.doi.org/10.1097/SCS.0b013e3180690182.

25. Naraghi M, Atari M. Comparison of patterns of psychopathology in aesthetic rhinoplasty patients versus functional rhinoplasty patients. *Otolaryngol Head Neck Surg.* 2015;152(2):244–249. http://dx.doi.org/10.1177/0194599814560139.

26. Fung E, Hong P, Moore C, Taylor SM. The effectiveness of modified Cottle maneuver in predicting outcomes in functional rhinoplasty. *Plast Surg Int.* 2014;2014:e618313. http://dx.doi.org/10.1155/2014/618313.

27. Garcia GJM, Rhee JS, Senior BA, Kimbell JS. Septal deviation and nasal resistance: an investigation using virtual surgery and computational fluid dynamics. *Am J Rhinol Allergy.* 2010;24(1):e46–e53. http://dx.doi.org/10.2500/ajra.2010.24.3428.

28. Sharp HR, Tingay RS, Coman S, Mills V, Roberts DN. Computer imaging and patient satisfaction in rhinoplasty surgery. *J Laryngol Otol.* 2002;116(12):1009–1013. http://dx.doi.org/10.1258/002221502761698748.

29. Rhee JS, Arganbright JM, McMullin BT, Hannley M. Evidence supporting functional rhinoplasty or nasal valve repair: a 25-year systematic review. *Otolaryngol Head Neck Surg.* 2008;139(1):10–20. http://dx.doi.org/10.1016/j.otohns.2008.02.007.

30. Lam DJ, James KT, Weaver EM. Comparison of anatomic, physiological, and subjective measures of the nasal airway. *Am J Rhinol.* 2006;20(5):463–470.

31. Hilberg O, Jackson AC, Swift DL, Pedersen OF. Acoustic rhinometry: evaluation of nasal cavity geometry by acoustic reflection. *J Appl Physiol Bethesda Md 1985.* 1989;66(1):295–303.

32. Clement PA, Gordts F, Standardisation Committee on Objective Assessment of the Nasal Airway, IRS, and ERS. Consensus report on acoustic rhinometry and rhinomanometry. *Rhinology.* 2005;43(3):169–179.

33. Cakmak O, Celik H, Ergin T, Sennaroglu L. Accuracy of acoustic rhinometry measurements. *Laryngoscope.* 2001;111(4Pt1):587–594. http://dx.doi.org/10.1097/00005537-200104000-00007.

34. Terheyden H, Maune S, Mertens J, Hilberg O. Acoustic rhinometry: validation by three-dimensionally reconstructed computer tomographic scans. *J Appl Physiol Bethesda Md 1985.* 2000;89(3):1013–1021.

35. Bermüller C, Kirsche H, Rettinger G, Riechelmann H. Diagnostic accuracy of peak nasal inspiratory flow and rhinomanometry in functional rhinosurgery. *Laryngoscope.* 2008;118(4):605–610. http://dx.doi.org/10.1097/MLG.0b013e318161e56b.

36. Tsounis M, Swart KMA, Georgalas C, Markou K, Menger DJ. The clinical value of peak nasal inspiratory flow, peak oral inspiratory flow, and the nasal patency index. *Laryngoscope.* 2014;124(12):2665–2669. http://dx.doi.org/10.1002/lary.24810.

37. Menger DJ, Swart KMA, Nolst Trenité GJ, Georgalas C, Grolman W. Surgery of the external nasal valve: the correlation between subjective and objective measurements. *Clin Otolaryngol.* 2014;39(3):150–155. http://dx.doi.org/10.1111/coa.12243.

38. Rhee JS, Pawar SS, Garcia GJM, Kimbell JS. Toward personalized nasal surgery using computational fluid dynamics. *Arch Facial Plast Surg.* 2011;13(5):305–310. http://dx.doi.org/10.1001/archfacial.2011.18.

39. Ellegård E. Mechanical nasal alar dilators. *Rhinology.* 2006;44(4):239–248.

40. Motamedi KK, Stephan SJ, Ries WR. Innovations in nasal valve surgery. *Curr Opin Otolaryngol Head Neck Surg.* 2016;24(1):31–36. http://dx.doi.org/10.1097/MOO.0000000000000217.

41. Zoumalan RA, Larrabee WF, Murakami CS. Intraoperative suction-assisted evaluation of the nasal valve in rhinoplasty. *Arch Facial Plast Surg.* 2012;14(1):34–38. http://dx.doi.org/10.1001/archfacial.2011.1111.

42. Georgiou I, Farber N, Mendes D, Winkler E. The role of antibiotics in rhinoplasty and septoplasty: a literature review. *Rhinology.* 2008;46(4):267–270.

43. Andrews PJ, East CA, Jayaraj SM, Badia L, Panagamuwa C, Harding L. Prophylactic vs postoperative antibiotic use in complex septorhinoplasty surgery: a prospective, randomized, single-blind trial comparing efficacy. *Arch Facial Plast Surg.* 2006;8(2):84–87. http://dx.doi.org/10.1001/archfaci.8.2.84.

44. Ong AA, Farhood Z, Kyle AR, Patel KG. Interventions to decrease postoperative edema and ecchymosis after rhinoplasty: a systematic review of the literature. *Plast Reconstr Surg.* 2016;137(5):1448–1462. http://dx.doi.org/10.1097/PRS.0000000000002101.

45. Sheen JH. Spreader graft: a method of reconstructing the roof of the middle nasal vault following rhinoplasty. *Plast Reconstr Surg.* 1984;73(2):230–239.

46. Kim L, Papel ID. Spreader grafts in functional rhinoplasty. *Facial Plast Surg.* 2016;32(1):29–35. http://dx.doi.org/10.1055/s-0035-1570127.

47. Samaha M, Rassouli A. Spreader graft placement in endonasal rhinoplasty: technique and a review of 100 cases. *Plast Surg Oakv Ont.* 2015;23(4):252–254.

48. Bewick JC, Buchanan MA, Frosh AC. Internal nasal valve incompetence is effectively treated using batten graft functional rhinoplasty. *Int J Otolaryngol.* 2013;2013:734795. http://dx.doi.org/10.1155/2013/734795.

49. Sufyan AS, Hrisomalos E, Kokoska MS, Shipchandler TZ. The effects of alar batten grafts on nasal airway obstruction and nasal steroid use in patients with nasal valve collapse and nasal allergic symptoms: a prospective study. *JAMA Facial Plast Surg.* 2013;15(3):182–186. http://dx.doi.org/10.1001/jamafacial.2013.974.

50. Troell RJ, Powell NB, Riley RW, Li KK. Evaluation of a new procedure for nasal alar rim and valve collapse: nasal alar rim reconstruction. *Otolaryngol Head Neck Surg.* 2000;122(2):204–211. http://dx.doi.org/10.1016/S0194-5998(00)70240-3.

51. Guyuron B, Bigdeli Y, Sajjadian A. Dynamics of the alar rim graft. *Plast Reconstr Surg.* 2015;135(4):981–986. http://dx.doi.org/10.1097/PRS.0000000000001128.

52. Ilhan AE, Saribas B, Caypinar B. Aesthetic and functional results of lateral crural repositioning. *JAMA Facial Plast Surg.* 2015;17(4):286–292. http://dx.doi.org/10.1001/jamafacial.2015.0590.

53. Constantian MB. The boxy nasal tip, the ball tip, and alar cartilage malposition: variations on a theme–a study in 200 consecutive primary and secondary rhinoplasty patients. *Plast Reconstr Surg.* 2005;116(1):268–281.

54. Toriumi DM, Asher SA. Lateral crural repositioning for treatment of cephalic malposition. *Facial Plast Surg Clin North Am.* 2015;23(1):55–71. http://dx.doi.org/10.1016/j.fsc.2014.09.004.

55. Gunter JP, Friedman RM. Lateral crural strut graft: technique and clinical applications in rhinoplasty. *Plast Reconstr Surg.* 1997;99(4). 943–952.955.

56. Gassner HG, Maneschi P, Haubner F. The stairstep graft: an alternative technique in nasal valve surgery. *JAMA Facial Plast Surg.* 2014;16(6):440–443. http://dx.doi.org/10.1001/jamafacial.2014.586.

57. Barham HP, Knisely A, Christensen J, Sacks R, Marcells GN, Harvey RJ. Costal cartilage lateral crural strut graft vs cephalic crural turn-in for correction of external valve dysfunction. *JAMA Facial Plast Surg.* 2015;17(5):340–345. http://dx.doi.org/10.1001/jamafacial.2015.0925.

58. Sazgar AA, Amali A, Peyvasty MN. Value of cephalic part of lateral crus in functional rhinoplasty. *Eur Arch Otorhinolaryngol.* 2016;273(12):4053–4059. http://dx.doi.org/10.1007/s00405-015-3866-4.

59. Oneal RM, Berkowitz RL. Upper lateral cartilage spreader flaps in rhinoplasty. *Aesthet Surg J.* 1998;18(5):370–371.

60. Sowder JC, Thomas AJ, Gonzalez CD, Limaye NS, Ward PD. Use of spreader flaps without dorsal hump reduction and the effect on nasal function. *JAMA Facial Plast Surg.* 2017. http://dx.doi.org/10.1001/jamafacial.2016.2057.

61. Clark JM, Cook TA. The "butterfly" graft in functional secondary rhinoplasty. *Laryngoscope.* 2002;112(11):1917–1925. http://dx.doi.org/10.1097/00005537-200211000-00002.

62. Friedman O, Cook TA. Conchal cartilage butterfly graft in primary functional rhinoplasty. *Laryngoscope.* 2009;119(2):255–262. http://dx.doi.org/10.1002/lary.20079.

63. Stacey DH, Cook TA, Marcus BC. Correction of internal nasal valve stenosis: a single surgeon comparison of butterfly versus traditional spreader grafts. *Ann Plast Surg.* 2009;63(3):280–284. http://dx.doi.org/10.1097/SAP.0b013e31818d45fb.

64. Chaiet SR, Marcus BC. Nasal tip volume analysis after butterfly graft. *Ann Plast Surg.* 2014;72(1):9–12. http://dx.doi.org/10.1097/SAP.0b013e3182586b5d.

65. Park SS. The flaring suture to augment the repair of the dysfunctional nasal valve. *Plast Reconstr Surg.* 1998;101(4):1120–1122.

66. Rasic I, Pegan A, Kosec A, Ivkic B, Bedekovic V. Use of intranasal flaring suture for dysfunctional nasal valve repair. *JAMA Facial Plast Surg.* 2015;17(6):462–463. http://dx.doi.org/10.1001/jamafacial.2015.1116.

67. Jalali MM. Comparison of effects of spreader grafts and flaring sutures on nasal airway resistance in rhinoplasty. *Eur Arch Otorhinolaryngol.* 2015;272(9):2299–2303. http://dx.doi.org/10.1007/s00405-014-3327-5.

68. Manuel CT, Leary R, Protsenko DE, Wong BJF. Nasal tip support: a finite element analysis of the role of the caudal septum during tip depression. *Laryngoscope.* 2014;124(3):649–654. http://dx.doi.org/10.1002/lary.24321.

69. Toriumi DM. Subtotal septal reconstruction: an update. *Facial Plast Surg.* 2013;29(6):492–501. http://dx.doi.org/10.1055/s-0033-1360600.

70. Kim DW, Gurney T. Management of naso-septal L-strut deformities. *Facial Plast Surg.* 2006;22(1):9–27. http://dx.doi.org/10.1055/s-2006-939948.

71. Britt CJ, Marcus B. Energy-based facial rejuvenation: advances in diagnosis and treatment. *JAMA Facial Plast Surg.* 2017;19(1):64–71. http://dx.doi.org/10.1001/jamafacial.2016.1435.

72. Harrill WC, Pillsbury HC, McGuirt WF, Stewart MG. Radiofrequency turbinate reduction: a NOSE evaluation. *Laryngoscope.* 2007;117(11):1912–1919. http://dx.doi.org/10.1097/MLG.0b013e3181271414.

73. Saban Y, Javier DB, Massa M. Nasal lift-nasal valve lift and nasal tip lift-preliminary results of a new technique using noninvasive self-retaining unidirectional nasal suspension with threads. *Facial Plast Surg.* 2014;30(6):661–669. http://dx.doi.org/10.1055/s-0034-1396526.

74. Seren E. A new surgical method of dynamic nasal valve collapse. *Arch Otolaryngol Head Neck Surg.* 2009;135(10):1010–1014. http://dx.doi.org/10.1001/archoto.2009.135.

75. Weissman JD, Most SP. Radiofrequency thermotherapy vs bone-anchored suspension for treatment of lateral nasal wall insufficiency: a randomized clinical trial. *JAMA Facial Plast Surg.* 2015;17(2):84–89. http://dx.doi.org/10.1001/jamafacial.2014.1384.

76. Dolan RW. Minimally invasive nasal valve repair: an evaluation using the NOSE scale. *Arch Otolaryngol Head Neck Surg.* 2010;136(3):292–295. http://dx.doi.org/10.1001/archoto.2010.1.

77. O'Halloran LR. The lateral crural J-flap repair of nasal valve collapse. *Otolaryngol Head Neck Surg.* 2003;128(5):640–649. http://dx.doi.org/10.1016/S0194-59980300096-2.

78. Dutton JM, Neidich MJ. Intranasal Z-plasty for internal nasal valve collapse. *Arch Facial Plast Surg.* 2008;10(3):164–168. http://dx.doi.org/10.1001/archfaci.10.3.164.

79. Nyte CP. Spreader graft injection with calcium hydroxylapatite: a nonsurgical technique for internal nasal valve collapse. *Laryngoscope.* 2006;116(7):1291–1292. http://dx.doi.org/10.1097/01.mlg.0000218047.06639.eb.

80. Spielmann PM, White PS, Hussain SSM. Surgical techniques for the treatment of nasal valve collapse: a systematic review. *Laryngoscope.* 2009;119(7):1281–1290. http://dx.doi.org/10.1002/lary.20495.

81. Rhee JS, McMullin BT. Outcome measures in facial plastic surgery: patient-reported and clinical efficacy measures. *Arch Facial Plast Surg.* 2008;10(3):194–207. http://dx.doi.org/10.1001/archfaci.10.3.194.

82. Rhee JS, Poetker DM, Smith TL, Bustillo A, Burzynski M, Davis RE. Nasal valve surgery improves disease-specific quality of life. *Laryngoscope.* 2005;115(3):437–440. http://dx.doi.org/10.1097/01.mlg.0000157831.46250.ad.

83. Most SP. Analysis of outcomes after functional rhinoplasty using a disease-specific quality-of-life instrument. *Arch Facial Plast Surg.* 2006;8(5):306–309. http://dx.doi.org/10.1001/archfaci.8.5.306.

84. Fuller JC, Levesque PA, Lindsay RW. Assessment of the EuroQol 5-dimension questionnaire for detection of clinically significant global health-related quality-of-life improvement following functional septorhinoplasty. *JAMA Facial Plast Surg.* 2017;19(2):95–100. http://dx.doi.org/10.1001/jamafacial.2016.1410.

85. Floyd EM, Ho S, Patel P, Rosenfeld RM, Gordin E. Systematic review and meta-analysis of studies evaluating functional rhinoplasty outcomes with the NOSE score. *Otolaryngol Neck Surg.* 2017;156(5):809–815. http://dx.doi.org/10.1177/0194599817691272.

86. Stewart MG, Smith TL, Weaver EM, et al. Outcomes after nasal septoplasty: results from the nasal obstruction septoplasty effectiveness (NOSE) study. *Otolaryngol Head Neck Surg.* 2004;130(3):283–290. http://dx.doi.org/10.1016/j.otohns.2003.12.004.

87. Ponsky D, Eshraghi Y, Guyuron B. The frequency of surgical maneuvers during open rhinoplasty. *Plast Reconstr Surg.* 2010;126(1):240–244. http://dx.doi.org/10.1097/PRS.0b013e3181dc54da.

88. Spataro E, Piccirillo JF, Kallogjeri D, Branham GH, Desai SC. Revision rates and risk factors of 175 842 patients undergoing septorhinoplasty. *JAMA Facial Plast Surg.* 2016;18(3):212–219. http://dx.doi.org/10.1001/jamafacial.2015.2194.

89. Paun SH, Nolst Trenité GJ. Revision rhinoplasty: an overview of deformities and techniques. *Facial Plast Surg.* 2008;24(3):271–287. http://dx.doi.org/10.1055/s-0028-1083082.

90. Thomas WW, Bucky L, Friedman O. Injectables in the nose: facts and controversies. *Facial Plast Surg Clin North Am.* 2016;24(3):379–389. http://dx.doi.org/10.1016/j.fsc.2016.03.014.

CHAPTER 7

Evidence-Based Practice: Sublingual Immunotherapy for Allergic Rhinitis

JOSHUA M. LEVY, MD, MPH • SARAH K. WISE, MD, MSCR

KEY POINTS

- Sublingual immunotherapy (SLIT) reduces symptoms and medication use in allergic rhinitis. Subgroup analysis shows benefit for seasonal and perennial antigens, adults and children, and higher antigen doses (evidence grade = 1a).
- The benefits of SLIT may persist for up to 4 years following completion of a 4-year treatment protocol (evidence grade = 1b).
- Most well-designed, controlled SLIT trials have been performed with single antigen therapy (evidence grade = 1b). Controlled trials of multiple-antigen SLIT are lacking.
- The safety profile of SLIT for the treatment of allergic rhinitis remains excellent (evidence grade = 1a).

DISEASE OVERVIEW—ALLERGIC RHINITIS

Allergic rhinitis (AR) has significant public health and quality of life impact in the United States. Using data extracted from the Agency for Healthcare Research and Quality 2007 Medical Expenditure Panel Survey, Bhattacharyya et al. reported that 17.8 million adults in the United States (7.9% of the US population) sought care for AR in 2007.[1] Patients with AR were older, were more commonly female, had three more physician office visits, filled nine more prescriptions, and had an overall annual healthcare expenditure totaling $1492 per person over persons without AR.[1] Much of the increased healthcare expenditure for AR is allocated to pharmacotherapy, including antihistamines, decongestants, topical and oral corticosteroids, and others. Allergen avoidance measures are often advocated as an adjunct to the overall treatment plan for AR or perhaps as the sole treatment when a single antigen trigger can be identified and avoided appropriately. Strong evidence for avoidance measures in controlling allergy symptoms is lacking, however.

Allergen-specific immunotherapy is frequently employed as part of the treatment paradigm for AR. Although the first application of antigen drops applied to the oral cavity (perhaps a form of sublingual immunotherapy [SLIT]) was reported around 1900 by Curtis et al., subcutaneous immunotherapy (SCIT) has remained the primary modality of allergen-specific immunotherapy in the United States.[2] The benefits of SCIT for seasonal allergic rhinitis (SAR) and perennial allergic asthma have been demonstrated in numerous randomized controlled trials, as well as recent Cochrane reviews.[3,4] However, safety concerns with SCIT remain. A North American surveillance study evaluated systemic reactions (SRs) associated with SCIT, with inclusion of 344,480 patients receiving 28.9 million injections from 2008 to 2013.[5] SRs occurred in 1.9% of patients, with 0.08% and 0.02% experiencing grade 3 and 4 SRs, with four reported deaths. This contrasts with retrospective reviews before 2002, which reported a rate of 3.4 SCIT-related deaths per year.[6–8]

Concerns regarding life-threatening SRs with SCIT led the British Committee on the Safety of Medicines to question the safety of this immunotherapy modality in 1986.[9] A surge of interest in alternative methods of allergen-specific immunotherapy followed. Immunotherapy methods such as intranasal,[10] bronchial,[11] and oral/gastrointestinal[12–14] administration have been investigated, but because of intolerable side effects or lack of efficacy have been largely abandoned in favor of SLIT.

SLIT has been a predominant immunotherapy modality in Europe for many years.[15] However, over the last decade, clinical interest in SLIT has been growing rapidly in North America. This increased interest and employment of SLIT in clinical practice worldwide has also been accompanied by numerous randomized clinical trials assessing the efficacy of SLIT. This chapter reviews the evidence behind diagnostic testing for AR, followed by a discussion of the current evidence supporting SLIT for AR.

EVIDENCE-BASED CLINICAL ASSESSMENT AND DIAGNOSTIC TESTING FOR ALLERGIC RHINITIS

AR is preliminarily diagnosed based upon history, symptom complex, and physical examination.[16] Common symptoms of AR include intermittent clear rhinorrhea, sneezing, and pruritus of the nose. This may be accompanied by nasal congestion or obstruction, as well as associated itching of the eyes and throat, watery eyes, and skin or pulmonary symptoms, among others. In the assessment of patients suspected of having AR, it is important to evaluate potential triggers by inquiring about seasonality of symptoms, exacerbating environments or situations, family history of allergy or asthma, and other associated diseases, such as rhinosinusitis, otitis media, and dermatitis. Certain risk factors for developing AR have been described and may provide useful information as part of the history. These include family history of atopy, first born child or only child, cigarette smoke exposure, higher socioeconomic status, and total serum IgE over 100 IU/L before age 6 years.[17] Physical findings associated with AR are relatively nonspecific and may also be seen with a number of other sinonasal conditions. Edema of the nasal mucosa, inferior and middle turbinate hypertrophy, and lymphoid hypertrophy of Waldeyer ring may be seen with AR but may also be present in other inflammatory conditions of the upper respiratory system, including acute upper respiratory infections, rhinosinusitis, and nasal obstructive conditions. In short, physical examination findings may support the diagnosis of AR but owing to low positive predictive values should not be the sole diagnostic factor for this condition.

This chapter is not intended to be a comprehensive review of items necessary for a complete allergy history and physical examination, and portions of these vary depending upon the environment and geographic location in which the patient with AR is being evaluated. However, it is important to remember that much of the initial assessment and treatment plan for AR is dependent upon patient history and environmental triggers. A thorough history and physical examination leading to a diagnosis of AR are often sufficient to guide initial avoidance measures and pharmacotherapy. However, if the diagnosis is in question, or allergen immunotherapy is being considered, specific antigen reactivity with skin or in vitro allergy testing should be undertaken.

Skin testing for inhalant allergy is based on the principle that once an antigen crosses the intact skin or mucosal barrier, the antigen interacts with mast cells in the tissue and cross-links adjacent specific IgE molecules.[18] Depolarization of the mast cell ensues, and histamine is released in a dose-dependent fashion with respect to the antigen administered. This histamine release results in the classic wheal and flare reaction characteristic of the allergy skin test.[19] Measurement of the wheal size allows a semiquantitative assessment of allergen reactivity. In vitro testing for IgE-mediated allergy may be undertaken as an alternative to skin testing. The first in vitro test for specific IgE was the radio-allergosorbent test, or RAST test, reported in *Lancet* in 1967.[20,21] Other examples of in vitro methods for the detection of allergen-specific IgE include ImmunoCAP and enzyme allergosorbent tests.[18,22] Although the specific techniques employed in each of these in vitro methods vary to some degree, a common principle involves exposure of the patient's serum to typical antigens in the test assay. The patient's IgE binds to these antigens and is then quantified via labeling and detection techniques specific to the individual assay. Owing to the techniques employed for in vitro allergy testing, quantification of allergen-specific IgE is possible.

In the late 1980s and early 1990s, several articles were published comparing the advantages and disadvantages of skin testing and in vitro testing for inhalant allergy. In 1988, Ownby commented that the results of both skin and in vitro tests depend largely on the quality of the extracts used to perform the tests.[23] Furthermore, this article concluded that appropriately performed skin tests represent the best testing modality for the detection of allergen-specific IgE, whereas in vitro tests may be used in circumstances in which the skin is not appropriate for testing, anaphylaxis is expected to occur with skin testing, or the patient cannot discontinue medications that interfere with skin testing. With either skin or in vitro testing, the results of the test must be correlated with the patient's history before making a decision regarding treatment. Although in vitro allergy tests are noted to be less sensitive than skin testing methods, the employment of in vitro test results for allergen-specific immunotherapy has been shown to be safe in large clinical series.[24] Furthermore, although much of this literature dates back 20 or more years, many of the same arguments are used in comparisons of skin versus in vitro allergy testing today.

More recent evaluations of skin testing methods question certain aspects of testing protocols. In a 2008 review,

Calabria and Hagan reported that the available literature at that time indicated that, when a skin prick test is negative, a positive intradermal skin test did not correlate well with in vitro and challenge test results, therefore providing little additional information for overall diagnosis.[25] However, these authors note that a negative intradermal skin test result appears to have a high negative predictive value. Krouse and colleagues generally agree that negative allergy screens by prick/puncture techniques are typically reliable with regard to the presence or absence of allergy.[26] These authors do note, however, that intradermal testing following a negative skin prick test may provide useful information if clinical suspicion for allergy remains high, especially in the case of mold antigens or unusual inhalant reactivity. Finally, special consideration should be given to skin testing for inhalant allergy when SLIT is planned. Owing to the high safety profile associated with SLIT, in combination with short SLIT escalation protocols, quantification (or semiquantification) of allergy skin test reactivity is often unnecessary. Compared with skin testing for patients planning to undergo SCIT, in which otolaryngic allergists often use intradermal dilutional testing to determine a patient's specific end point for each antigen and shorten the escalation period as much as possible, patients on aqueous SLIT protocols have short escalation protocols with all antigens typically starting at the same dilution, thus obviating the need for extensive dilutional skin testing.[19]

EVIDENCE-BASED MEDICAL MANAGEMENT—SUBLINGUAL IMMUNOTHERAPY FOR ALLERGIC RHINITIS

Efficacy of Sublingual Immunotherapy

SLIT is recognized as an efficacious treatment option for AR and recommended by both the World Allergy Organization[15,27] and Allergic Rhinitis and its Impact on Asthma initiative.[28] The 2013 update of the World Allergy Organization Position Paper on Sublingual Immunotherapy reviewed the findings of 77 randomized, double-blind, placebo-controlled trials.[27] Study findings included the overall efficacy of SLIT for the control of AR symptoms and reduction of medication use, with heterogeneous study protocols and variability in allergen-specific outcomes. The sustained benefits of SLIT for the treatment of AR have been demonstrated in several trials with prolonged follow-up, with reduced disease-specific symptom scores, medication use, and heightened allergen-specific antibody response for up to 4 years following completion of a 4-year treatment protocol.[29-31]

Based upon the availability of well-conducted, randomized, placebo-controlled trials of SLIT efficacy, it is not surprising that meta-analyses have also been undertaken in this realm. The most recent Cochrane systematic review and meta-analysis of SLIT efficacy for AR was performed by Radulovic and colleagues in 2010[32] and is an update of the highly cited Wilson et al. Cochrane review and meta-analysis initially published in 2003.[33] The updated analysis pooled 49 randomized controlled trials of SLIT, involving 2333 actively treated and 2256 placebo participants. Using standard mean difference (SMD) methodology, significant symptom reduction (SMD −0.49, $P < .001$) and significant reduction in medication requirements (SMD −0.32, $P < .001$) were noted, favoring SLIT over placebo.[32] Subgroup analysis revealed benefit for seasonal and perennial allergens, as well as significant benefit for pediatric and adult patients. In children, a meta-analysis of SLIT for SAR was published in 2006 by Penagos et al.[34] This analysis included 10 randomized, double-blind, placebo-controlled trials and a total of 484 participants. A significant reduction was seen for AR symptoms (SMD 0.56, $P = .02$) and medication use (SMD 0.76, $P = .03$) with SLIT treatment. Active treatment for greater than 18 months and treatment with pollen extracts showed benefit in subgroup analyses. With a plethora of randomized controlled SLIT trials available, meta-analyses have also been published for specific individual antigens. In these meta-analyses, significant benefit has been shown in AR symptom reduction and medication reduction for seasonal grass pollen[35] and house dust mite (HDM)[36] SLIT treatment. Although systematic reviews and meta-analyses are highly regarded as representing the highest levels of evidence, one should remember that many such meta-analyses have some degree of heterogeneity among the trials that are included. Upon reading any of these systematic reviews or meta-analyses, it is important for the reader to determine how meaningful this heterogeneity is and to what degree it should be considered in the overall interpretation of the study conclusions.

Allergen-Specific Immunotherapy

One of the first documented benefits of SLIT is for the treatment of grass-pollen sensitivity. Early studies largely evaluated timothy grass,[37,38] with a subsequent study demonstrating the safety and efficacy of a five-grass pollen tablet.[39] The 2006 study by Durham et al. was a multinational, multicenter, randomized, double-blind, placebo-controlled study of SLIT in which 855 patients were randomized to three timothy grass tablet dosing regimens or placebo.[37] Seven-hundred ninety patients completed this trial, which employed a pre- and coseasonal dosing schedule. The highest dose regimen (15 µg major allergen) resulted in a significant reduction of allergy symptoms and medication use. These benefits were seen over both the entire and peak season. Likewise, Dahl and colleagues published a multicenter, multinational, randomized, double-blind, placebo-controlled timothy grass SLIT trial that included 634 randomized patients (546 completed).[38] This study also showed a significant reduction in allergy symptoms and medication use and a significant increase in well days with SLIT, as compared with placebo. In 2010, Durham et al. reported on the long-term effects of timothy grass SLIT in patients with AR.[40] In a double-blind, randomized, placebo-controlled trial of 257 participants, significant benefits in symptom control and medication use were seen at the 1-year follow-up time point after 3 years of active SLIT treatment. Furthermore, the sustained benefits were the same as during the active treatment phase.

A recently published pooled analysis by Durham et al. evaluated treatment outcomes of SLIT tablets and pharmacotherapies for AR, with separate analyses of timothy grass, ragweed, and HDM trials.[41] A fixed-effect meta-analysis method was used to estimate differences in total nasal symptom score (TNSS) outcome measures. Six timothy grass SLIT-tablet trials (n = 3094), two ragweed SLIT-tablet trials (n = 658), and two HDM SLIT-tablet trials (n = 1768) were included, with overall improvement in TNSS scores of 16.3, 17.1, and 16.1% relative to placebo. Reduction in TNSS among patients who received montelukast, desloratadine, and mometasone furoate nasal spray was 5.4%, 8.5%, and 22.2%, demonstrating statistically similar outcomes in pharmacotherapy and SLIT treatment groups. As with other meta-analyses, comparison was limited by heterogeneous trial designs.

Randomized placebo-controlled trials by Nolte et al.[42] and Creticos et al.[43] have evaluated the safety and efficacy of ragweed-specific SLIT tablets for the treatment of AR. Nolte et al.[42] evaluated the outcomes of daily short ragweed SLIT over a 52-week ragweed season, with evaluation of peak and entire season total combined score (TCS), comprising daily symptom scores and medication usage. Five hundred sixty-five patients demonstrated significant improvement in all outcome measures versus placebo, with comparable efficacy during the peak and entire ragweed season. Creticos et al.[43] further demonstrated the efficacy of ragweed-specific SLIT. Seven hundred eighty-four adults self-administering daily short ragweed SLIT were followed up over a 52-week ragweed season, with primary end points of

peak and entire season TCS. The greatest efficacy was seen in patients who received 12 units of *Ambrosia artemisiifolia* major antigen 1 (Amb a 1-U), with reduced TCS of 24% during the peak and 27% during the entire ragweed season versus placebo (P < .005). No systemic allergic reactions were reported in either study. HDM-specific SLIT has been evaluated by three randomized, double-blind, placebo-controlled Phase III trials.[44–46] The EudraCT (MT-02) trial evaluated safety and change in combined rhinitis symptom and medications score, presented as the total combined rhinitis score (TCRS), following 1 year of therapy with Standardized quality (SQ)-HDM SLIT.[46] Significant findings include a 28.8% reduction in TCRS and rhinitis quality-of-life questionnaire (RQLQ) scores following treatment with 6 SQ-HDM. Interestingly, the greatest change in quality of life was found in the sleep impairment domain of the RQLQ, which improved by 50%. Significant change was not found when treated with lower dose (1 or 3 SQ-HDM) SLIT. Onset of clinical efficacy was evaluated by the P003 trial, wherein HDM-sensitized patients underwent a series of controlled environmental challenges during a 24-week trial of SQ-HDM SLIT.[44] After 8 weeks of treatment, the 12 SQ-HDM group reported significantly lower TNSS following allergen challenge, with a 48.6% reduction versus placebo after 24 weeks of treatment. Onset duration extended to 16 weeks among patients who received 6 SQ-HDM, demonstrating higher efficacy and faster onset with 12 SQ-HDM. Finally, the EudraCT (MT-06) trial evaluated clinically relevant symptom improvement (defined as change in TCRS ≥ 1) among 992 adults who received daily SLIT with 6 or 12 SQ-HDM. Clinically relevant improvements in rhinitis symptoms and pharmacotherapy use were reported in both groups after 14 weeks of treatment, with only the 12 SQ-HDM group demonstrating significant improvements in RQLQ scores. Klimek et al.[47] pooled safety data from these clinical trials and found a higher percentage of treatment-related adverse reactions among patients who received the higher 12 SQ-HDM dosage. These largely consisted of localized allergic reactions that resolved with continued administration. Most commonly reported reactions include oral pruritus, throat irritation, and oral edema, occurring in 20%, 19%, and 11% of patients, respectively.

Pediatric Populations

The efficacy of SLIT for the treatment of SAR has been demonstrated in the pediatric population, a group in which SLIT is very attractive owing to its safety, convenience, and avoidance of needles. A recently published systematic review by Kim et al.[48] evaluated the results of 18 studies, wherein 1583 children received SLIT or usual care, and found a moderate level of evidence that SLIT improves rhinitis and conjunctivitis symptoms as well as medication usage. A high level of evidence was cited for the treatment of asthma. A multicenter, randomized, double-blind, placebo-controlled study published by Bufe and colleagues in 2009 included 253 children aged 5–16 years with grass pollen allergy.[49] With pre- and coseasonal administration of timothy grass tablets, there were significant reductions in AR symptom and medication scores, as well as a significant reduction in asthma symptoms. Observed immunologic changes were similar to those seen in adults. Similarly, Wahn et al. showed a significant reduction in AR symptoms and medication use in 266 children aged 5–17 years with a five-grass tablet in a multicenter, multinational, randomized, double-blind, placebo-controlled trial.[50]

Single- Versus Multiantigen Sublingual Immunotherapy

One aspect of SLIT efficacy that is often discussed is treatment with a single antigen versus multiple antigens. The vast majority of controlled SLIT trials are performed with single-antigen therapy (i.e., grass pollen, HDM, or birch only). This occurs for several reasons. First, compared with practices in the United States, there is a general tendency in European countries to test and treat with fewer antigens for allergic disease, and most of the available SLIT efficacy studies are performed in European countries. Second, to perform a well-designed clinical trial, it is important to control as many extraneous factors as possible. In this vein, a trial that treats only timothy grass allergy with SLIT is able to measure timothy grass pollen counts and correlate patient symptoms over the course of the season, without the need to account for overlapping seasonal symptoms from other tree or weed antigens or year-round symptoms from perennial antigens. Third, designing a clinical trial that incorporates multiple antigen treatment requires all participants to have a similar antigen reactivity and symptom pattern for multiple antigens, which may lead to substantial problems with study enrollment.

The issues with single- versus multiple-allergen SLIT intuitively make sense when considering a randomized placebo-controlled trial design, but translation to clinical practice in the United States is somewhat problematic. In the United States, general immunotherapy practice incorporates testing for a panel of 8–12 (and often more) common antigens. Treatment vials are then mixed according to the patient's individual pattern

of reactivity and symptoms, which most often incorporates multiple antigens. However, direct translation of single-antigen efficacy studies to multiple-allergen therapy is questioned. Very few studies have evaluated the efficacy of SLIT with multiple allergens, and even these are often limited to only two antigens, rather than 10 antigens, which is the mean number included on an immunotherapy prescription in the United States.[51]

The safety of multiantigen SLIT has been demonstrated in an open-label, multicenter trial by Maloney et al.[52] wherein 102 patients received daily SLIT with sequential (within 5 min) administration of short ragweed and timothy grass tablets following a 4-week initiation period. Overall compliance was 96.1% with no reported asthma attacks or SRs.[52] Although there is evidence supporting the safety of multiantigen SLIT, a high level of evidence supporting the efficacy of this treatment approach has not been reliably demonstrated.

Conflicting findings prevent consensus recommendations regarding the efficacy of multiantigen SLIT. For example, a 2009 US study by Amar and colleagues was unable to demonstrate significant benefit of multiple-antigen SLIT over single-antigen SLIT or placebo.[53] Interestingly, in this study, the pollen counts were particularly low for timothy grass, the common allergen included in all immunotherapy prescriptions for both single- and multiallergen groups. In contrast, in a small open-label controlled study of 58 patients with grass and birch sensitization, Marogna and colleagues found that patients treated with both grass and birch antigens had significant clinical improvement over those treated with a single antigen or placebo.[54] Based upon the current available evidence, treatment with multiantigen SLIT needs additional investigation before solid clinical treatment recommendations can be made.

Safety of Sublingual Immunotherapy

SLIT has an extremely high safety profile. The safety of SLIT, which gives rise to its tendency to be dosed at home rather than in the physician's office, is one of the reasons this modality of allergy immunotherapy is so attractive for working individuals and children. Among 60 trials in the 2010 Cochrane systematic review and meta-analysis by Radulovic and colleagues, no cases of anaphylaxis occurred and no patient required epinephrine for treatment of SRs.[32] In this meta-analysis, a total of 53 participants discontinued treatment because of adverse reactions (41 of 824 SLIT patients and 12 of 861 placebo patients), with treatment discontinuation for local reactions being the most common.

In children, Penagos and colleagues also reported no lethal or severe reactions in the 2006 meta-analysis of 10 pediatric SLIT studies for AR, with the exception of three patients with onset of severe asthma that was thought to be caused by SLIT overdose.[34] In the 2009 study by Bufe and colleagues, six subjects withdrew from the study because of a total of 15 adverse events.[49] Two of these withdrawals were in the placebo group, and three in the active group were due to local reactions without sequelae. There was one withdrawal due to a serious systemic reaction that was judged as likely related to active treatment—tongue swelling and itching, shortness of breath, and tightness. This event did not require the administration of epinephrine. The pediatric SLIT study by Wahn and colleagues, also published in 2009, reported no serious adverse events related to active treatment with the five-grass pollen tablet, although nine patients in the active treatment group withdrew from the study because of adverse events.[50] Risk factors associated with SRs to SLIT include allergen overdose, first-dose SLIT therapy, multiallergen SLIT, and previous asthma exacerbation or SR with SCIT.[55]

At this time, 11 cases of anaphylaxis have been reported during SLIT treatment, with a calculated risk of one case of anaphylaxis per 100 million SLIT doses.[55,56] No SLIT-related deaths have been reported. Nonetheless, practitioners prescribing SLIT should be aware of the potential for anaphylaxis with any form of immunotherapy. In reporting these episodes of SLIT-related anaphylaxis, some have speculated on the potential causes for the incitement of such severe reactions. Potential causes include prior systemic reaction or intolerance to immunotherapy, noncompliance and interruptions in immunotherapy treatment, severe or uncontrolled asthma, high pollen counts, use of nonstandardized extracts, and little to no escalation phase.[56] Although a diagnosis of asthma has been suggested as a risk-factor for severe adverse reactions, an ad hoc analysis of timothy grass SLIT tablets demonstrated no such association.[52] Randomized, blinded research is unethical in this realm, and therefore, we remain reliant on case reports and small case series to advise us of SLIT anaphylaxis potential.

Sublingual Immunotherapy Dosing

The most advantageous SLIT dose has not yet been determined for most antigens. Evidence supports an optimal SCIT maintenance dose of 5–20 μg of major allergen per injection for most allergens, which is commonly defined as "the dose of an allergen vaccine inducing a clinically relevant effect in the majority of patients without causing unacceptable side effects."[57,58] However, the desired SLIT maintenance dose to achieve

an appropriate effect while remaining free of side effects has not been fully resolved, with dose findings studies currently available for HDM,[59,60] timothy grass,[37] and five-grass pollen tablets.[61] An evidence-based review with recommendations by Leatherman et al.[62] reports recommended sublingual dosing ranges for several allergens, including HDM, timothy/Bermuda grasses, ragweed, cat, dog, pollen, mold/fungi, and cockroach extracts. Larenas-Linnemann et al.[63] reviewed dosing recommendations for children and found generally equivalent recommendations for adults and children receiving SLIT/SCIT. It is noted that the maximum tolerated SLIT dose may be lower for smaller children, with a clear dose-response relationship.[63]

SLIT maintenance doses are up to 500 times higher than SCIT maintenance doses but administered on a different schedule, with SLIT administered daily and SCIT monthly.[64] Owing to these differences, it is best to compare the median monthly dose for each approach. Using this measure, the median monthly SLIT maintenance dose is approximately 49 times higher than the median monthly dose for SCIT maintenance.

Emerging Therapies

Oral mucosal immunotherapy (OMIT) is an emerging form of Allergen immunotherapy (AIT) that is similar to, but distinctly different from, SLIT. Utilizing a toothpaste vehicle, OMIT introduces allergen to high-density antigen-processing oral Langerhans cells in the oral vestibular and buccal mucosa.[65] Patients therefore introduce allergen while brushing their teeth, with theoretical benefits of induction of immune tolerance with lower antigen concentrations, decreased local side effects, and higher adherence rates versus SLIT.[27] A recently completed open-label, 12-month pilot study of patients electing OMIT versus SLIT identified clinically meaningful improvements in rhinoconjunctivitis quality-of-life scores with a significant rise in specific immunoglobulin G4 over the first 6 months of treatment.[66] No adverse events were reported, with adherence rates of 80% for patients electing OMIT versus 62% for SLIT ($P = .61$).[66] Additional study is needed to further explore the role of OMIT for the treatment of AR.

BOTTOM LINE: WHAT DOES THE EVIDENCE TELL US?

There is strong evidence to support allergy skin testing and SLIT for the treatment of recalcitrant AR. However, evidence is lacking in other aspects of this treatment paradigm. First, available evidence supports the fact that AR has significant public health and economic impact, with nearly 8% of adults in the United States seeking care for AR and patients with AR spending nearly $1500 more in healthcare costs than those without.[1] Second, when evaluating a patient for possible AR, allergy skin testing is often undertaken in association with a thorough history and physical examination that guides the diagnosis. In proceeding through the allergy skin testing procedure, the practitioner should remain aware that with negative skin prick test results, a subsequent positive intradermal skin test does not correlate well with in vitro or challenge tests and provides little additional information in the diagnosis of allergy, whereas a negative intradermal skin test result has a high negative predictive value.[25]

Multiple large-scale single-antigen SLIT efficacy studies have been performed and show significant reduction in allergy symptoms and medication use.[32,35,41,47] These studies are largely well designed, randomized, double blind, and placebo controlled. In support of the evidence from individual randomized controlled trials, a number of systematic reviews and meta-analyses have also been performed. The evidence supporting SLIT for seasonal and perennial AR, and for adults and pediatric patients, is strong.[32,34] In addition, the clinical benefits of SLIT beyond the active treatment period have been documented,[54] as have dosage recommendations for several allergens.[62] Less clear, however, is the translation of single-antigen SLIT efficacy results to clinical practice that incorporates multiple-antigen SLIT prescriptions. These are areas that deserve future investigation before we have solid evidence to support clinical treatment decisions.

The safety of SLIT is well documented, with anaphylaxis risks distinctly lower than those historically quoted for SCIT. In addition, no lethal events have been reported related to SLIT. However, SLIT-related anaphylaxis events have been documented in case reports and small case series,[55] and we must remain vigilant of the safety concerns with any form of immunotherapy.

REFERENCES

1. Bhattacharyya N. Incremental healthcare utilization and expenditures for allergic rhinitis in the United States. *Laryngoscope.* 2011;121(9):1830–1833.
2. Curtis H. The immunizing cure of hay fever. *Med News.* 1900;77(16).
3. Calderon MA, Alves B, Jacobson M, Hurwitz B, Sheikh A, Durham S. Allergen injection immunotherapy for seasonal allergic rhinitis. *Cochrane Database Syst Rev.* 2007;(1):CD001936.
4. Abramson MJ, Puy RM, Weiner JM. Injection allergen immunotherapy for asthma. *Cochrane Database Syst Rev.* 2010;(8):CD001186.
5. Epstein TG, Liss GM, Murphy-Berendts K, Bernstein DI. Risk factors for fatal and nonfatal reactions to subcutaneous immunotherapy: national surveillance study on allergen immunotherapy (2008-2013). *Ann Allergy Asthma Immunol.* 2016;116(4): 354–359.e2.
6. Lockey RF, Benedict LM, Turkeltaub PC. Fatalities from immunotherapy (IT) and skin testing (ST). *J Allergy Clin Immunol.* 1987;79.
7. Reid MJ, Lockey RF, Turkeltaub PC. Survey of fatalities from skin testing and immunotherapy 1985–1989. *J Allergy Clin Immunol.* 1993;92.
8. Bernstein DI, Wanner M, Borish L, Liss GM. Immunotherapy Committee, American Academy of Allergy, Asthma and Immunology. Twelve-year survey of fatal reactions to allergen injections and skin testing: 1990-2001. *J Allergy Clin Immunol.* 2004;113(6):1129–1136.
9. Committee on the Safety of Medicines update: desensitizing vaccines. *Br Med J.* 1986;293:948.
10. Passalacqua G, Albano M, Ruffoni S, et al. Nasal immunotherapy to *Parietaria*: evidence of reduction of local allergic inflammation. *Am J Respir Crit Care Med.* 1995;152(2):461–466.
11. Tari MG, Mancino M, Monti G. Immunotherapy by inhalation of allergen in powder in house dust allergic asthma – a double-blind study. *J Investig Allergol Clin Immunol.* 1992;2(2):59–67.
12. Taudorf E, Laursen LC, Lanner A, et al. Oral immunotherapy in birch pollen hay fever. *J Allergy Clin Immunol.* 1987;80(2):153–161.
13. Oppenheimer J, Areson JG, Nelson HS. Safety and efficacy of oral immunotherapy with standardized cat extract. *J Allergy Clin Immunol.* 1994;93(1 Pt 1):61–67.
14. Van Deusen MA, Angelini BL, Cordoro KM. Efficacy and safety of oral immunotherapy with short ragweed extract. *Ann Allergy.* 1997;78(6):573–580.
15. Bousquet P-J, Cox LS, Durham SR, Nelson HS. *Sub-Lingual Immunotherapy: World Allergy Organization Position Paper 2009.* 2009.
16. Seidman MD, Gurgel RK, Lin SY, et al. Clinical practice guideline: allergic rhinitis. *Otolaryngol Head Neck Surg.* 2015;152(1 suppl):S1–S43.
17. Skoner DP. Allergic rhinitis: definition, epidemiology, pathophysiology, detection, and diagnosis. *J Allergy Clin Immunol.* 2001;108(1 suppl):S2–S8.
18. Shearer WT. Specific diagnostic modalities: IgE, skin tests, and RAST. *J Allergy Clin Immunol.* 1989;84(6 Pt 2):1112–1116.
19. Cox L, Nelson H, Lockey R, et al. Allergen immunotherapy: a practice parameter third update. *J Allergy Clin Immunol.* 2011;127(1 suppl):S1–S55.
20. Wide L, Bennich H, Johansson SG. Diagnosis of allergy by an in-vitro test for allergen antibodies. *Lancet.* 1967;2(7526):1105–1107.

21. Kemeny DM. Tests for immune reactivity in allergy. *Curr Opin Immunol.* 1989;2(6):910–916.

22. Ewan PW, Coote D. Evaluation of a capsulated hydrophilic carrier polymer (the ImmunoCAP) for measurement of specific IgE antibodies. *Allergy.* 1990;45.

23. Ownby DR. Allergy testing: in vivo versus in vitro. *Pediatr Clin North Am.* 1988;35.

24. Yeoh KH, Wang D-Y, Gordon BR. Safety and efficacy of radioallergosorbent test-based allergen immunotherapy in treatment of perennial allergic rhinitis and asthma. *Otolaryngol Head Neck Surg.* 2004;131(5):673–678.

25. Calabria CW, Hagan L. The role of intradermal skin testing in inhalant allergy. *Ann Allergy.* 2008;101.

26. Krouse JH, Stachler RJ, Shah A. Current in vivo and in vitro screens for inhalant allergy. *Otolaryngol Clin North Am.* 2003;36(5):855–868.

27. Canonica GW, Cox L, Pawankar R, et al. Sublingual immunotherapy: World Allergy Organization position paper 2013 update. *World Allergy Organ J.* 2014;7(1):1–52.

28. Brozek JL, Bousquet J, Baena-Cagnani CE, et al. Allergic rhinitis and its impact on asthma (ARIA) guidelines: 2010 revision. *J Allergy Clin Immunol.* 2010;126(3):466–476.

29. Durham SR, Emminger W, Kapp A, et al. SQ-standardized sublingual grass immunotherapy: confirmation of disease modification 2 years after 3 years of treatment in a randomized trial. *J Allergy Clin Immunol.* 2012;129(3). 717–725.e5.

30. Didier A, Malling H-J, Worm M, Horak F, Sussman GL. Prolonged efficacy of the 300IR 5-grass pollen tablet up to 2 years after treatment cessation, as measured by a recommended daily combined score. *Clin Transl Allergy.* 2015;5(1):12.

31. Marogna M, Spadolini I, Massolo A, Canonica GW, Passalacqua G. Long-lasting effects of sublingual immunotherapy according to its duration: a 15-year prospective study. *J Allergy Clin Immunol.* 2010;126(5):969–975.

32. Radulovic S, Calderon MA, Wilson D, Durham S. Sublingual immunotherapy for allergic rhinitis. *Cochrane Database Syst Rev.* 2010;(12):CD002893.

33. Wilson DR, Torres LI, Durham SR. Sublingual immunotherapy for allergic rhinitis. Wilson D, ed. *Cochrane Database Syst Rev.* 2003;57(2):CD002893.

34. Penagos M, Compalati E, Tarantini F, et al. Efficacy of sublingual immunotherapy in the treatment of allergic rhinitis in pediatric patients 3 to 18 years of age: a meta-analysis of randomized, placebo-controlled, double-blind trials. *Ann Allergy Asthma Immunol.* 2006;97(2): 141–148.

35. Di Bona D, Plaia A, Leto-Barone MS, La Piana S, Di Lorenzo G. Efficacy of grass pollen allergen sublingual immunotherapy tablets for seasonal allergic rhinoconjunctivitis: a systematic review and meta-analysis. *JAMA Intern Med.* 2015;175(8):1301–1309.

36. Compalati E, Passalacqua G, Bonini M, Canonica GW. The efficacy of sublingual immunotherapy for house dust mites respiratory allergy: results of a GA2LEN meta-analysis. *Allergy.* 2009;64(11):1570–1579.

37. Durham SR, Yang WH, Pedersen MR, Johansen N, Rak S. Sublingual immunotherapy with once-daily grass allergen tablets: a randomized controlled trial in seasonal allergic rhinoconjunctivitis. *J Allergy Clin Immunol.* 2006;117(4):802–809.

38. Dahl R, Kapp A, Colombo G, et al. Efficacy and safety of sublingual immunotherapy with grass allergen tablets for seasonal allergic rhinoconjunctivitis. *J Allergy Clin Immunol.* 2006;118(2):434–440.

39. Nelson H, Cartier S, Allen-Ramey F, Lawton S, Calderon MA. Network meta-analysis shows commercialized subcutaneous and sublingual grass products have comparable efficacy. *J Allergy Clin Immunol Pract.* 2015;3(2): 256–266.e3.

40. Durham SR, Emminger W, Kapp A, et al. Long-term clinical efficacy in grass pollen-induced rhinoconjunctivitis after treatment with SQ-standardized grass allergy immunotherapy tablet. *J Allergy Clin Immunol.* 2010;125(1): 131–138.e1-7.

41. Durham SR, Creticos PS, Nelson HS, et al. Treatment effect of sublingual immunotherapy tablets and pharmacotherapies for seasonal and perennial allergic rhinitis: pooled analyses. *J Allergy Clin Immunol.* 2016;138(4): 1081–1088.e1084.

42. Nolte H, Hébert J, Berman G, et al. Randomized controlled trial of ragweed allergy immunotherapy tablet efficacy and safety in North American adults. *Ann Allergy Asthma Immunol.* 2013;110(6): 450–456.e454.

43. Creticos PS, Maloney J, Bernstein DI, et al. Randomized controlled trial of a ragweed allergy immunotherapy tablet in North American and European adults. *J Allergy Clin Immunol.* 2013;131(5): 1342–1349.e1346.

44. Nolte H, Maloney J, Nelson HS, et al. Onset and dose-related efficacy of house dust mite sublingual immunotherapy tablets in an environmental exposure chamber. *J Allergy Clin Immunol.* 2015;135(6): 1494–1501.e1496.

45. Demoly P, Emminger W, Rehm D, Backer V, Tommerup L, Kleine-Tebbe J. Effective treatment of house dust mite-induced allergic rhinitis with 2 doses of the SQ HDM SLIT-tablet: results from a randomized, double-blind, placebo-controlled phase III trial. *J Allergy Clin Immunol.* 2016;137(2): 444–451.e448.

46. Mosbech H, Canonica GW, Backer V, et al. SQ house dust mite sublingually administered immunotherapy tablet (ALK) improves allergic rhinitis in patients with house dust mite allergic asthma and rhinitis symptoms. *Ann Allergy Asthma Immunol.* 2015;114(2):134–140.

47. Klimek L, Mosbech H, Zieglmayer P, Rehm D, Stage BS, Demoly P. SQ house dust mite (HDM) SLIT-tablet provides clinical improvement in HDM-induced allergic rhinitis. *Expert Rev Clin Immunol.* 2016;12(4):369–377.

48. Kim JM, Lin SY, Suarez-Cuervo C, et al. Allergen-specific immunotherapy for pediatric asthma and rhinoconjunctivitis: a systematic review. *Pediatrics.* 2013;131(6):1155–1167.

49. Bufe A, Eberle P, Franke-Beckmann E, et al. Safety and efficacy in children of an SQ-standardized grass allergen tablet for sublingual immunotherapy. *J Allergy Clin Immunol.* 2009;123(1): 167–173.e167.

50. Wahn U, Tabar A, Kuna P, et al. Efficacy and safety of 5-grass-pollen sublingual immunotherapy tablets in pediatric allergic rhinoconjunctivitis. *J Allergy Clin Immunol.* 2009;123(1): 160–166.e163.

51. Nelson HS. Multiallergen immunotherapy for allergic rhinitis and asthma. *J Allergy Clin Immunol.* 2009;123(4): 763–769.

52. Maloney J, Durham S, Skoner D, et al. Safety of sublingual immunotherapy Timothy grass tablet in subjects with allergic rhinitis with or without conjunctivitis and history of asthma. *Allergy.* 2015;70(3):302–309.

53. Amar SM, Harbeck RJ, Sills M, Silveira LJ, O'Brien H, Nelson HS. Response to sublingual immunotherapy with grass pollen extract: monotherapy versus combination in a multiallergen extract. *J Allergy Clin Immunol.* 2009;124(1): 150–156.e1–5.

54. Marogna M, Spadolini I, Massolo A, Zanon P. Effects of sublingual immunotherapy for multiple or single allergens in polysensitized patients. *Ann Allergy.* 2007.

55. Epstein TG, Calabria CW, Cox LS, Dreborg S. Current evidence on safety and practical considerations for administration of sublingual allergen immunotherapy (SLIT) in the United States. *J Allergy Clin Immunol Pract.* 2017;5(1): 34–40.e2.

56. Calderon MA, Simons FER, Malling H-J, Lockey RF, Moingeon P, Demoly P. Sublingual allergen immunotherapy: mode of action and its relationship with the safety profile. *Allergy.* 2012;67(3):302–311.

57. van Ree R. Indoor allergens: relevance of major allergen measurements and standardization. *J Allergy Clin Immunol.* 2007;119(2):270–277. quiz 278–9.

58. Bousquet J, Lockey R, Malling H-J. Allergen immunotherapy: therapeutic vaccines for allergic diseases. A WHO position paper. *J Allergy Clin Immunol.* 1998;102:558–562.

59. Roux M, Devillier P, Yang WH, et al. Efficacy and safety of sublingual tablets of house dust mite allergen extracts: results of a dose-ranging study in an environmental exposure chamber. *J Allergy Clin Immunol.* 2016;138(2): 451–458.e455.

60. Hüser C, Dieterich P, Singh J, et al. A 12-week DBPC dose-finding study with sublingual monomeric allergoid tablets in house dust mite-allergic patients. *Allergy.* 2017;72(1):77–84.

61. Didier A, Malling H-J, Worm M, et al. Optimal dose, efficacy, and safety of once-daily sublingual immunotherapy with a 5-grass pollen tablet for seasonal allergic rhinitis. *J Allergy Clin Immunol.* 2007;120(6):1338–1345.

62. Leatherman BD, Khalid A, Lee S, et al. Dosing of sublingual immunotherapy for allergic rhinitis: evidence-based review with recommendations. *Int Forum Allergy Rhinol.* 2015;5(9):773–783.

63. Larenas-Linnemann D. Direct comparison of efficacy of sublingual immunotherapy tablets for rhinoconjunctivitis. *Ann Allergy Asthma Immunol.* 2016;116(4):274–286.

64. Cox LS, Larenas-Linnemann D, Nolte H, Weldon D, Finegold I, Nelson HS. Sublingual immunotherapy: a comprehensive review. *J Allergy Clin Immunol.* 2006;117(5):1021–1035.

65. Allam JP, Stojanovski G, Friedrichs N, et al. Distribution of Langerhans cells and mast cells within the human oral mucosa: new application sites of allergens in sublingual immunotherapy? *Allergy.* 2008;63(6):720–727.

66. Reisacher WR, Suurna MV, Rochlin K, Bremberg MG, Tropper G. Oral mucosal immunotherapy for allergic rhinitis: a pilot study. *Allergy Rhinol (Providence).* 2016;7(1):21–28.

CHAPTER 8

Evidence-Based Practice: Pediatric Obstructive Sleep Apnea

DAVID CONRAD, MD, FAAP • KRISTINA ROSBE, MD, FAAP

OVERVIEW

Obstructive sleep apnea (OSA) of childhood is a common disorder with a prevalence of 1%–5%.[1] Although the frequency of adenoidectomy and tonsillectomy for sleep-disordered breathing (SDB) has decreased since the 1970's, there are still over 500,000 tonsillectomies performed per year in the United States.[2] Global assessment of the child and patient selection are valued, and more stringent evidence-based guidelines and surgical criteria have been thoughtfully instituted to maximize patient benefit. Moreover, management of obstructive sleep apnea syndromes (OSASs) encourages a personalized approach to medical decision-making. Given that OSAS is common in any otolaryngology setting, it is important to incorporate evidence-based medicine into everyday practice.

SDB is an encompassing term, describing a spectrum of disorders ranging from primary snoring to severe OSA. Because habitual snoring is present in nearly 10%–20% of children, it is often challenging to determine if a given patient requires intervention from the history and physical examination alone.[1] Multiple clinicians and investigators have tried to develop clinical tools that have better correlation with disease severity, but these efforts are ongoing. Although polysomnography (PSG) is our currently best objective assessment of SDB, there are still challenges in offering this to every patient, including cost, a limited number of pediatric sleep laboratories, and reliability of one night's sleep in a foreign setting for a child, especially for those patients with developmental or cognitive delays. Given that snoring is not synonymous with OSA, it is important to understand the differences among sleep disorders and the management options available.

Use of evidence-based medicine is particularly important in children with OSAS, as this is a common diagnosis of many otolaryngology practice. In a study examining gaps in evidence, Ishman and colleagues determined that up to 61% of decisions made in their clinical setting were not evidence based.[3] This chapter aims to provide the most current literature review and discussion of evidence-based guidelines and analysis for pediatric OSAS.

Common definitions of SDB and associated terms are listed in Box 8.1.

EPIDEMIOLOGY OF PEDIATRIC SLEEP DISORDERS

Prevalence rates of pediatric sleep diagnoses vary across the spectrum of disorders. It is estimated that 5%–27% of patients have primary snoring, whereas 1%–4% of the general pediatric population have OSA.[4,5] Sleep-disordered breathing is an umbrella term that includes a spectrum of severity; several of these can be found in Fig. 8.1. Evidence varies in the frequency of OSAS with regard to age, race, and gender. Snoring prevalence has been shown to decrease between ages 4 and 12 years, and a bimodal prevalence has been suspected because of initiation of school and exposure to sick contacts.[6,7] SDB has also been shown to be more common in boys than in girls, especially following puberty.[6]

Nonrespiratory disorders also may present with common parental complaints of sleep disturbances. Behavioral insomnia of childhood, which involves night waking and aversion to being put to bed, affects 20%–30% of infants and toddlers.[8–10] In adolescents and youths with developmental disorders, primary psychophysiologic insomnia ranges from 5% to 20%.[11] Periodic limb movement disorder is characterized by repetitive limb jerking, which can be diagnosed during PSG, is observed. Alternatively, restless leg syndrome (RLS) is characterized by the urge to continuously move one's legs during wakefulness. These symptoms must be distressing enough to impair sleep and cannot be attributable to any other conditions. Risk factors for RLS include history of prematurity, caffeine, iron deficiency, and family history. Children suspected of having periodic limb movement disorder or RLS should undergo appropriate workup to rule out contributing factors, and PSG is often helpful in establishing a diagnosis.[12]

BOX 8.1
Sleep Disorders and Definitions

SLEEP-DISORDERED BREATHING

- Primary snoring—may present with apnea hypopnea index (AHI) < 1/h.
- Upper airway resistance syndrome (UARS).
- Obstructive sleep apnea (OSA)—absence or reduction in airflow despite respiratory effort.[1]

    Mild: AHI 1–5/h;

    Moderate: AHI 5.1–10/h;

    Severe: AHI >10/h.

- Congenital central hypoventilation syndrome—rare disorder associated with *PHOX2B* (paired-like homeobox 2B gene) chr 4p12 mutation. Patients often present with sleep-related central apneas, increased risk of Hirschsprung disease, and neural crest tumors such as neuroblastoma and ganglioneuroma.[2]

SLEEP DISORDERS

OSA—Episodes of complete or partial airway obstruction associated with sleep disturbances, including brief arousals, restless sleep, daytime hyperactivity or sleepiness and fatigue. Severity is based on PSG and AHI > 1 is abnormal.

Parasomnia—sleepwalking (somnambulism), sleeptalking (somniloquy), nocturnal groaning (catathrenia), and night terror (pavor nocturnus), often occur in the first one-third of the night during nonrapid eye movement (NREM) sleep.

Apnea—cessation of airflow or 90% or greater reduction in airflow for a minimum of 10 seconds.

Hypopnea—reduction in airflow over two or more respiratory cycles accompanied by a 3% reduction in oxygen saturation and/or resulting in EEG arousal.[3]

Central apnea—cessation of airflow due to lack of respiratory effort.

Nocturnal hypoxemia—oxygen saturation <89% for >5% of total sleep time.

Hypoventilation—persistent $EtCO_2$ > 50 Torr for more than 10% of total sleep time.

INDICES

Apnea Hypopnea Index (AHI)

1. Bluestone CD. *Pediatric Otolaryngology*. 4th ed. Philadelphia: Saunders; 2003.

2. Weese-Mayer DE, et al. An official ATS clinical policy statement: congenital central hypoventilation syndrome: genetic basis, diagnosis, and management. *Am J Respir Crit Care Med*. 2010;181(6): 626–644.

Hypopnea

3. American Academy of Sleep Medicine. International Classification of Sleep Disorders: Diagnostic and Coding Manual. 2nd ed. Westchester, IL: American Academy of Sleep Medicine—USA; 2005.

POTENTIAL CONSEQUENCES OF OBSTRUCTIVE SLEEP APNEA SYNDROMES
Cardiometabolic Health

There is strong evidence that shows physiologic and cardiovascular changes in children with even moderate SDB. Although the severity of cardiopulmonary sequelae is likely reduced in comparison with adults, more investigation into the long-term morbidity is necessary, given these findings are likely common in the general pediatric population.

Heart rate has been found to be a sensitive indicator of pediatric SDB severity.[13] A randomized controlled clinical trial by Quante and colleagues associated with the Childhood Adenotonsillectomy (CHAT) study compared metabolic parameters and cardiac changes in children over the age of 5 years who received surgery versus observation. They found an average heart rate increase of 3 beats per minute (bmp) for an apnea hypopnea index (AHI) of 2 versus 10 (standard error = 0.60).[13] Likewise, they found that heart rate could be lowered by 1 and 1.5 bmp with a 5-unit reduction in AHI and a 5-mmHg improvement in peak end-tidal CO_2 ($EtCO_2$), respectively. Other than heart rate, AHI, and $EtCO_2$ being measures of OSA severity between groups, there was no change in the levels of fasting glucose, insulin, lipids, and C-reactive protein (CRP). A summary of key discovery of the AHI normalization rates before and after AD can be found in Fig. 8.2. Although the long-term impact of heart rate remains unclear, it demonstrates the effect of even mild SDB on the cardiac and circulatory system, which merits further investigation.

The cardiovascular burden of SDB is more pronounced in children with obesity. Untreated sleep apnea results in repetitive arousals, hypoxemia, hypercapnia, increased sympathetic activation, and an increase in renin-angiotensin system.[14] As a result, children with severe SDB may present with hypertension and need routine monitoring by their otolaryngologist and primary care provider. Blood pressure elevation may be observed in children who are nonobese as well. A study of nonpubertal children with SDB found an elevation of blood pressure by 10–15 mmHg independent of their body mass index (BMI).[15,16]

Systemic effects of OSA can also manifest increased cardiac afterload, resulting in left ventricular remodeling. In one study, children with OSA and obesity had an odds ratio of 11.2 for a left ventricular mass index > 95th percentile.[17] Another study showed relief of these parameters following AD, suggesting this process is reversible with adequate therapy.[17] The long-term impact and reversibility of cardiovascular morbidity needs further investigation but provides an insight into systemic effects of OSA in children.

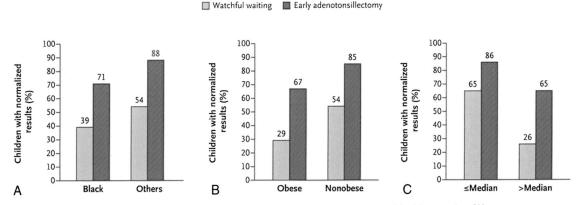

Sleep-disordered breathing

Primary snoring	Upper airway resistance syndrome	OSAS	Obesity-hypoventilation syndrome
Noisy breathing Stertor quality No interruptions in sleep quality	Absence of O_2 desaturation Absence of apnea, hypopnea RERAs EDS	PSG with AHI > 1/h Obstructive hypoventilation Daytime impairment	Obesity Hypoventilation ($P_aCO_2 \geq$ 45 mm Hg) Presence of OSA

FIG. 8.1 Sleep-disordered breathing and associated syndromes. *EDS*, excessive daytime sleepiness; *OSA*, obstructive sleep apnea; *RERA*, respiratory effort-related arousal.

FIG. 8.2 Percentage of children with normalized results (defined <2 events/h) with regard to **(A)** race; **(B)** obesity; and **(C)** apnea hypopnea index (AHI) score. (From Marcus CL, Moore RH, Rosen CL, et al. A randomized trial of adenotonsillectomy for childhood sleep apnea. *N Engl J Med.* 2013;368(25):2366–2376, with permission.)

Hyperactivity and Daytime Disturbances

Attention-deficit/hyperactivity disorder (ADHD) is characterized by hyperactive behavior, inattention, and impulsivity, affecting 3%–5% of school-aged children.[18] The effects of this disorder on executive and social functioning are pervasive, affecting working memory, self-regulation of affect/arousal, internalization of speech, and reconstitution.[19] Because hyperactivity behavior can be present in nearly a third of children with snoring or SDB, it is important to consider the presence of underlying sleep-related disorders in children with ADHD.

The association of ADHD and SDB in children has been well demonstrated. In animal models, episodic hypoxia has been found to cause sex-dependent behavioral hyperactivity and impaired spatial learning in rats.[20] O'Brien and colleagues found that SDB is significantly prevalent among children with parentally reported mild hyperactive behaviors. However, they also demonstrated that the prevalence of SDB in children with significant ADHD was not different than in the general population.[18]

The long-term consequences of SDB on behavior also require further investigation. A large, population-based longitudinal study of more than 11,000 patients studied the presence of behavioral issues in children who had parental perception of snoring, mouth breathing, and apnea. It was found that SDB was associated with 40%–60% more behavioral difficulties at 4 and 7 years of age, respectively. Peer difficulty, conduct disorder, and hyperactivity have also been found to be prevalent in children with SDB, in other studies.[21]

Effects on Academic Performance and Learning

SDB has been associated with cognitive impairment in children.[22] Although parameters such as inattentiveness, daytime hyperactivity, and difficulty performing in a classroom setting have been studied, the effects on cognitive development in children less than 5 years of age have not been fully evaluated. More research is needed to determine if surgical intervention is a particularly time-critical intervention and if younger children receive greater benefit from surgery than older patients.

SDB in preschool-aged childhood has gained increased attention in particular. Intelligence quotient (IQ), attention, and executive functioning have been shown to be negatively affected by SDB.[18] Vigilance, sustained attention, and visual sequencing have been examined through standardized testing, but the inherent subjectivity of these assessments has not shown a significant difference before and after surgery.[23] Lau and colleagues used a Baddeley's working memory model that showed impaired basic storage and executive components of memory in the verbal domain when compared with controls.[23] These findings are in agreement with several other studies that also showed improved sustained attention and working memory but did not show that verbal knowledge, language development, visuospatial ability, and generalized intelligence improve posttreatment.[24–26] Although many of these studies vary widely in their findings, there is some evidence to support the notion that surgery may improve cognitive effects of SDB, and more studies are needed to determine if the therapy is time sensitive.

School performance and intelligence before and after adenotonsillectomy (AD) have also been examined by several authors. Biggs and colleagues studied the improvements in neurocognition and behavioral changes after treatment in school-aged children. In contrast to other studies, they found improvements in tasks associated with spatial visualization, visual-motor coordination, abstract thought, and nonverbal fluid reasoning (collectively categorized as Performance IQ) when children were treated for SDB.[27] School performance is closely linked to Verbal IQ, which did not improve after treatment. Improvements in attention span after surgery in children older than 5 years has not been reliably found. The CHAT study published in the *New England Journal of Medicine* did show improvements in AHI, behavior, and quality of life but did not find significant benefit in attention or executive function as measured by neuropsychological testing.[25] Data remain mixed about the effects of tonsil and adenoid surgery on school performance and IQ, but these studies provide impetus to examine the benefits of surgery.

UTILITY OF POLYSOMNOGRAPHY

Laboratory PSG is an indispensable tool for confirming and quantifying the severity of sleep-related disorders. The American Academy of Pediatrics currently recommends PSG for any child with a history of snoring. If PSG is unavailable, it is recommended that a child should be evaluated by an otolaryngologist or should undergo alternative testing with nocturnal video recording and nocturnal oximetry. Although sleep studies are commonly obtained by pulmonologists, otolaryngologists, and pediatricians, poor access to such studies can often delay treatment, and a careful history and physical examination are equally important critical steps in the initial workup.

The sensitivity and accuracy of laboratory PSG has been well established. There is more than adequate evidence to support the need for PSG, as clinical evaluation alone is inaccurate to determine the presence of apnea. In the CHAT study, 49% of children with SDB on clinical evaluation had a normal sleep study.[25] Another study found that history alone was not sufficient to predict the abnormal polysomnographic parameters in children.[28] It is therefore generally recommended to obtain a sleep study, especially if moderate or severe disease is suspected. There are challenges with this, however, including costs and availability of pediatric sleep laboratories.

Alternative diagnostic modalities may be useful when access to PSG is limited. Nocturnal oximetry has been shown to be a sensitive modality for differentiating snoring from OSAS. Several studies have shown significant positive predictive value in nocturnal oximetry, which approaches that of formal PSG evaluation. The McGill oximetry score was developed and validated by several authors and has been shown to have a 97% positive predictive value when compared with PSG.[29,30] Home oximetry hastened the time to treatment, and about one-fourth of patients avoided PSG as part of their workup. Pulse oximetry has been shown to be an acceptable alternative to PSG for the initial workup of sleep apnea; however, more studies are needed to create a standardized approach to preoperative evaluation.

OBESITY AND SLEEP-DISORDERED BREATHING

Although childhood obesity rates have been tripled since 1980, childhood obesity has remained stable over the past decade, with rates declining in ages 2–5 years, stable in ages 6–11 years, and increasing among children older than 12 years.[31] Childhood obesity can be defined as >95th percentile and overweight as >85th percentile. OSA often accompanies obesity, with abnormal PSG findings occurring in up to 60% of patients.[14] Morbidities such as hypertension, type II diabetes, dyslipidemia, and left ventricular abnormalities can be confounded by chronic intermittent hypoxemia during sleep. Dietary modification and support with structured comprehensive preventative therapies are essential, as approximately 75% of obese children will become obese adults.[32]

The success rate for cure of OSAS of adenotonsillectomy is reduced in obese patients because of several anatomic and metabolic factors. Increased mechanical load on the chest wall and central adiposity reduce lung compliance and lead to hypoventilation of distal alveoli and an increase in pulmonary arterial pressures. OSA persists in approximately 50% of obese children.[14] It is therefore important to counsel parents on the reduced efficacy of surgery and how multimodality therapy is often indicated after the removal of hypertrophied tonsils and adenoids. Nonetheless, evidence supports that tonsil size is an important predictor of SDB severity, and obese children should be considered for surgery after PSG and preoperative health assessment.

Referral to a bariatric surgeon should be considered for morbid obesity, defined as BMI ≥40 or 35–40 kg/m^2, where surgery is unlikely to reduce sleep study parameters to acceptable levels. A study assessing gastric bypass and sleeve gastrectomy in adolescents and teenagers found a significant and early decline in AHI postoperatively.[33] It is generally recommended that a child performs at least 60 min of moderate intense activity daily. Although weight loss is challenging for any child, it is recommended to refer patients for comprehensive nutritional evaluation and consider all possible therapies for morbid obesity.

MEDICAL MANAGEMENT OF SLEEP-DISORDERED BREATHING

Medical management continues to have an important role in treatment of primary snoring and mild SDB. A variety of studies have examined the efficacy of both topical and systemic medications that reduce mucosal swelling and tissue inflammation. With adequate analysis and low morbidity, it is possible to incorporate these evidence-based recommendations into practice.

Topical nasal steroids have been investigated as a medical modality for SDB in children younger than 16 years. Two randomized clinical trial studies were adequate in a Cochrane Review, showing success in reducing AHI following treatment with intranasal fluticasone and budesonide for at least 6 weeks.

However, results should be interpreted with caution because of a lack of complete randomization in a study and evidence lacking in long-term benefit and therapy duration.[34] Fluticasone propionate gained FDA approval for use in children older than 2 years of age and in children with concomitant allergic rhinitis and is generally safe.

Montelukast, a leukotriene receptor antagonist, has been shown to be effective in affecting adenotonsillar tissue because of the elevated human cysteinyl leukotrienes receptor 1 expression.[35] It has been shown to significantly improve AHI score following surgery in patients who had persistent AHI elevation following surgery.[36] A prospective randomized controlled trial (RCT) was performed in 57 children aged 2–10 years who completed a 16-week trial of therapy with montelukast versus placebo. 71.4% of patients showed statistically significant reduction in AHI score.[37] In another double-blind placebo-controlled study, Goldbart and colleagues found significant improvements in obstructive apnea index, symptoms, and adenoid size.[38] Although these medications are not first-line therapy for severe symptoms, they should be considered for patients with mild-moderate symptoms or patients who have failed to normalize their symptoms after AD.

A variety of other adjuvant treatment modalities have been examined. It is important to consider referring children with retrognathia, excessive palatal narrowing, or crossbite to be evaluated for orthodontics. Positional changes and sleeping upright has been shown to improve AHI in patients who are younger, have thin body habitus, and have less severe OSA.[39] Decongestants and antihistamines may be indicated for concurrent allergic rhinitis, but studies are lacking in their role in long-term therapy. It is important to caution parents that symptoms of SDB will likely worsen during upper respiratory infection.

SLEEP ENDOSCOPY

Localizing the anatomic sites of obstruction is important in patients who have not responded adequately to first-line management of SDB. Drug-induced sleep endoscopy (DISE) or sleep nasoendoscopy is used to visualize and study the dynamic changes of the combined upper airway during a sleeplike state while the patient is spontaneously breathing. First described in 1991 by Croft and Pringle, DISE has increasing utility in pediatric SDB, strengthened by greater standardization and analysis of various pharmacologic agents. DISE offers an individualized approach to the surgical management of residual sleep apnea. It is easy to learn and has been proven effective at identifying the site(s) of obstruction in children who have failed first-line therapy or do not have adenotonsillar hypertrophy.

DISE is most often performed using a flexible nasolaryngoscope to systematically examine from the nasal cavity to the vocal cords. Adjuvant maneuvers may be performed, including chin lift to replicate mouth breathing and jaw thrust to study tongue-base position. Other than adenotonsillar hypertrophy, the areas of concern are, namely, lingual tonsillar hypertrophy, hypotonia and lateral pharyngeal wall collapse, laryngomalacia, vocal fold dysfunction, and baseline patency of the airway during sleep. The subglottis and trachea may be evaluated if concomitant tracheomalacia is suspected.

A variety of pharmacologic induction agents have been studied in children and adults. Pediatric DISE most often uses a combination of induction agents, such as dexmedetomidine and ketamine. Ehsan and Ishman conducted a review of the effects of various anesthetics and opioids on airway collapse.[40] Dexmedetomidine and ketamine had the least effect on airway collapsibility, compared with propofol, inhalational anesthetic agents, midazolam, and pentobarbital. Propofol is often favored in adults, and slower target-controlled infusion has been shown to be a safe alternative to manual bolus injection.[41]

The reliability of DISE has been studied in adults and children through validated classification systems. Interrater reliability and test-test reliability have been shown by several studies in adults.[42-44] Chang and Parikh developed and validated a scoring system in children, assessing five areas of obstruction: adenoid, velum, lateral pharyngeal walls, tongue base, and supraglottis.[45] They also found a correlation between multilevel score severity and polysomnographic parameters. Greater standardization in the future will facilitate communication between examiners and reliability in clinical research.

Although the utility of DISE has been embraced by many tertiary centers, there has been less consensus on the indication for DISE, the role of PSG in decision-making to perform DISE, and the pharmacologic agents used and the method of endoscopy.[46] A multi-institutional survey investigating DISE practices found that most patients who undergo DISE no longer have their tonsils, and there is still less agreement on anesthesia protocols. More analysis is needed to provide standardization, but there is more than adequate evidence to support the safety and efficacy of DISE. The two main indications for DISE are (1) children who

have persistent SDB after adenotonsillectomy and (2) children with examination findings inconsistent with adenotonsillar hypertrophy as the site of obstruction. Children with Down syndrome, craniofacial abnormalities, Beckwith-Wiedemann syndrome, and mucopolysaccharidosis also deserve DISE because of the higher likelihood of synchronous airway obstruction.

RESIDUAL OBSTRUCTIVE SLEEP APNEA AFTER ADENOTONSILLECTOMY

Given that up to 30%–40% of patients who undergo surgery will fail to respond, it is important to have a treatment plan for patients who have persistent symptoms. This approach may encompass multiple therapy modalities, including medical management, consideration of continuous positive airway pressure (CPAP), lifestyle modification, orthodontia, DISE, and/or revision surgery.

Predicting which patients may have persistent symptoms is useful when counseling parents. Children with small tonsils preoperatively particularly pose a challenge. Imanguli and Ulualp found that children with Brodsky Score 1 tonsils had a residual AHI of 2.2 after surgery, and the majority of these patients had persistent obstructions despite therapy.[47] A study of 154 patients with small tonsils, who underwent DISE, revealed that the tongue base and adenoids were the most common sites of obstruction.[46] Children with obesity also have a much higher failure rate of 60%. Facial dysmorphisms, such as midface hypoplasia, retrognathia, and reduced palatal width, may also be contributing factors.

In general, it is reasonable to consider medical management with nasal steroids and leukotriene antagonist therapy because of their low side effect profile and efficacy in treatment of residual disease. The majority of patients with convincing symptoms of persistent SDB should be evaluated with a postoperative sleep study. Central apneas and hypoventilation should be ruled out as well with PSG. Patients who have persistent AHI elevation may be candidates considered for DISE to localize the area of obstruction. Likewise, patients should be evaluated for comorbidities, such as obesity, dental crowding, and palatal disposition. Although CPAP compliance remains challenging in adults and children, it may be indicated for persistently elevated AHI in the absence of obstructive pathology. Depending on the severity of residual disease, follow-up should be provided, and caregivers should be counseled on all available options.

ANALGESIA FOLLOWING ADENOTONSILLECTOMY

Analgesia after surgery has changed over recent years to encompass greater use of nonsteroidal antiinflammatory drugs (NSAIDS) over opioid medications in children. Opioids have been associated with respiratory suppression, and there is ample evidence to consider avoidance in children younger than 6 years. Various risk factors for opioid-associated complications have been identified, including age <1 year, obesity, OSA, underweight, history of prematurity, and developmental delay.[48] Rapid metabolization of codeine through the cytochrome P450 family 2 subfamily D type 6 (CYP2D6) has been studied, and this medication should generally be avoided in children and is not recommended by the FDA in 2012. Many institutions will avoid opioids altogether in children younger than 6 years and instead use a combination of acetaminophen and ibuprofen, with oral dexamethasone on postoperative days 1 and 2 as an option. Hydrocodone is a potential alternative to codeine due to its less variable analgesic effects but is similarly associated with respiratory depression and added risk in younger children. Future directions of research may help establish routine CYP2D6 genotyping for prescription oral opioids.

NSAID mechanism of action is through inhibition of cyclooxygenase activity and yields antiinflammatory and antipyretic effects. Ibuprofen has been the most studied and found to have the most suitable profile for analgesia. The primary concern for its use has been an increased risk of posttonsillectomy hemorrhage. A Cochrane Review of 15 studies that involved 1101 children found insufficient evidence to support that NSAIDs result in higher bleeding risk.[49] There is sufficient evidence to support the safety and efficacy of ibuprofen and acetaminophen following AD.

Additional pain reduction through modalities such as antibiotics and steroids has been evaluated. Postsurgical antibiotics have not been shown to reduce pain or the risk of posttonsillectomy hemorrhage.[50] A single dose of dexamethasone 0.5 mg/kg has been shown to be associated with faster diet advancement on postoperative day 1 and improve postoperative pain overall.[51]

METHOD OF TONSILLECTOMY

The introduction of intracapsular tonsillectomy (IT) provides an alternative surgical approach to one of the most common surgeries performed in any otolaryngology practice. This technique affords adequate reduction in tonsillar tissue while sparing underlying tonsil capsule and pharyngeal musculature. Subtotal tonsil removal results in an increased risk of lymphoid regrowth but a reduction in postsurgical pain and bleeding risk. There is sufficient evidence to support this alternative method for tonsillectomy, which is easily learned and safe to perform in any otolaryngology surgical setting.

First reported by Koltai and colleagues in 2003,[52] IT may be performed using a microdebrider or coblator to reduce tonsil tissue to a depth perceived to be. Suction monopolar cautery is often applied to remaining tonsil tissue using a separate instrument or a function built into the apparatus. Care is taken to avoid violation of the tonsil capsule and underlying musculature during cautery. The resulting eschar acts as a biologic dressing within the tonsillar fossae.

IT has been shown to have a lower risk of bleeding and postoperative pain, presumably due to less disruption of underlying tissue via selective tonsil parenchyma ablation.[53] A systematic review of RCTs comparing IT found an overall reduction in pain by 2–2.5 days when compared with total tonsillectomy methods.

A review of literature comparing microdebridement versus coblation found that microdebridement was the lowest-cost modality but took longer to perform.[54] The coblator system, which uses bipolar radio frequency energy to deliver heat at lower temperatures, can also be used as a cutting instrument to perform a total tonsillectomy. A study examining the pain following coblation via IT versus total tonsillectomy method found less pain when coblation was used only in an intracapsular technique.[55]

The IT is a safe and effective alternative to conventional total tonsillectomy. Caregivers should be advised of a risk of bleeding and lymphoid regrowth, although the need for revision AD is rare. Although there are several surgical instruments available for IT, the concept of intracapsular tonsil ablation remains the same. Further studies are needed to determine the efficacy of IT through tonsil crypt exteriorization for patients with chronic tonsillitis. A shared decision making model is ideal for deciding on total tonsillectomy vs intracapsular tonsillectomy in an individual patient.

CONCLUSIONS

Evidence-based medicine is particularly important in children with OSAS, as AD remains a common aspect of any otolaryngology practice. In a study examining gaps in evidence, Ishman and colleagues determined that up to 61% of decisions made in their clinical setting were not evidence based.[3] A review of the evidence reaffirms that clinical history alone is not reliable in distinguishing snoring from OSA, and DISE may be indicated in patients with small tonsils or those who have failed first-line therapies. There continues to be a role for medical management of mild OSAS or snoring, with nasal steroids and leukotriene receptor antagonists showing efficacy. Although more studies are needed to evaluate the differences in pain and bleed rate, intracapsular and total tonsillectomy are equivocal, and both are accepted methods for tonsil removal. NSAIDs and acetaminophen are efficacious in children younger than 6 years, and caution is advised in the use of opioids. Although there is evidence to support the negative consequences of SDB on the developing brain, more data are needed to determine if younger children benefit more than school-aged children. The approach to a child with OSAS affords the personalization of medical and surgical management, and applying an evidence-based medication remains important in everyday practice.

REFERENCES

1. Bluestone CD. *Pediatric Otolaryngology*. 4th ed. Philadelphia: Saunders; 2003.
2. Hall MJ, et al. Ambulatory surgery data from hospitals and ambulatory surgery centers: United States, 2010. *Natl Health Stat Rep*. 2017;(102):1–15.
3. Tang A, et al. Gaps in evidence: management of pediatric obstructive sleep apnea without tonsillar hypertrophy. *Laryngoscope*. 2016;126(3):758–762.
4. Meltzer LJ, et al. Prevalence of diagnosed sleep disorders in pediatric primary care practices. *Pediatrics*. 2010;125(6):e1410–e1418.
5. Johnson CR. Sleep problems in children with mental retardation and autism. *Child Adolesc Psychiatr Clin North Am*. 1996;5:673–681.
6. Lumeng JC, Chervin RD. Epidemiology of pediatric obstructive sleep apnea. *Proc Am Thorac Soc*. 2008;5(2):242–252.
7. Rosen CL, et al. Prevalence and risk factors for sleep-disordered breathing in 8- to 11-year-old children: association with race and prematurity. *J Pediatr*. 2003;142(4):383–389.
8. Owens JA, et al. Sleep habits and sleep disturbance in elementary school-aged children. *J Dev Behav Pediatr*. 2000;21(1):27–36.
9. Blader JC, et al. Sleep problems of elementary school children. A community survey. *Arch Pediatr Adolesc Med*. 1997;151(5):473–480.
10. Mindell JA, et al. Behavioral treatment of bedtime problems and night wakings in infants and young children. *Sleep*. 2006;29(10):1263–1276.
11. Roberts RE, Roberts CR, Duong HT. Chronic insomnia and its negative consequences for health and functioning of adolescents: a 12-month prospective study. *J Adolesc Health*. 2008;42(3):294–302.
12. Cielo CM, et al. Periodic limb movements and restless legs syndrome in children with a history of prematurity. *Sleep Med*. 2017;30:77–81.
13. Quante M, et al. The effect of adenotonsillectomy for childhood sleep apnea on cardiometabolic measures. *Sleep*. 2015;38(9):1395–1403.
14. Narang I, Mathew JL. Childhood obesity and obstructive sleep apnea. *J Nutr Metab*. 2012;2012:134202.
15. Amin RS, Carroll JL, Jeffries JL, et al. Twenty-four-hour ambulatory blood pressure in children with sleep disordered breathing. *Am J Respir Crit Care Med*. 2004;169(8):950–956.
16. Horne RS, Yang JS, Walter LM, et al. Elevated blood pressure during sleep and wake in children with sleep disordered breathing. *Pediatrics*. 2011;128(1):e85–e92.
17. Attia G, Ahmad MA, Saleh AB, Elsharkawy A. Impact of obstructive sleep apnea on global myocardial performance in children assessed by tissue doppler imaging. *Pediatr Cardiol*. 2010;31(7):1025–1036.
18. O'Brien LM, Holbrook CR, Mervis CB, et al. Sleep and neurobehavioral characteristics of 5- to 7-year-old children with parentally reported symptoms of attention-deficit/hyperactivity disorder. *Pediatrics*. 2003;111;(3):554–563.
19. Ali NJ, Pitson DJ, Stradling JR. Snoring, sleep disturbance and behaviour in 4–5 year olds. *Arch Dis Child*. 1993;68:360–366.
20. Row BW, Kheirandish L, Neville JJ, Gozal D. Impaired spatial learning and hyperactivity in developing rats exposed to intermittent hypoxia. *Pediatr Res*. 2002;52(3):449–453.
21. Bonuck K, et al. Sleep-disordered breathing in a population-based cohort: behavioral outcomes at 4 and 7 years. *Pediatrics*. 2012;129(4):e857–e865.
22. Marcus CL, Brooks LJ, Ward SD, et al. Diagnosis and management of childhood obstructive sleep apnea syndrome. *Pediatrics*. 2012;130(3).
23. Lau EY, Choi EW, Lai ES, et al. Working memory impairment and its associated sleep-related respiratory parameters in children with obstructive sleep apnea. *Sleep Med*. 2015;16(8):1109–1115.
24. Friedman BC, et al. Adenotonsillectomy improves neurocognitive function in children with obstructive sleep apnea syndrome. *Sleep*. 2003;26(8):999–1005.
25. Marcus CL, et al. A randomized trial of adenotonsillectomy for childhood sleep apnea. *N Engl J Med*. 2013;368(25):2366–2376.
26. Jackman AR, et al. Sleep-disordered breathing in preschool children is associated with behavioral, but not cognitive, impairments. *Sleep Med*. 2012;13(6):621–631.
27. Biggs SN, et al. Long-term cognitive and behavioral outcomes following resolution of sleep disordered breathing in preschool children. *PLoS One*. 2015;10(9):e0139142.
28. Carroll JL, et al. Inability of clinical history to distinguish primary snoring from obstructive sleep apnea syndrome in children. *Chest*. 1995;108(3):610–618.
29. Pavone M, et al. At-home pulse oximetry in children undergoing adenotonsillectomy for obstructive sleep apnea. *Eur J Pediatr*. 2017;176(4):493–499.

30. Pavone M, et al. Night-to-night consistency of at-home nocturnal pulse oximetry testing for obstructive sleep apnea in children. *Pediatr Pulmonol.* 2013;48(8):754–760.

31. Ogden CL, et al. Trends in obesity prevalence among children and adolescents in the United States, 1988-1994 through 2013-2014. *JAMA.* 2016;315(21):2292–2299.

32. Whitaker RC, et al. Predicting obesity in young adulthood from childhood and parental obesity. *N Engl J Med.* 1997;337(13):869–873.

33. Amin R, et al. Early improvement in obstructive sleep apnea and increase in orexin levels after bariatric surgery in adolescents and young adults. *Surg Obes Relat Dis.* 2017;13(1):95–100.

34. Kuhle S, Urschitz M. Anti-inflammatory drugs for the treatment of obstructive sleep apnea in children. *Cochrane Database Syst Rev.* 2011;(1).

35. Kaditis AG, et al. Sleep-disordered breathing in 3,680 Greek children. *Pediatr Pulmonol.* 2004;37(6):499–509.

36. Wang B, Liang J. The effect of montelukast on mild persistent OSA after adenotonsillectomy in children: a preliminary study. *Otolaryngol Head Neck Surg.* 2017;156(5):952–954.

37. Kheirandish-Gozal L, Bandla HP, Gozal D. Montelukast for children with obstructive sleep apnea: results of a double-blind, randomized, placebo-controlled trial. *Ann Am Thorac Soc.* 2016;13(10):1736–1741.

38. Goldbart AD, Greenberg-Dotan S, Tal A. Montelukast for children with obstructive sleep apnea: a double-blind, placebo-controlled study. *Pediatrics.* 2012;130(3):e575–e580.

39. Morgenthaler TI. Practice parameters for the medical therapy of obstructive sleep apnea. *Sleep.* 2006;29(8).

40. Ehsan Z, et al. The effects of anesthesia and opioids on the upper airway: a systematic review. *Laryngoscope.* 2016;126(1):270–284.

41. De Vito A, et al. Drug-induced sleep endoscopy: conventional versus target controlled infusion techniques–a randomized controlled study. *Eur Arch Otorhinolaryngol.* 2011;268(3):457–462.

42. Gillespie MB, et al. A trial of drug-induced sleep endoscopy in the surgical management of sleep-disordered breathing. *Laryngoscope.* 2013;123(1):277–282.

43. Vicini C, et al. The nose oropharynx hypopharynx and larynx (NOHL) classification: a new system of diagnostic standardized examination for OSAHS patients. *Eur Arch Otorhinolaryngol.* 2012;269(4):1297–1300.

44. Kezirian EJ, Hohenhorst W, de Vries N. Drug-induced sleep endoscopy: the VOTE classification. *Eur Arch Otorhinolaryngol.* 2011;268(8):1233–1236.

45. Chan DK, et al. A new scoring system for upper airway pediatric sleep endoscopy. *JAMA Otolaryngol Head Neck Surg.* 2014;140(7):595–602.

46. Miller C, et al. Clinically small tonsils are typically not obstructive in children during drug-induced sleep endoscopy. *Laryngoscope.* 2016;127.

47. Imanguli M, Ulualp SO. Risk factors for residual obstructive sleep apnea after adenotonsillectomy in children. *Laryngoscope.* 2016;126(11):2624–2629.

48. Chidambaran V, Sadhasivam S, Mahmoud M. Codeine and opioid metabolism: implications and alternatives for pediatric pain management. *Curr Opin Anaesthesiol.* 2017;30.

49. Lewis SR, et al. Nonsteroidal anti-inflammatory drugs and perioperative bleeding in paediatric tonsillectomy. *Cochrane Database Syst Rev.* 2013;(7):CD003591.

50. Dhiwakar M, et al. Antibiotics to reduce post-tonsillectomy morbidity. *Cochrane Database Syst Rev.* 2012;(12):CD005607.

51. Steward DL, Grisel J, Meinzen-Derr J. Steroids for improving recovery following tonsillectomy in children. *Cochrane Database Syst Rev.* 2011;(8):CD003997.

52. Koltai PJ. Capsule sparing in tonsil surgery: the value of intracapsular tonsillectomy. *Arch Otolaryngol Head Neck Surg.* 2003;129(12):1357.

53. Walton J, Ebner Y, Stewart MG, April MM. Systematic review of randomized controlled trials comparing intracapsular tonsillectomy with total tonsillectomy in a pediatric population. *Arch Otolaryngol Head Neck Surg.* 2012;138.

54. Windfuhr JP, et al. Tonsillotomy: facts and fiction. *Eur Arch Otorhinolaryngol.* 2015;272(4):949–969.

55. Duarte VM, Liu YF, Shapiro NL. Coblation total tonsillectomy and adenoidectomy versus coblation partial intracapsular tonsillectomy and adenoidectomy in children. *Laryngoscope.* 2014;124(8):1959–1964.

CHAPTER 9

Evidence-Based Practice: Pediatric Tonsillectomy

ALISON MARESH, MD • VIKASH K. MODI, MD, FAAP • MICHAEL G. STEWART, MD, MPH

OVERVIEW

Tonsillectomy is one of the most common surgical procedures performed in children in the United States, with more than 530,000 procedures performed annually.[1] Tonsillectomy is defined as a surgical procedure that removes the pharyngeal tonsils. Removal of the tonsil may be specified as complete, in which the tonsil is removed via a dissection through the peritonsillar space, or partial, in which tonsil tissue is removed within the capsule, leaving behind the capsule and varying amounts of tonsil tissue overlying the muscle bed.[2] Although tonsillectomy is common, there are associated risks including but not limited to anesthesia risks, postoperative respiratory risks, throat pain, dehydration, and postoperative bleeding. These risks should be taken into consideration when considering surgical intervention.[3] Some patient populations are at higher risk for complications as well as residual/recurrent pathology after surgery, and many studies have attempted to clarify how to best identify and manage these patients.

There exist a significant number of publications regarding patient assessment, indications for surgery, tonsillectomy technique, perioperative management, and outcomes assessment; however, the quality of studies is variable and there is still a lack of consensus regarding many of these topics. This article provides an evidence-based perspective on indications, technique, and perioperative decision making for tonsillectomy in children.

EVIDENCE-BASED CLINICAL ASSESSMENT
Indications for Tonsillectomy

Indications for tonsillectomy are multiple, the most common and generally accepted of which are sleep-disordered breathing (SDB) and recurrent throat infections. Although recurrent pharyngitis used to be the main indication for surgery,[4] there has been a gradual incidence shift toward SDB over the past several decades[5]; 85% of tonsillectomy or adenotonsillectomy procedures are currently performed for an indication of obstruction, with only 13% being performed for infection.[6]

SDB is the most common indication for tonsillectomy with or without adenoidectomy; SDB constitutes a range of disorders from snoring and restless sleep to obstructive sleep apnea (OSA).[7] There are multiple factors that contribute to SDB, and large tonsils and adenoids are the most common cause in healthy normal-weight children. A prospective randomized study by Marcus et al.[8] comparing adenotonsillectomy with watchful waiting demonstrated benefit to early surgical intervention with improved behavior, quality of life, and polysomnography (PSG) outcomes. This hallmark study showed that patients with mild OSA were more likely to show improvement without intervention within 7 months compared with subjects with more severe disease; however, patients with symptomatic mild OSA had significant improvement with adenotonsillectomy compared with observation based on symptoms and quality-of-life surveys suggesting that symptomatic patients with even mild disease benefit from intervention. An additional finding of this study was that residual disease was more likely in patients with severe OSA, obesity, and black ethnicity.

A meta-analysis in 2017 of tonsillectomy for patients with SDB demonstrated improved sleep, decreased apnea-hypopnea index (AHI) on PSG, improved quality of life, and improved behavior for patients undergoing surgery compared with watchful waiting[9] and the American Academy of Otolaryngology–Head and Neck Surgery (AAO-HNS) guidelines recommend tonsillectomy for children with tonsillar hypertrophy and SDB.[2] These guidelines were developed in 2011 with the goal of providing evidence-based guideline statements about performing tonsillectomy in children; Table 9.1 summarizes these recommendations, which are also discussed throughout this review.

TABLE 9.1
AAO-HNS Clinical Practice Guideline Statements

Statement 1	Clinicians should recommend watchful waiting for recurrent throat infection if there have been fewer than seven episodes in the past year or fewer than five episodes per year in the last 2 years or fewer than three episodes per year in the past 3 years.
Statement 2	Clinicians may recommend tonsillectomy for recurrent throat infection with a frequency of at least seven episodes in the past year, five episodes per year for 2 years, or three episodes per year for 3 years with documentation in the medical record for each episode of sore throat and one or more of the following: temperature >38.3°C, cervical adenopathy, tonsillar exudate, or positive test for GABHS.
Statement 3	Clinicians should assess the child with recurrent throat infection who does not met criteria in Statement 2 for modifying factors that may nonetheless favor tonsillectomy, which may include but are not limited to multiple antibiotic allergy/intolerance, PFAPA, or history of peritonsillar abscess.
Statement 4	Clinicians should ask caregivers of children with sleep-disordered breathing and tonsil hypertrophy about comorbid conditions that might improve after tonsillectomy, including growth retardation, poor school performance, enuresis, and behavioral problems.
Statement 5	Clinicians should counsel caregivers about tonsillectomy as a means to improve health in children with abnormal polysomnography who also have tonsil hypertrophy and sleep-disordered breathing.
Statement 6	Clinicians should counsel caregivers and explain that SDB may persist or recur after tonsillectomy and may require further management.
Statement 7	Clinicians should administer a single, intraoperative dose of intravenous dexamethasone to children undergoing tonsillectomy
Statement 8	Clinicians should not routinely administer or prescribe perioperative antibiotics to children undergoing tonsillectomy.
Statement 9	The clinician should advocate for pain management after tonsillectomy and educate caregivers about the importance of managing and reassessing pain.
Statement 10	Clinicians who perform tonsillectomy should determine their rate of primary and secondary posttonsillectomy hemorrhage at least annually.

PFAPA, periodic fever, aphthous stomatitis, pharyngitis, and adenitis; *SDB*, sleep-disordered breathing; *GABHS*, Group A beta-hemolytic Streptococcus.
From Baugh RF, Archer SM, Mitchell RB, et al. Clinical practice guideline: tonsillectomy in children. *Otolaryngol Head Neck Surg*. 2011;144(1 suppl):S1-S30, with permission.

Strength of evidence for specific interventions and outcomes is based on the type and quality of scientific studies used to assess them. Box 9.1 summarizes the grades of evidence quality, which are referenced throughout this review. Evidence supporting tonsillectomy for patients with OSA is grade A.

The other most common intervention for tonsillectomy is recurrent throat infections, as caused by viral or bacterial infections of the pharynx, palatine tonsils, or both. Infections are documented as episodes of sore throat with one or more of the following: temperature higher than 38.3 °C, cervical adenopathy, tonsillar exudates, or positive results from a group A B-hemolytic streptococcus test.[2] The benefit of tonsillectomy in patients with recurrent strep infections compared with observation remains controversial. The most commonly used criteria for intervention are based on a 1984 study by Paradise et al.,[10] which showed a reduction in

BOX 9.1
Quality of Evidence

A—Well-designed randomized controlled trials or diagnostic studies performed on a population similar to the guideline's target population

B—Randomized controlled trials of diagnostic studies with minor limitations; overwhelmingly consistent evidence from observational studies

C—Observational studies (case-control and cohort design)

D—Case reports, reasoning from first principles (bench research or animal studies)

X—Exceptional situations in which validating studies cannot be performed and there is a clear preponderance of benefit over harm frequency and severity of infections in severely affected children. In moderately affected children there was only a modest benefit, which was not believed to justify the risks, morbidity, and cost of surgery.[11,12] There is a high 91% rate of parental satisfaction after tonsillectomy for those with severe disease based on surveys 1 year after surgery.[13] A systematic review of tonsillectomy for recurrent sore throats by Barraclough et al. in 2014[14] confirms benefit based on sore-throat episodes for those with severe disease but not for those with milder disease. This review also demonstrated improved quality of life based on validated measures; several of these studies included patients with disease severity that did not meet criteria for severe disease,[15,16] which raises the possibility that previous work showing less benefit for patients with milder disease may have overlooked important outcome measures that affect quality of life, which may be relevant in surgical decision making. Another systematic review in 2017[17] similarly identified fewer sore throat episodes, fewer streptococcal infections, and fewer school absences in the 12 months following tonsillectomy compared with observation-only controls. The 2011 AAO-HNS guideline[2] recommends the option of surgical intervention for patients with seven infections in the prior year, five infections per year for the past 2 years, or three infections per year for the past three or more years, the "Paradise criteria" (grade B and C). It also recommends tonsillectomy for patients who do not meet criteria for severe disease based on the number of infections but who have qualifying factors that worsen disease morbidity, including peritonsillar abscess, antibiotic intolerance, or allergy, as the potential benefits outweigh potential risks in these groups of patients (grade C).

Specific clinical syndromes may affect clinical decision making for tonsillectomy. Periodic fever, aphthous stomatitis, pharyngitis, and adenitis (PFAPA) is a syndrome generally seen in younger children diagnosed with at least three documented episodes of recurring fevers at 3- to 6-week intervals associated with pharyngitis, tender cervical lymphadenopathy, and aphthous stomatitis. Tonsillectomy has been shown to be beneficial in randomized control trials[18,19] and can be considered in patients with PFAPA (grade B).

Pediatric autoimmune neuropsychiatric disorders associated with streptococcal infection (PANDAS) is another syndrome for which tonsillectomy is sometimes performed. Although some studies suggest benefit to surgical intervention,[20] a systematic review of the literature does not show tonsillectomy as any more beneficial than alternative medical therapies.[21] Studies are limited by small numbers; at this time the benefit of tonsillectomy for PANDAS remains unproven.

Other more rare indications for surgery include orthognathic concerns, tonsiliths, and halitosis, all for which substantial evidence is currently not available or of lesser quality.[12,22,23]

Patient Assessment

Careful history taking in children for whom tonsillectomy is being considered should include symptoms of:
- Throat infections including school absences, antibiotic tolerance, history of peritonsillar abscess
- Snoring
- Apneas
- Restless sleep
- Nocturnal enuresis
- Growth retardation
- Daytime somnolence
- Poor school performance
- Behavior problems
- Attention deficit hyperactivity disorder

Physical examination should focus on the anatomy, including size of the tonsils in relation to the position and size of the palate and oropharynx. The classic four-point grading scale[24] is commonly used but does not provide a three-dimensional assessment of tonsil size, which is more accurate in quantifying tonsillar hypertrophy. Tonsil size alone does not correlate with the severity of SDB; the combined volume of the tonsils and adenoids more accurately correlates with the severity of SDB.[25] Even patients with small tonsils and OSA improve after surgery, and sleep apnea is more likely resolved in those with large tonsils graded as 3+ or 4+.[26]

Outcomes after tonsillectomy are generally favorable for otherwise healthy, normal-weight children with SDB; however, persistent disease and postoperative complications are more prevalent in certain populations. These are discussed in greater depth later in this review; however, preoperative assessments should include assessing patients for these comorbidities, including obesity, trisomy 21, craniofacial abnormalities, neuromuscular disorders, sickle cell disease, mucopolysaccharidosis, failure to thrive, respiratory disease, and cardiac disease.[27-30] This allows for appropriate preoperative counseling and surgical planning.

Polysomnography

Although there are aspects of patient history and physical examination that are suggestive of SDB, relying on history and physical examination alone has been shown to be a poor predictor of the presence and severity of OSA.[31] PSG is the gold standard for diagnosing and quantifying OSA. Burdens of obtaining sleep studies include cost, emotional distress for pediatric patients and families, as well as practical and logistical barriers, as sleep laboratories are not easily available for many practitioners and wait times are typically long. A 2015 review[32] identified multiple feasibility studies that demonstrate the ability to perform home PSG using portable monitors (PMs) on patients 5 years and older; however, there are no studies that have validated the results of these PMs compared with formal PSG. The American Academy of Pediatrics (AAP) practice guidelines recommend overnight PSG in all patients with suspicion of SDB (grade A).[27] The AAO-HNS has attempted to define more specific populations in which PSG is most beneficial. The guidelines recommend that patients who are high risk for surgery and anesthesia should undergo PSG. This improves diagnostic accuracy and better defines the need for surgical intervention, as well as defines the severity of OSA to optimize perioperative planning and safety in these at-risk populations.[7] Based on current observational studies, patients with the following comorbidities are recommended to undergo PSG (grade C)[28–30]:

- Obesity
- Trisomy 21
- Craniofacial abnormalities
- Neuromuscular disorders
- Sickle cell disease
- Mucopolysaccharidoses

In addition, patients might benefit from PSG if the need for intervention is unclear based on history or physical examination or when there is discordance between the reported history and physical examination findings. As further described later, patients with severe OSA with AHI greater than 10 or nadir oxygen saturations below 80% are recommended for admission postoperatively for monitoring.

EVIDENCE-BASED SURGICAL TECHNIQUE FOR TONSILLECTOMY
Instrumentation
Traditionally tonsillectomy is performed with cold dissection with metal instruments such as knife, scissor, or snare. The tonsil is removed completely by dissecting under the capsule through the peritonsillar space. Hemostasis is obtained by ligation of vessels or cauterization. Cold steel techniques are the standards by which the effectiveness and safety of other techniques are measured.

New surgical approaches to tonsillectomy have been explored with goals of improving surgical time, ease and safety of technique, and perioperative morbidity. Electrosurgical dissection and coblation are the most common techniques currently used for total

tonsillectomy (TT).[33] Other techniques include radiofrequency, harmonic scalpel, bipolar cautery, and PEAK PlasmaBlade. A systematic review assessing randomized controlled trials that compared instrumentation for tonsillectomy[34–38] did not demonstrate differences in postoperative pain, and there is no consensus regarding the best instrumentation for this procedure (grade A).

Technique: Partial Intracapsular Tonsillectomy Versus Total Tonsillectomy
Partial intracapsular tonsillectomy (IT), also referred to as tonsillotomy, involves removal of most tonsil tissue, leaving a small amount of tonsil tissue in the tonsillar fossa.[39–41] The residual tissue prevents exposure of pharyngeal musculature, with the goal of decreasing postoperative hemorrhage as well as decreasing the severity and duration of postoperative pain. Several instruments have been used to perform IT, including the microdebrider, the Coblator, and cold steel. The effectiveness in terms of resolving SDB symptoms is equivalent to TT.[42–44] Postoperatively, several randomized controlled trials and two systematic reviews of these studies have shown less postoperative pain, shorter pain symptoms, less use of pain medication, earlier return to normal diet, and earlier return to normal activity.[43,45,46] In addition, there is decreased postoperative bleeding compared with TT techniques.[45,46] Evidence supporting the short-term effectiveness and decreased morbidity of IT is grade B.

The long-term effectiveness of IT given the risk for regrowth warrants further investigation. Studies have shown that the rates of revision surgery performed because of recurrent symptoms and regrowth range from 0.8% to 6% with variability in technique[47,48]; a large database study of 27,535 patients showed a reoperation rate of 0.2% for TT and 1.6% for IT.[49] The study with the longest follow-up was 6 years and demonstrated equal rates of SDB symptom recurrence after IT compared with TT; however, this was based on telephone questionnaires without objective assessment.[50] Also unknown is the benefit of the IT technique for recurrent throat infections. Although limited evidence suggests equal improvements in episodes of pharyngitis after IT and TT,[51] a systematic review of randomized controlled trials comparing these techniques demonstrated increased sore throat episodes in patients undergoing IT.[43]

EVIDENCE-BASED PERIOPERATIVE MANAGEMENT FOR TONSILLECTOMY
Dexamethasone
Current guidelines recommend the administration of a single dose of intravenous dexamethasone at the

time of tonsillectomy.[2] Studies demonstrate benefit in decreasing postoperative nausea and vomiting.[52,53] In addition, there are improvements in pain and oral intake (grade A).[54] Although there is some concern for an increased risk of bleeding caused by steroids, studies including a recent randomized, prospective, double-blind, placebo-controlled study have demonstrated no increased risk.[55]

Perioperative Antibiotics

Although it is common practice to prescribe perioperative antibiotics, such practice is not supported by the literature. There is no benefit in pain management, diet, and activity based on multiple systemic reviews and meta-analyses.[56-58] Based on known risks of antibiotic administration, including cost, rash, allergy, gastrointestinal upset, promotion of resistance, and additional burden of administration, current AAO-HNS guidelines recommend strongly against the routine use of antibiotics (grade A).[2]

Postoperative Hospitalization

Several studies have established the safety of performing pediatric tonsillectomy in an outpatient setting.[59-61] However, several populations of patients have been identified to be at higher risk for postoperative respiratory complications, and for these patients monitoring as inpatients after surgery is recommended. The AAP guideline on pediatric OSA syndrome identified the following patients as at risk (grade B)[27]:

- Age less than 3 years
- Severe OSA
- Cardiac disease
- Failure to thrive
- Obesity
- Craniofacial anomalies
- Neuromuscular disorders
- Respiratory disease

Although subsequent research has supported these guidelines,[62-66] the actual admission practices among practitioners are quite variable.[67] Even though surgery improves or resolves sleep apnea in the long term, in the immediate postoperative period patients with OSA may continue to experience upper airway obstruction and oxygen desaturations until the pharyngeal neuromotor response recovers.[68,69] Although studies agree that there is a correlation between increased severity of OSA and increased postoperative risk (grade C), there is some controversy as to what specific PSG findings should constitute criteria for admission; current AAO-HNS guidelines recommend admission for patients with AHI greater than 10 and/or oxygen saturation

nadir less than 80%.[2] In addition, although postoperative risk has been identified for patients younger than 3 years undergoing TT, a study by Bent et al. in 2004[70] of patients undergoing partial tonsillectomy did not identify complications in groups younger than 3 years compared with patients older than 3 years, suggesting that, when this technique is used, this patient group may be safely monitored on an outpatient basis (grade C).

Pain Control

Pain after TT lasts 7–14 days[71,72] and can cause morbidity, including decreased oral intake, dysphagia, dehydration, and weight loss. Postoperative pain is responsible for a 3.5%–6.2% rate of Emergency Department visits and hospital readmissions in postoperative tonsillectomy patients.[72-74] Although there is a large body of literature assessing pain management regimens after tonsillectomy, there is no consensus regarding the best regimen (grade B).[2]

Codeine used to be the mainstay of therapy for pain after pediatric tonsillectomy because of wide availability and ease of prescribing; previously codeine was thought to have a reassuring safety profile. However, independent investigations by the Patient Safety and Quality Improvement Committee of the AAO-HNS and the US Food and Drug Administration (FDA) in 2011–12 identified 10 deaths and 3 life-threatening events in children given appropriate codeine doses; the majority were in patients after adenotonsillectomy. Codeine is metabolized in the liver to its active metabolite, morphine, by a P450 isoenzyme CYP2D6. Over 100 genetic variations are known to exist for this enzyme, causing a range of activities within the population from poor metabolizers who get little to no benefit from codeine to extensive and ultrafast metabolizers who produce significantly more morphine and are at risk for adverse reactions.[75,76] Because of these findings, codeine received a safety warning from the FDA, contraindicating its use in pediatric patients undergoing adenotonsillectomy.[77,78] Codeine is therefore no longer an appropriate medication choice for pain control for these patients.

Other narcotic medications also have risks in unmonitored pediatric patients, especially in the specific populations that undergo surgery for SDB. Children with severe OSA, patients who are overweight, and patients who are younger than 3 years are already at high risk for respiratory complications following surgery.[79] Opioid medications decrease the ventilatory response to hypercarbia and hypoxemia, blunt arousal responses during obstruction, and depress upper airway musculature, adding additional risk of respiratory complications to these already high-risk patients.[80,81] Patients with OSA have an increased sensitivity to opioids and decreased opioid requirements by up to 50%; based on animal models, this is thought to be caused by an altered balance between the μ-opioid and neurokinin-1 system due to hypoxemia.[82,83]

All narcotic medications, including morphine, have variability in bioavailability, enzyme conversions to metabolites, and transport to the central nervous system.[80] There are very narrow therapeutic indexes in small children. There are additional dosing challenges in obese children, because these drugs should be dosed on ideal body weight, and children with OSA have an increased sensitivity to narcotics. Finally, there are very limited high-quality studies regarding dosing protocols in pediatric patients. For these reasons caution is recommended for outpatient narcotic use in children after tonsillectomy.

Ibuprofen is a nonsteroidal antiinflammatory medication with the greatest evidence and experience to support safe use in children. The combination use of ibuprofen and acetaminophen is more effective for analgesia than the individual drugs alone. There is concern for postoperative bleeding given the antiplatelet activity of this class of medication; however, a systematic review and meta-analysis from 2013 based on 36 randomized control trials concluded there is no significant risk for bleeding when given after tonsillectomy (grade A).[84] It is also an effective analgesic in this population. A randomized trial of morphine compared with ibuprofen demonstrated equivalent pain control with no increased risk of bleeding in the ibuprofen group; it also demonstrated increased desaturations in the morphine group.[85]

An important component to pain management includes family counseling to ensure compliant caregivers.[86] Local anesthesia injections have not been proved beneficial based on a Cochrane review (grade B).[87] Maintaining hydration helps with pain control (grade C).[88] Intraoperative dexamethasone as discussed earlier also helps with postoperative pain (grade A).[54] Although some practitioners routinely prescribe a course of prednisone postoperatively as well, a randomized, placebo-controlled, double-blind trial did not demonstrate any improvements in pain, nausea/vomiting, diet, activity, or sleep in these patients.[89]

Outcomes Assessment

A critical component for practitioners who perform tonsillectomy is assessing outcomes. Main points of consideration include quantifying the rates of postoperative hemorrhage and assessing for symptom resolution.

Primary hemorrhage is defined as bleeding within the first 24 h, and secondary hemorrhage is defined as bleeding after this time, usually seen 5–10 days after surgery as a result of sloughing of eschar. Bleeding in some cases can be associated with high-volume blood loss; occasionally, transfusions or reoperation for control of bleeding may be required. Primary bleeding occurs in 0.2%–2.2% of postoperative tonsillectomy patients,[2] and secondary hemorrhage occurs in 0.1%–3%.[90] Clinicians who perform tonsillectomy are recommended to always inquire about bleeding after surgery and determine their rate of primary and secondary hemorrhage at least annually (grade C).[2]

Increasing age has been found to be a risk factor for an increased rate of bleeding.[91–93] As previously discussed, steroid and ibuprofen have not been found to be associated with an increased risk of postoperative bleeding.

Many studies have attempted to determine whether surgical instrumentation can affect postoperative bleeding. Comparisons of "hot" (electrosurgery or electrocautery techniques) and cold tonsillectomy have demonstrated similar outcomes.[34–38] Systematic reviews summarizing randomized controlled trials on cold steel tonsillectomy, diathermy, monopolar cautery, coblation, or harmonic scalpel techniques have also shown no difference in postoperative hemorrhage rates (grade A). However, as previously reviewed, significant differences seem to exist in postoperative hemorrhage rates when comparing the technique of TT with partial IT.

In patients with SDB it is important to assess for resolution of symptoms. In normal-weight healthy children, 70%–80% will have symptom resolution after tonsillectomy.[94] Several populations have been defined to have a higher risk for persistent disease. In obese patients, defined as those with a body mass index greater than the 95th percentile, symptoms completely resolve in only 10%–20% of posttonsillectomy patients, with 51% having persistent moderate or severe OSA.[95] With increasing severity of obesity there is decreasing effectiveness of tonsillectomy.[94,96] There is also an increased risk of incomplete resolution in patients with severe OSA[97] and patients with trisomy 21.[98,99] Other at-risk populations likely include patients with craniofacial or neurologic disorders; however, there are no high-quality studies that have assessed this. Lack of snoring after tonsillectomy is predictive of resolution of OSA.[94] For patients who have persistent symptoms or patients who are at risk for persistent disease follow-up PSG is recommended based on the 2012 AAP guidelines (grade B).[27] Better definition of at-risk patients will help define patients for whom postoperative PSG is beneficial.

Recent evidence shows that patients who undergo tonsillectomy are at risk for postoperative weight gain. A

> **BOX 9.2**
> **Key Points—Pediatric Tonsillectomy**
>
> - Outcome measures in sleep-disordered breathing and recurrent throat infections should focus both on recurrence of disease and also on quality of life and school performance as indicators of well-being
> - Preoperative PSG is recommended for patients who have comorbidities that put them at increased risk for surgery
> - Reported success rates of tonsillectomy in curing sleep-disordered breathing in normal-weight children are 70%–80%; in obese children success rates are 10%–20%
> - Weight gain after tonsillectomy poses risks for recurrence of sleep-disordered breathing symptoms and warrants counseling
> - Based on FDA recommendations codeine is contraindicated for pain management in pediatric patients after tonsillectomy. Other narcotic medications are controversial. No consensus exists on the best regimen for postoperative pain management.
> - Intracapsular tonsillectomy represents an alternative surgical strategy that has immediate postoperative benefits regarding pain and bleeding risks compared to total tonsillectomy; further studies are warranted regarding long-term outcomes.

FDA, US Food and Drug Administration; *PSG*, polysomnography.

prospective randomized trial comparing adenotonsillectomy with watchful waiting in patients with OSA showed there was significant weight gain in the surgery group compared with the observation group over a 7-month follow-up.[100] A 2016 systematic review also concluded that adenotonsillectomy patients were at risk for increased weight gain.[101] As just discussed, obese patients are at a higher risk for SDB after tonsillectomy and there are additional health concerns in overweight children; the risk of weight gain should be discussed with patients and families before surgery, especially for those patients who are already overweight (grade B).

CONCLUSIONS

This review attempts to address the current state of knowledge regarding pediatric tonsillectomy. There is a large amount of literature describing indications, techniques/instrumentation, perioperative management, and outcomes of tonsillectomy. Several high-quality studies have significantly advanced our knowledge in these areas; however, gaps in knowledge do exist; Box 9.2 summarizes these key points as described in this review.

Continued efforts to produce high-quality studies will allow for better clinical management of tonsillectomy patients. Specific goals include:

- Updated data regarding the effectiveness of tonsillectomy for recurrent throat infections, including both disease recurrence outcomes and quality of life/school performance outcomes
- Evaluation of long-term SDB outcomes after IT
- Effectiveness of IT in treating recurrent throat infections
- Better understanding of safety profiles for narcotic use in pediatric patients
- What is the ideal posttonsillectomy pain regimen for IT and TT?
- Clarification of benefit of preoperative PSG in patients with SDB, especially in patients without comorbidities
- Necessity of postoperative PSG in specific patient populations
- Validation of accuracy of PMs in pediatric patients
- Indications and effectiveness of tonsillectomy in patients with obesity and other comorbidities

REFERENCES

1. Cullen KA, Hall MJ, Golosinskiy A. Ambulatory surgery in the United States. *Natl Health Stat Rep.* 2006;2009(11): 1–25.
2. Baugh RF, Archer SM, Mitchell RB, et al. Clinical practice guideline: tonsillectomy in children. *Otolaryngol Head Neck Surg.* 2011;144(1 suppl):S1–S30.
3. Johnson LB, Elluru RG, Myer CM. Complications of adenotonsillectomy. *Laryngoscope.* 2002;112(8 Pt 2 suppl 100):35–36.
4. Gates GA, Folbre TW. Indications for adenotonsillectomy. *Arch Otolaryngol Head Neck Surg.* 1986;112(5): 501–502.
5. Erickson BK, Larson DR, St Sauver JL, Meverden RA, Orvidas LJ. Changes in incidence and indications of tonsillectomy and adenotonsillectomy, 1970-2005. *Otolaryngol Head Neck Surg.* 2009;140(6):894–901.
6. Parker NP, Walner DL. Trends in the indications for pediatric tonsillectomy or adenotonsillectomy. *Int J Pediatr Otorhinolaryngol.* 2011;75(2):282–285.
7. Roland PS, Rosenfeld RM, Brooks LJ, et al. Clinical practice guideline: polysomnography for sleep-disordered breathing prior to tonsillectomy in children. *Otolaryngol Head Neck Surg.* 2011;145(1 suppl):S1–S15.
8. Marcus CL, Moore RH, Rosen CL, et al. A randomized trial of adenotonsillectomy for childhood sleep apnea. *N Engl J Med.* 2013;368(25):2366–2376.
9. Chinnadurai S, Jordan AK, Sathe NA, Fonnesbeck C, McPheeters ML, Francis DO. Tonsillectomy for obstructive sleep-disordered breathing: a meta-analysis. *Pediatrics.* 2017;139(2).

10. Paradise JL, Bluestone CD, Bachman RZ, et al. Efficacy of tonsillectomy for recurrent throat infection in severely affected children. Results of parallel randomized and nonrandomized clinical trials. *N Engl J Med.* 1984;310(11):674–683.

11. Paradise JL, Bluestone CD, Colborn DK, Bernard BS, Rockette HE, Kurs-Lasky M. Tonsillectomy and adenotonsillectomy for recurrent throat infection in moderately affected children. *Pediatrics.* 2002;110(1 Pt 1):7–15.

12. Burton MJ, Glasziou PP. Tonsillectomy or adeno-tonsillectomy versus non-surgical treatment for chronic/recurrent acute tonsillitis. *Cochrane Database Syst Rev.* 2009;(1):CD001802.

13. Wolfensberger M, Haury JA, Linder T. Parent satisfaction 1 year after adenotonsillectomy of their children. *Int J Pediatr Otorhinolaryngol.* 2000;56(3):199–205.

14. Barraclough J, Anari S. Tonsillectomy for recurrent sore throats in children: indications, outcomes, and efficacy. *Otolaryngol Head Neck Surg.* 2014;150(5):722–729.

15. Goldstein NA, Stewart MG, Witsell DL, et al. Quality of life after tonsillectomy in children with recurrent tonsillitis. *Otolaryngol Head Neck Surg.* 2008;138(1 suppl):S9–S16.

16. Schwentner I, Schmutzhard J, Schwentner C, Abraham I, Höfer S, Sprinzl GM. The impact of adenotonsillectomy on children's quality of life. *Clin Otolaryngol.* 2008;33(1):56–59.

17. Morad A, Sathe NA, Francis DO, McPheeters ML, Chinnadurai S. Tonsillectomy versus watchful waiting for recurrent throat infection: a systematic review. *Pediatrics.* 2017;139(2).

18. Renko M, Salo E, Putto-Laurila A, et al. A randomized, controlled trial of tonsillectomy in periodic fever, aphthous stomatitis, pharyngitis, and adenitis syndrome. *J Pediatr.* 2007;151(3):289–292.

19. Garavello W, Romagnoli M, Gaini RM. Effectiveness of adenotonsillectomy in PFAPA syndrome: a randomized study. *J Pediatr.* 2009;155(2):250–253.

20. Demesh D, Virbalas JM, Bent JP. The role of tonsillectomy in the treatment of pediatric autoimmune neuropsychiatric disorders associated with streptococcal infections (PANDAS). *JAMA Otolaryngol Head Neck Surg.* 2015;141(3):272–275.

21. Farhood Z, Ong AA, Discolo CM. PANDAS: a systematic review of treatment options. *Int J Pediatr Otorhinolaryngol.* 2016;89:149–153.

22. Morawska A, Łyszczarz J, Składzień J. An analysis of indications orthodontic for surgical treatment of Waldeyer ring hyperplasia in pediatric patients of the Otolaryngology and Stomatology department of the University Hospital of Krakow. *Otolaryngol Pol.* 2008;62(3):272–277.

23. Tanyeri HM, Polat S. Temperature-controlled radiofrequency tonsil ablation for the treatment of halitosis. *Eur Arch Otorhinolaryngol.* 2011;268(2):267–272.

24. Brodsky L. Modern assessment of tonsils and adenoids. *Pediatr Clin North Am.* 1989;36(6):1551–1569.

25. Arens R, McDonough JM, Corbin AM, et al. Upper airway size analysis by magnetic resonance imaging of children with obstructive sleep apnea syndrome. *Am J Respir Crit Care Med.* 2003;167(1):65–70.

26. Tang A, Benke JR, Cohen AP, Ishman SL. Influence of tonsillar size on OSA improvement in children undergoing adenotonsillectomy. *Otolaryngol Head Neck Surg.* 2015;153(2):281–285.

27. Marcus CL, Brooks LJ, Draper KA, et al. Diagnosis and management of childhood obstructive sleep apnea syndrome. *Pediatrics.* 2012;130(3):576–584.

28. Messner AH. Evaluation of obstructive sleep apnea by polysomnography prior to pediatric adenotonsillectomy. *Arch Otolaryngol Head Neck Surg.* 1999;125(3):353–356.

29. Mitchell RB, Kelly J. Outcome of adenotonsillectomy for severe obstructive sleep apnea in children. *Int J Pediatr Otorhinolaryngol.* 2004;68(11):1375–1379.

30. Rhodes SK, Shimoda KC, Waid LR, et al. Neurocognitive deficits in morbidly obese children with obstructive sleep apnea. *J Pediatr.* 1995;127(5):741–744.

31. Brietzke SE, Katz ES, Roberson DW. Can history and physical examination reliably diagnose pediatric obstructive sleep apnea/hypopnea syndrome? A systematic review of the literature. *Otolaryngol Head Neck Surg.* 2004;131(6):827–832.

32. Tan HL, Kheirandish-Gozal L, Gozal D. Pediatric home sleep apnea testing: slowly getting there!. *Chest.* 2015;148(6):1382–1395.

33. Setabutr D, Adil EA, Adil TK, Carr MM. Emerging trends in tonsillectomy. *Otolaryngol Head Neck Surg.* 2011;145(2):223–229.

34. Alexiou VG, Salazar-Salvia MS, Jervis PN, Falagas ME. Modern technology-assisted vs conventional tonsillectomy: a meta-analysis of randomized controlled trials. *Arch Otolaryngol Head Neck Surg.* 2011;137(6):558–570.

35. Parsons SP, Cordes SR, Comer B. Comparison of posttonsillectomy pain using the ultrasonic scalpel, coblator, and electrocautery. *Otolaryngol Head Neck Surg.* 2006;134(1):106–113.

36. Stoker KE, Don DM, Kang DR, Haupert MS, Magit A, Madgy DN. Pediatric total tonsillectomy using coblation compared to conventional electrosurgery: a prospective, controlled single-blind study. *Otolaryngol Head Neck Surg.* 2004;130(6):666–675.

37. Bäck L, Paloheimo M, Ylikoski J. Traditional tonsillectomy compared with bipolar radiofrequency thermal ablation tonsillectomy in adults: a pilot study. *Arch Otolaryngol Head Neck Surg.* 2001;127(9):1106–1112.

38. Philpott CM, Wild DC, Mehta D, Daniel M, Banerjee AR. A double-blinded randomized controlled trial of coblation versus conventional dissection tonsillectomy on post-operative symptoms. *Clin Otolaryngol.* 2005;30(2):143–148.

39. Wilson YL, Merer DM, Moscatello AL. Comparison of three common tonsillectomy techniques: a prospective randomized, double-blinded clinical study. *Laryngoscope.* 2009;119(1):162–170.

40. Ericsson E, Graf J, Hultcrantz E. Pediatric tonsillotomy with radiofrequency technique: long-term follow-up. *Laryngoscope.* 2006;116(10):1851–1857.

41. Bitar MA, Rameh C. Microdebrider-assisted partial tonsillectomy: short- and long-term outcomes. *Eur Arch Otorhinolaryngol.* 2008;265(4):459–463.

42. Chang DT, Zemek A, Koltai PJ. Comparison of treatment outcomes between intracapsular and total tonsillectomy for pediatric obstructive sleep apnea. *Int J Pediatr Otorhinolaryngol.* 2016;91:15–18.

43. Sathe N, Chinnadurai S, McPheeters M, Francis DO. Comparative effectiveness of partial versus total tonsillectomy in children. *Otolaryngol Head Neck Surg.* 2017;156(3):456–463.

44. Mukhatiyar P, Nandalike K, Cohen HW, et al. Intracapsular and extracapsular tonsillectomy and adenoidectomy in pediatric obstructive sleep apnea. *JAMA Otolaryngol Head Neck Surg.* 2016;142(1):25–31.

45. Walton J, Ebner Y, Stewart MG, April MM. Systematic review of randomized controlled trials comparing intracapsular tonsillectomy with total tonsillectomy in a pediatric population. *Arch Otolaryngol Head Neck Surg.* 2012;138(3):243–249.

46. Kordeluk S, Goldbart A, Novack L, et al. Randomized study comparing inflammatory response after tonsillectomy versus tonsillotomy. *Eur Arch Otorhinolaryngol.* 2016;273(11):3993–4001.

47. Zhang Q, Li D, Wang H. Long term outcome of tonsillar regrowth after partial tonsillectomy in children with obstructive sleep apnea. *Auris Nasus Larynx.* 2014;41(3):299–302.

48. Doshi HK, Rosow DE, Ward RF, April MM. Age-related tonsillar regrowth in children undergoing powered intracapsular tonsillectomy. *Int J Pediatr Otorhinolaryngol.* 2011;75(11):1395–1398.

49. Odhagen E, Sunnergren O, Hemlin C, Hessén Söderman AC, Ericsson E, Stalfors J. Risk of reoperation after tonsillotomy versus tonsillectomy: a population-based cohort study. *Eur Arch Otorhinolaryngol.* 2016;273(10):3263–3268.

50. Wireklint S, Ericsson E. Health-related quality of life after tonsillotomy versus tonsillectomy in young adults: 6 years postsurgery follow-up. *Eur Arch Otorhinolaryngol.* 2012;269(8):1951–1958.

51. Schmidt R, Herzog A, Cook S, O'Reilly R, Deutsch E, Reilly J. Powered intracapsular tonsillectomy in the management of recurrent tonsillitis. *Otolaryngol Head Neck Surg.* 2007;137(2):338–340.

52. Czarnetzki C, Elia N, Lysakowski C, et al. Dexamethasone and risk of nausea and vomiting and postoperative bleeding after tonsillectomy in children: a randomized trial. *JAMA.* 2008;300(22):2621–2630.

53. Steward DL, Welge JA, Myer CM. Steroids for improving recovery following tonsillectomy in children. *Cochrane Database Syst Rev.* 2003;(1):CD003997.

54. Afman CE, Welge JA, Steward DL. Steroids for posttonsillectomy pain reduction: meta-analysis of randomized controlled trials. *Otolaryngol Head Neck Surg.* 2006;134(2):181–186.

55. Gallagher TQ, Hill C, Ojha S, et al. Perioperative dexamethasone administration and risk of bleeding following tonsillectomy in children: a randomized controlled trial. *JAMA.* 2012;308(12):1221–1226.

56. Dhiwakar M, Clement WA, Supriya M, McKerrow W. Antibiotics to reduce post-tonsillectomy morbidity. *Cochrane Database Syst Rev.* 2010;(7):CD005607.

57. Burkart CM, Steward DL. Antibiotics for reduction of posttonsillectomy morbidity: a meta-analysis. *Laryngoscope.* 2005;115(6):997–1002.

58. Dhiwakar M, Eng CY, Selvaraj S, McKerrow WS. Antibiotics to improve recovery following tonsillectomy: a systematic review. *Otolaryngol Head Neck Surg.* 2006;134(3):357–364.

59. Chan KH, Friedman NR, Allen GC, et al. Randomized, controlled, multisite study of intracapsular tonsillectomy using low-temperature plasma excision. *Arch Otolaryngol Head Neck Surg.* 2004;130(11):1303–1307.

60. Haberman RS, Shattuck TG, Dion NM. Is outpatient suction cautery tonsillectomy safe in a community hospital setting? *Laryngoscope.* 1990;100(5):511–515.

61. Helmus C, Grin M, Westfall R. Same-day-stay adenotonsillectomy. *Laryngoscope.* 1990;100(6):593–596.

62. Kieran S, Gorman C, Kirby A, et al. Risk factors for desaturation after tonsillectomy: analysis of 4092 consecutive pediatric cases. *Laryngoscope.* 2013;123(10):2554–2559.

63. Thongyam A, Marcus CL, Lockman JL, et al. Predictors of perioperative complications in higher risk children after adenotonsillectomy for obstructive sleep apnea: a prospective study. *Otolaryngol Head Neck Surg.* 2014;151(6):1046–1054.

64. Keamy DG, Chhabra KR, Hartnick CJ. Predictors of complications following adenotonsillectomy in children with severe obstructive sleep apnea. *Int J Pediatr Otorhinolaryngol.* 2015;79(11):1838–1841.

65. Kang KT, Chang IS, Tseng CC, et al. Impacts of disease severity on postoperative complications in children with sleep-disordered breathing. *Laryngoscope.* 2017.

66. Kasle D, Virbalas J, Bent JP, Cheng J. Tonsillectomies and respiratory complications in children: a look at pre-op polysomnography risk factors and post-op admissions. *Int J Pediatr Otorhinolaryngol.* 2016;88:224–227.

67. Goyal SS, Shah R, Roberson DW, Schwartz ML. Variation in post-adenotonsillectomy admission practices in 24 pediatric hospitals. *Laryngoscope.* 2013;123(10):2560–2566.

68. Nixon GM, Kermack AS, Davis GM, Manoukian JJ, Brown KA, Brouillette RT. Planning adenotonsillectomy in children with obstructive sleep apnea: the role of overnight oximetry. *Pediatrics.* 2004;113(1 Pt 1):e19–e25.

69. Marcus CL, Katz ES, Lutz J, Black CA, Galster P, Carson KA. Upper airway dynamic responses in children with the obstructive sleep apnea syndrome. *Pediatr Res.* 2005;57(1):99–107.

70. Bent JP, April MM, Ward RF, Sorin A, Reilly B, Weiss G. Ambulatory powered intracapsular tonsillectomy and adenoidectomy in children younger than 3 years. *Arch Otolaryngol Head Neck Surg.* 2004;130(10):1197–1200.

71. Stewart DW, Ragg PG, Sheppard S, Chalkiadis GA. The severity and duration of postoperative pain and analgesia requirements in children after tonsillectomy, orchidopexy, or inguinal hernia repair. *Paediatr Anaesth.* 2012;22(2):136–143.

72. Stanko D, Bergesio R, Davies K, Hegarty M, von Ungern-Sternberg BS. Postoperative pain, nausea and vomiting following adeno-tonsillectomy – a long-term follow-up. *Paediatr Anaesth.* 2013;23(8):690–696.

73. Sutters KA, Miaskowski C. Inadequate pain management and associated morbidity in children at home after tonsillectomy. *J Pediatr Nurs.* 1997;12(3):178–185.

74. Duval M, Wilkes J, Korgenski K, Srivastava R, Meier J. Causes, costs, and risk factors for unplanned return visits after adenotonsillectomy in children. *Int J Pediatr Otorhinolaryngol.* 2015;79(10):1640–1646.

75. Daly AK, Brockmöller J, Broly F, et al. Nomenclature for human CYP2D6 alleles. *Pharmacogenetics.* 1996;6(3):193–201.

76. Marez D, Legrand M, Sabbagh N, et al. Polymorphism of the cytochrome P450 CYP2D6 gene in a European population: characterization of 48 mutations and 53 alleles, their frequencies and evolution. *Pharmacogenetics.* 1997;7(3):193–202.

77. Racoosin JA, Roberson DW, Pacanowski MA, Nielsen DR. New evidence about an old drug – risk with codeine after adenotonsillectomy. *N Engl J Med.* 2013;368(23):2155–2157.

78. Kuehn BM. FDA: no codeine after tonsillectomy for children. *JAMA.* 2013;309(11):1100.

79. Lee PC, Hwang B, Soong WJ, Meng CC. The specific characteristics in children with obstructive sleep apnea and cor pulmonale. *Sci World J.* 2012;2012:757283.

80. Lauder G, Emmott A. Confronting the challenges of effective pain management in children following tonsillectomy. *Int J Pediatr Otorhinolaryngol.* 2014;78(11):1813–1827.

81. Strauss SG, Lynn AM, Bratton SL, Nespeca MK. Ventilatory response to CO_2 in children with obstructive sleep apnea from adenotonsillar hypertrophy. *Anesth Analg.* 1999;89(2):328–332.

82. Brown KA, Laferrière A, Lakheeram I, Moss IR. Recurrent hypoxemia in children is associated with increased analgesic sensitivity to opiates. *Anesthesiology.* 2006;105(4):665–669.

83. Brown KA, Laferrière A, Moss IR. Recurrent hypoxemia in young children with obstructive sleep apnea is associated with reduced opioid requirement for analgesia. *Anesthesiology.* 2004;100(4):806–810. Discussion 805A.

84. Riggin L, Ramakrishna J, Sommer DD, Koren GA. 2013 updated systematic review & meta-analysis of 36 randomized controlled trials; no apparent effects of non steroidal anti-inflammatory agents on the risk of bleeding after tonsillectomy. *Clin Otolaryngol.* 2013;38(2):115–129.

85. Kelly LE, Sommer DD, Ramakrishna J, et al. Morphine or ibuprofen for post-tonsillectomy analgesia: a randomized trial. *Pediatrics.* 2015;135(2):307–313.

86. Fortier MA, MacLaren JE, Martin SR, Perret-Karimi D, Kain ZN. Pediatric pain after ambulatory surgery: where's the medication? *Pediatrics.* 2009;124(4):e588–e595.

87. Hollis LJ, Burton MJ, Millar JM. Perioperative local anaesthesia for reducing pain following tonsillectomy. *Cochrane Database Syst Rev.* 2000;(2):CD001874.

88. Tabaee A, Lin JW, Dupiton V, Jones JE. The role of oral fluid intake following adeno-tonsillectomy. *Int J Pediatr Otorhinolaryngol.* 2006;70(7):1159–1164.

89. Macassey E, Dawes P, Taylor B, Gray A. The effect of a postoperative course of oral prednisone on postoperative morbidity following childhood tonsillectomy. *Otolaryngol Head Neck Surg.* 2012;147(3):551–556.

90. Windfuhr JP, Chen YS, Remmert S. Hemorrhage following tonsillectomy and adenoidectomy in 15,218 patients. *Otolaryngol Head Neck Surg.* 2005;132(2):281–286.

91. Spektor Z, Saint-Victor S, Kay DJ, Mandell DL. Risk factors for pediatric post-tonsillectomy hemorrhage. *Int J Pediatr Otorhinolaryngol.* 2016;84:151–155.

92. Kshirsagar R, Mahboubi H, Moriyama D, Ajose-Popoola O, Pham NS, Ahuja GS. Increased immediate postoperative hemorrhage in older and obese children after outpatient tonsillectomy. *Int J Pediatr Otorhinolaryngol.* 2016;84:119–123.

93. Pfaff JA, Hsu K, Chennupati SK. The use of ibuprofen in posttonsillectomy analgesia and its effect on posttonsillectomy hemorrhage rate. *Otolaryngol Head Neck Surg.* 2016;155(3):508–513.

94. Mitchell RB. Adenotonsillectomy for obstructive sleep apnea in children: outcome evaluated by pre- and postoperative polysomnography. *Laryngoscope.* 2007;117(10):1844–1854.

95. Costa DJ, Mitchell R. Adenotonsillectomy for obstructive sleep apnea in obese children: a meta-analysis. *Otolaryngol Head Neck Surg.* 2009;140(4):455–460.

96. Lennon CJ, Wang RY, Wallace A, Chinnadurai S. Risk of failure of adenotonsillectomy for obstructive sleep apnea in obese pediatric patients. *Int J Pediatr Otorhinolaryngol.* 2017;92:7–10.

97. Isaiah A, Hamdan H, Johnson RF, Naqvi K, Mitchell RB. Very severe obstructive sleep apnea in children: outcomes of adenotonsillectomy and risk factors for persistence. *Otolaryngol Head Neck Surg.* 2017. http://dx.doi.org/10.1177/0194599817700370.

98. Thottam PJ, Trivedi S, Siegel B, Williams K, Mehta D. Comparative outcomes of severe obstructive sleep apnea in pediatric patients with trisomy 21. *Int J Pediatr Otorhinolaryngol.* 2015;79(7):1013–1016.

99. Farhood Z, Isley JW, Ong AA, et al. Adenotonsillectomy outcomes in patients with Down syndrome and obstructive sleep apnea. *Laryngoscope.* 2017.

100. Katz ES, Moore RH, Rosen CL, et al. Growth after adenotonsillectomy for obstructive sleep apnea: an RCT. *Pediatrics.* 2014;134(2):282–289.

101. Van M, Khan I, Hussain SS. Short-term weight gain after adenotonsillectomy in children with obstructive sleep apnea: systematic review. *J Laryngol Otol.* 2016;130(3):214–218.

CHAPTER 10

Evidence-Based Practice: Evaluation and Management of Unilateral Vocal Fold Paralysis

STEPHANIE MISONO, MD, MPH • ALBERT L. MERATI, MD, FACS

KEY POINTS

- Unilateral vocal fold paralysis (uvfp) has a broad range of etiologies, including postsurgical, neoplasm-related, and idiopathic (Evidence Grade C).
- Workup should include computed tomography imaging but not serology. Electromyography is useful for predicting poor prognosis (Evidence Grade C).
- Voice therapy can be beneficial but is not sufficient for many patients with uvfp. In the short term, injection medialization can achieve comparable clinical results to medialization thyroplasty. Thyroplasty and reinnervation also achieve comparable voice outcomes (Evidence Grade B).

ABBREVIATIONS

CT   Computed tomography
CXR   Chest X-ray/radiograph
LEMG Laryngeal electromyography
uvfp Unilateral vocal fold paralysis

PROBLEM OVERVIEW

Unilateral vocal fold paralysis (uvfp) continues to command attention as a fundamental clinical problem in Otolaryngology. Its impact on voice, swallowing, and even airway function is notable. Fortunately, patients and their physicians have many helpful diagnostic and therapeutic options for treatment. In this chapter we aim to provide an evidence-based overview of (1) the etiology and symptomatology, (2) evaluation, and (3) management of uvfp. The number of publications addressing aspects of this topic number in the thousands, and therefore we have made an attempt to present selected papers that will provide the reader with a sense of how the evidence has been developed and assessed. The discussion focuses primarily on uvfp rather than on the broader topic of unilateral vocal fold immobility or the narrower topic of unilateral vocal fold paresis. For each topic, the Oxford Centre for Evidence-based Medicine Levels of Evidence are listed.

Etiology (Levels 3–4)

The list of potential etiologies of uvfp is long and includes iatrogenic, traumatic, pulmonary, neoplastic, and systemic. **Iatrogenic** injury is commonly related to retraction and/or dissection along the route of the recurrent laryngeal nerve or even the vagus itself. Procedures associated with risk of postoperative vocal fold paralysis include thyroidectomy (0.8%–≥7% rate of permanent uvfp and much higher rates of temporary impairment),[1–6] anterior cervical spine surgery (<1%–>20% risk),[7–11] esophagectomy (at least ~11%–25% risk),[11a,b] cardiac/aortic surgery (~2% risk),[12] mediastinoscopy (0.2%–6% risk),[13,14] and carotid endarterectomy (~4% risk).[15,16] Vagus nerve stimulators also carry a low risk (0.4%) of leading to uvfp, particularly when smaller coil sizes are used.[17]

Thyroid surgery is associated with the greatest proportion of uvfp, given its frequency, and therefore it bears mention that the risk of uvfp may be influenced by the presence of invasive cancer and anatomic variants of the course of the recurrent laryngeal nerve,[18] including nonrecurrent laryngeal nerves and extralaryngeal bifurcation of the recurrent laryngeal nerve.[19] Other factors, such as age and comorbidities,[5] may also play a role. Whether preoperative laryngoscopy should be performed routinely, performed systematically in selected higher risk cases (e.g., preexisting voice concern, revision surgery), or performed at the discretion of the provider is controversial.[2,20] Intraoperative nerve monitoring also remains controversial, with some studies suggesting an association with reduced rates of temporary but not permanent paralysis and others showing no significant difference.[21-23] Recent data suggest that if there is a nerve injury noted intraoperatively, immediate reconstruction is important and more predictive of recovery than a series of other potential predictors such as age, preoperative mobility, reconstruction, and surgeon experience.[24]

Interpretation of the risks of uvfp associated with surgical procedures can be murky because of the difficulty of determining the contribution of underlying pathology to the postoperative outcome. Without systematic pre- and postoperative assessment of laryngeal function, which may not be clinically feasible, precise risk of uvfp associated with a given surgical procedure can be difficult to estimate. The picture is further clouded by the association of endotracheal intubation[25] or laryngeal mask airway[26] with uvfp. Some work has shown that the risk of iatrogenic uvfp related to retraction may be decreased by ongoing monitoring and adjustment of endotracheal tube pressure, particularly when retractors are placed or repositioned,[11] and that cuff pressure monitoring may also reduce iatrogenic uvfp risk.[10]

Traumatic etiologies associated with uvfp include high vagus nerve injury caused by direct trauma, although vagus nerve injuries more commonly result from surgical removal of masses involving the vagus itself.[27] Arytenoid dislocation has been proposed as a cause of unilateral vocal fold immobility, but this topic remains controversial; some evidence suggests that the diagnosis cannot be made by laryngoscopy alone and that there is insufficient evidence in the literature to characterize arytenoid dislocation as a unique entity.[28]

Pulmonary diseases and **tumors** have been implicated in the pathophysiology of uvfp as well, including lung cancer, thoracic aortic aneurysm, metastases, pulmonary/mediastinal tuberculosis, esophageal cancer,[15] patent ductus arteriosus,[16] and laryngeal chondrosarcoma.[29] Direct infiltration of the recurrent laryngeal nerve can also occur with thyroid carcinomas in addition to lung carcinomas as mentioned earlier.[30] Uvfp has also been reported after iodine-131 treatment of thyrotoxicosis[31,32] or radiation of other types to the head and neck[33,36] or upper chest.[34-35] Tumors in the central nervous system can also cause uvfp, but these typically have a constellation of associated symptoms.

Systemic etiologies can be divided into a variety of categories. Infectious etiologies include West Nile,[37] varicella[38] and herpes, Lyme,[39] mucormycosis[40] and coccidiodomycosis,[41] and syphilis,[42] whereas inflammatory processes can include sarcoidosis,[43] lupus,[44] microscopic polyangiitis,[45] amyloidosis, polyarteritis nodosa, and silicosis. Neurologic diagnoses associated with vocal fold paralysis include myasthenia gravis,[46] severe degenerative spine disease[47] or masses of the cervical spine,[48] multiple sclerosis,[49] neurofibromatosis,[50] amyotrophic lateral sclerosis,[51] Guillain-Barré syndrome (although typically bilateral),[52] Parkinson disease (also more commonly described as bilateral),[53] Charcot-Marie-Tooth disease, and familial hypokalemic periodic paralysis. Diabetes[54] or malnutrition, such as B_{12} deficiency,[55] can contribute, as can other endocrine disturbances such as acromegaly[56] medications such as vinca alkaloids,[57] and unusual sources such as stingray tail venom.[58] "Idiopathic" uvfp is a diagnosis of exclusion, and in those cases the pathogenesis remains poorly understood.

Evolving Distribution of Etiologies (Levels 3–4)

Both in the United States and abroad, numerous studies have focused on the relative distribution of etiologies for uvfp. Neoplasm, trauma, and surgery had been the most consistently cited etiologies in the 1970s, but the distribution has evolved over time.[59-61] In 1998 a retrospective review by Ramadan et al. examined etiologies in 98 patients with uvfp; they were categorized as neoplastic in 32%, surgical in 30%, idiopathic in 16%, traumatic in 11%, central in 8%, and infectious in 3%.[62] Several years later, a large comparative retrospective analysis spanning a 20-year period was presented by Rosenthal et al., comprising 827 patients who were seen with vocal fold immobility. In the first decade, spanning 1985–95, the most common etiology was malignancy (mostly lung). By contrast, in the second decade, 1996–2005, the most common etiology was nonthyroid surgery (including anterior cervical spine, carotid).[63] A study of 938 patients seen with uvfp at a single US academic medical center in 2002–12 indicated that iatrogenic causes were the most common (56%, of which the largest single category was thyroidectomy); 44% had nonsurgical causes, including 13% whose uvfp was idiopathic.[64] Distributions are similar in Japan, where postsurgical (predominantly thyroid) etiologies increased and idiopathic cases increased over a 45-year period,[65] but slightly different in Italy, where they noted a decrease in postthyroidectomy etiologies and an increase in postthoracic and idiopathic etiologies over the past 25 years.[66]

Thus, although the distribution of etiologies has evolved over time and may vary depending on geographic location,[67-69] commonly reported etiologies include neoplasms, particularly lung and thyroid neoplasms, and postsurgical (commonly spine surgery, carotid surgery, and thyroidectomy), with a persistent minority remaining idiopathic after thorough evaluation.

Laterality and Natural History of Idiopathic Unilateral Vocal Fold Paralysis (Level 4)

Approximately two-thirds of patients with idiopathic uvfp have left-sided paralysis. The reason for this is unknown, but a potential role for dynamic changes in aortic arch size related to aortic arch compliance has been postulated.[70] Data from a small number of potential patients suggest that concurrent palsy of the external branch of the superior laryngeal nerve may occur more commonly in idiopathic right uvfp than left, although the reason for this also remains unknown.[71]

Observational studies have provided some insight into the natural history of uvfp. A retrospective review of 633 patients with vocal fold paralysis diagnosed in 1940–49 included 181 of unknown etiology. Of those, 31 had respiratory infection before the onset of symptoms and 29 had incidental findings such as goiter or pharyngoesophageal diverticulum, but the vast majority had no apparent predisposing factors. Long-term survival data suggested that patients with truly idiopathic uvfp seemed to have normal life spans with 33% chance of vocal improvement over time.[72] More recently, Sulica performed a review of the literature and identified 20 papers reporting 717 cases of idiopathic vocal fold paralysis. He reported that idiopathic vocal fold paralysis comprises $24 \pm 10\%$ of uvfp. When findings from all of the studies were summarized, complete recovery of motion was observed in $36 \pm 22\%$ and some recovery (complete and partial) in $39 \pm 20\%$. Complete recovery of voice was reported in $52 \pm 17\%$, and some recovery in $61 \pm 22\%$. Most recovered in well under a year, but a small minority (5/717) described recovery after more than a year. As noted in the review, the variable recovery rates reported in different studies likely relate to heterogeneity of timeframe as well as criteria for defining recovery,[73] but in summary, most patients with idiopathic uvfp demonstrated some vocal improvement, typically in well under a year.

Symptoms (Levels 3–4)

Although evaluation of uvfp is frequently focused on *voice* complaints (discussed later), *dysphagia* and other complaints seem to be fairly common. Studies soliciting patient perspectives through surveys or interviews have reported unanimous concerns about voice, approximately two-thirds with concerns about swallowing, and approximately three-fourths with concerns about breathing, particularly with exercise.[74,75] In patients with dysphagia and uvfp who underwent flexible endoscopic evaluation of swallowing studies, liquid bolus retention and penetration was associated with aspiration in nearly half,[76] and the pharyngeal residues were noted at the base of tongue, valleculae, and piriform sinuses.[77] When examination was limited only to patients with postsurgical or idiopathic etiologies, patients with uvfp demonstrated aspiration in 36% (compared with 0% of normal controls) and had weaker pharyngeal constriction.[78]

Quality of Life at Presentation (Levels 3–4)

Intuitively it makes sense that uvfp would have a considerable effect on quality of life given the findings described earlier, and indeed, multiple well-accepted scales have demonstrated this impact. In a study at Vanderbilt University, patients with uvfp prospectively completed SF-36 (The Medical Outcomes Study Short Form 36-Item Health Survey),[79] Voice Handicap Index (VHI),[80] and Voice Outcome Survey (VOS)[81] at presentation and at first postoperative visit after thyroplasty with or without arytenoid adduction. The SF-36 is a general health status measure, the VHI is a voice-specific handicap measure, and the VOS is a survey designed to assess vocal quality and life impact of voice-related problems *specifically* in patients with uvfp. At presentation, patients with uvfp were observed to have significantly lower (worse) scores than normal on all domains of the SF-36 and on the VOS. Postoperatively, acoustic and aerodynamic measures of voice were markedly improved. All domains of the SF-36 were observed to have a trend toward increased scores, with some domains demonstrating a statistically significant increase. The VHI and its subscales and the VOS were noted to have significant improvement.[82] Several other measures of voice-related patient-reported quality of life have been utilized, including the Voice-Related Quality of Life (VRQOL)[83] and a variety of study-specific scales. These and other studies[84] underscore the significant impact of uvfp on both voice-related and overall health-related quality of life.

EVIDENCE-BASED CLINICAL ASSESSMENT
Examination (Levels 3–5)

Examination of the patient who presents with suspected uvfp may include several components, including auditory-perceptual evaluation of voice, acoustic/aerodynamic measurements, evaluation of intensity measures, and laryngoscopy.

Auditory-perceptual evaluation using the "GRBAS" scale (Grade, Roughness, Breathiness, Asthenia, Strain) demonstrates that patients with uvfp are rated *significantly worse than normal*.[85] More recently, a Consensus Auditory Perceptual Evaluation of Voice (CAPE-V) was developed for voice disorders in general. Relatively little information is available in the literature about CAPE-V evaluation of uvfp, but work in postthyroidectomy patients at Walter Reed Hospital suggest that overall severity, habitual loudness, habitual pitch, and roughness are parameters that may be affected.[86] The challenges with auditory-perceptual evaluation of voice are well-documented and include issues of inter- and intrarater reliability[87,88] as well as the impact of listener experience[89] and knowledge of the patient's history and/or diagnosis.[90] In addition, patients' perceptual self-ratings seemed to be distinct from those of trained listeners.[91] It is well established that patient ratings of the impact of vocal problems on quality of life do not correlate well with auditory-perceptual judgments.[92] Nonetheless, these judgments do allow raters to follow voice changes over time.

Acoustic and aerodynamic evaluation in uvfp demonstrates worse jitter, shimmer, noise to harmonic ratio, and maximum phonation time as compared with normal voices.[85] As noted by Behrman, acoustic and aerodynamic measures, although sometimes seen as "objective," are not truly so, because of the need for behavioral investment on the part of both patient and clinician to obtain representative phonatory samples and the challenge of performing some of these measurements when vocal fold vibration is irregular.[93] The relevance and validity of measures such as maximum phonation time and s to z ratio are also questioned, because in some cases suboptimal techniques such as excessive supraglottic recruitment can lead to apparently improved maximum vocal performance measures. Nonetheless, these measures are frequently reported. Development of nonlinear, random time-series analysis may provide further information, but it is in its early stages.[94] Another potentially promising technique is spectral moment analysis.[95] Assessment incorporating *cepstral measures*, such as cepstral peak prominence[96] and the multidimensional Cepstral

Spectral Index of Dysphonia,[97] also successfully detect voice quality abnormalities associated with uvfp. These measures are not pathognomonic or diagnostic for uvfp but are helpful in offering an instrumental perspective that corroborates perceptual assessments. *Intensity* has been occasionally used as a measure of vocal function, particularly habitual speaking intensity (loudness) and/or maximum physiologic dynamic range; these measures may be more closely related to the patient's assessment of vocal impact of vocal fold paralysis.[93] *Average airflow* has also been shown to be a useful measure in uvfp and is responsive to treatment.[98]

Laryngoscopy is an essential part of the evaluation of uvfp. Per a consensus statement from the American Head and Neck Society, laryngoscopy is the gold standard for diagnosis of uvfp following thyroid and parathyroid surgery.[99] Laryngoscopy has also been shown to have excellent intra- and interrater reliability for assessing for the presence of purposeful motion.[100] The importance of precise terminology (e.g., distinguishing paresis from paralysis) has been emphasized by a recent expert panel.[101]

The most common laryngoscopic findings beyond vocal fold motion impairment include bowing, incomplete glottal closure, and phase asymmetry on videostroboscopy.[85] Interestingly, the position of the vocal fold (paramedian vs. lateral) does not necessarily clarify the location of the lesion along the neurologic pathway from brain to motion of vocal fold.[102] However, the paralyzed side does tend to be shortened and arytenoid is commonly anteriorly rotated.[102] No definitive signs on laryngoscopy have been identified to predict recovery, but interarytenoid paralysis and posterolateral tilt of arytenoid may portend worse recovery.[103] Passive gliding motion of arytenoid is seen in 91% patients with uvfp examined by 3-D computed tomography (CT); caudal displacement in 100%.[104] Some have suggested that the position and shape of the false vocal fold may be informative, but this is controversial.[105] The specific value of stroboscopy over routine flexible fiberoptic laryngoscopy has also been debated, and its use is limited by challenges in capturing an adequate signal in profoundly dysphonic patients.[106] More recently, noninvasive laryngeal ultrasonography has been reported to detect uvfp after total thyroidectomy,[107] but its utility may be limited in overweight patients.[108] In addition, different approaches may be needed for male versus female[109] due in part to calcification of the larynx.[110]

Imaging (Levels 3–5)

A variety of imaging techniques have been utilized in the workup of patients with suspected uvfp. In a survey of members of the American Broncho-Esophagological Association, respondents indicated that chest X-ray (CXR) and/or neck/chest CT is always or often necessary (69%–72%). MRI was felt to be always or often necessary by 39%, sometimes by 51%.[111]

CXR can detect important diagnoses such as goiter and pulmonary fibrosis[72] but may miss findings detected by CT,[112] particularly those in the left aortopulmonary window.[113] It has also been suggested that MRI is more sensitive but carries a higher rate of false positives.[114] Because of the false-negative rate seen on CXR, several algorithms have been proposed for imaging used as part of the workup of uvfp. Altman and Benninger described starting with CXR and proceeding with CT or MRI if the CXR is negative. The CT is performed from the skull base to thoracic inlet for right uvfp and skull base to aortic triangle for left uvfp.[115] In contrast, El Badawey et al. described primary use of CT, without routine use of CXR.[67] Liu et al. have described stratification of patients with newly diagnosed uvfp using clinical findings (such as a history of malignancy) to divide them into high-suspicion and low-suspicion groups. They then examined costs associated with imaging for each group. The high-suspicion group workup (which included MRI and/or CT) cost $2304 per true positive, whereas low-suspicion group cost $10,849 per true positive case.[114] An implication of these findings is that perhaps imaging could be deferred for the low-suspicion group, but the associated risks and costs of delayed diagnosis would need to be evaluated thoroughly before making such a recommendation. Consistent with this, others have shown that routine CT in patients with uvfp is cost-effective when added to laryngoscopy, even without stratifying by suspicion level, as its cost is below most willingness-to-pay levels.[116] Some authors have raised consideration of repeated CT imaging after initial imaging has been negative because of concern for a low rate of subsequent detection of contributory findings[117]; others have concluded that this is not necessary.[118] These types of decisions may also depend on factors such as baseline prevalence of potentially contributing findings, availability of imaging, and medicolegal climate.

Although the use of CT imaging is generally accepted, some have pointed to the relatively low "hit" rate and the radiation exposure associated with CT as a reason to consider other imaging modalities as a first step.[119] There is growing evidence in support of using neck ultrasound imaging in the detection and workup of uvfp. Neck ultrasonography has also been used to identify contributing etiologies such as thyroid carcinoma, vagal schwannoma, and metastatic cervical lymphadenopathy.[69,120] More research is required to determine the optimal role of ultrasonography in the workup for uvfp etiology.

Although positron emission tomography (PET) scanning is not routinely used in the diagnosis of uvfp, it is important to be aware of the potential for misleading results on PET that are related to the presence of uvfp. Several studies have demonstrated that when uvfp is present, the contralateral normal side can have high fludeoxyglucose uptake thought to be secondary to attempted compensatory motion, potentially raising misleading concern for malignancy.[121,122] These findings have most commonly been described in patients with primary lung malignancies who had secondary unilateral recurrent laryngeal nerve paralysis. Other potentially misleading findings arise from the treatment of uvfp; Teflon granulomas that arise from the use of Teflon (polytetrafluoroethylene, DuPont, Wilmington, DE) for injection medialization can lead to false-positive findings on PET,[123] as can an elastomer suspension (trade name Vox, Uroplasty Inc., Minnetonka, MN) implant.[124]

Ultimately, the ideal algorithm for imaging in the workup of uvfp remains controversial. Evidence in the literature is inadequate to make a blanket recommendation, but numerous studies have reported the use of imaging to identify significant abnormalities in patients who present with idiopathic vocal fold paralysis, and *cross-sectional imaging is likely indicated*. It can be difficult to directly synthesize across studies given different recruitment and/or inclusion criteria. Prospective controlled studies are necessary for further evaluation. Other factors to consider include cost and exposure to radiation.[125]

Serology (Levels 3–5)

Use of serology as part of the evaluation of patients with uvfp has been described in a variety of studies. A survey of American Broncho-Esophagological Association members indicated that 54% of respondents felt serum tests could be considered as part of a workup, but the majority (80%) of these indicated the tests were appropriate only occasionally or rarely. The most commonly mentioned tests were rheumatoid factor (RF) (38%), Lyme titer (36%), erythrocyte sedimentation rate (ESR) (34%), and anti-nuclear antibody (ANA) (33%).[111] Review of the literature at that time demonstrated mostly case reports with one case-control study on diabetes[54,111]; sarcoidosis and ANA were also frequently addressed, but there remains no population-based information. Some authors advocate for using a comprehensive laboratory evaluation in the setting of uvfp, because of the possibility of detecting medically important conditions,[126] but neither the pretest likelihood of positive findings nor the cost-effectiveness has been incorporated into existing analyses. There remains *no definite evidence to support routine serology* in patients with uvfp who do not have signs/symptoms of underlying disease, and practitioners will likely be best served by ordering serology only if they have a clinical index of suspicion for particular associated diseases.

Laryngeal Electromyography (Levels 2–5)

The inclusion of laryngeal electromyography (LEMG) in the evaluation of patients with uvfp has garnered attention as a technique that could evaluate the current neurologic status of the affected vocal fold and provide prognostic information. Although the advent of injection medialization has in some ways tempered the impact of LEMG because immediate and temporary intervention is now available, interest in electromyography (EMG) continues.

A variety of findings on LEMG have been examined as potentially important prognostic characteristics, including fibrillations, positive sharp waves, and absent or reduced voluntary motor unit potentials.[127] Other proposed methods for LEMG interpretation include interference pattern analysis, which allows description of motor unit recruitment[128] in patients with uvfp and the use of the ratio of mean peak-to-peak amplitude comparing motor unit amplitude on sniff versus sustained phonation for evaluation of synkinesis and associated poor prognosis for recovery.[129]

A 2016 consensus statement from an expert panel convened by the American Association of Neuromuscular & Electrodiagnostic Medicine indicated that LEMG can be useful for prognostic information particularly for patients whose symptom duration is 4 weeks–6 months. Polyphasic motor unit potentials and active voluntary motor unit potential recruitment were the most positive prognostic signs for recovery.[130]

The current evidence indicates that LEMG with negative prognostic factors is likely to predict a poor functional outcome, but the optimal timing of LEMG in relation to symptom onset remains unclear, and improved diagnostic accuracy is still needed. Prospective blinded studies are needed to confirm these and

other potential ways to utilize LEMG in a quantitative, objective, and reproducible fashion.

EVIDENCE-BASED MEDICAL MANAGEMENT AND SURGICAL TECHNIQUE

The natural history of recovery from uvfp can vary depending on the etiology and severity of recurrent laryngeal nerve injury. This can be further complicated by the fact that motion recovery and vocal handicap are not necessarily concurrent. For example, in a sample of 72 patients with uvfp with a mean follow-up of 9 months, 35% experienced motion recovery, but a minority of those with some motion recovery still had significant voice handicap, and conversely, 21% without motion recovery had no significant voice handicap.[131] Although conventional wisdom has been to allow 12 months for spontaneous recovery, it has been demonstrated that those who experience recovery may be divided into two subgroups: one with neuropraxic injury that experiences early recovery and another with more severe injury requiring neuronal recovery that leads to late recovery. In a paper incorporating mathematical models of the probability of recovery, Mau et al. reported that among those who recovered, 85% recovered within 6 months and 96% within 9 months, suggesting that 9 months may be a sufficient period of time to await motion recovery for most patients.[132]

Speech Pathology
Voice therapy (level 4)

Several studies have described the use of voice therapy in the management of uvfp, although there is an opportunity in the literature for further examination of this issue. Although swallowing therapy is outside the scope of this review, techniques may include chin tuck, neck extension, head turn, supraglottic and suprasupraglottic swallow and/or dietary modification. Some patients also benefit from oral motor exercises, vocal adduction exercises, Valsalva swallow, and Mendelsohn maneuvers.[133]

Voice therapy in uvfp is typically directed at abdominal breathing and humming/resonant voice with the goal of improving closure of the glottis, encouraging abdominal breath support, and improving vocal fold function while avoiding supraglottic hyperfunction. Depending upon the study, significant proportions of patients with uvfp who opted for voice therapy reported vocal improvement subjectively or as measured by glottal closure, acoustic measurements, pitch range, and/or patient-reported voice handicap,[134,135] even in patients who have had long-standing uvfp.[136] Voice therapy may particularly affect factors associated with the functional and emotional items in the VHI.[137] Interpretation of the impact of voice therapy in uvfp may be obscured by returning neurologic function,[138] and it is unknown whether there is a relationship between voice therapy and neurologic recovery.

Other studies have also suggested the utility of voice therapy in the management of uvfp,[139,140] but there is often no comparison group, making it difficult to assess whether voice therapy affected the likelihood of these improvements. Randomized controlled studies may be difficult to perform in this area, as patients who desire surgery may not be receptive to randomization into voice therapy and vice versa, but controlled studies may be possible using alternate study designs. An additional challenge to study of this topic is the variability of therapy techniques across institutions or across individual therapists. A recent systematic review by Walton et al. offers additional insights into challenges of assessing the impact of speech therapy on uvfp.[141]

Surgical Techniques
Medialization
One of the mainstays of surgical treatment for uvfp is the concept of medialization, in which the paralyzed vocal fold is displaced toward midline to facilitate glottal closure. This can improve voice quality as well as dysphagia symptoms[142] and, less commonly, odynophonia.[143] The ideal timing for medialization remains unclear. Some have postulated that over time, the immobile cricoarytenoid joint may become fixed, whereas other studies suggest that joint mobility may remain intact even many years after the onset of paralysis.[144-146] Other studies examine voice and other functional outcomes after early medialization versus late medialization—these are discussed under the contexts of different types of medialization techniques.

Injection medialization (levels 1–4). Injection medialization of the vocal fold was first performed in 1911 by Brunings via peroral injection using paraffin. This fell out of favor until the development of other injectables that were felt to be less reactogenic. A retrospective review from multiple institutions summarized characteristics and complications of 460 injections for augmentation of the vocal folds. There was essentially an even split between awake injections performed in clinic versus those performed under general anesthesia. About 54% of the injections were performed for vocal fold paralysis. The majority of awake injections

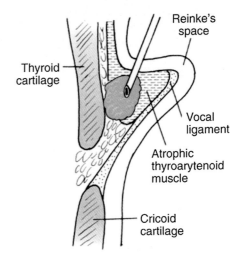

FIG. 10.1 Injection medialization. This figure shows a hemicoronal section through the larynx, demonstrating the placement of an injectable material to medialize the affected vocal fold. (From *Cummings Otolaryngology*. 5th ed. Mosby: Elsevier, Fig. 66-4A, with permission.)

were performed via the transcricothyroid approach (47%); also frequent were peroral (23%) and transthyrohyoid (21%). Reported success rates were ≥97% and complication rates were ≤3%, with no difference between awake and asleep techniques. Injection augmentation is increasing both in awake patients[147] and in the operating room.[148] The goal of injection medialization is to reposition the vocal fold medially (Fig. 10.1), allowing better contact between the affected side and the normal side. Injection medialization causes passive medial rotation and translation of the arytenoid cartilage.[149]

A variety of materials is now available for use in injection medialization. The literature was summarized by Paniello,[150] who examined findings from 42 papers describing up to 30 patients each with follow-up time up to 1 year, describing injection medialization and voice outcomes as reflected by a variety of measures. All studies demonstrated vocal improvement after injection medialization. There were two level 1 studies, both by Hertegard et al., describing the use of hyaluronan versus collagen for injection; their findings suggested better vibratory function and less resorption of hyaluronan over time. The remainder of the studies described injection with fat, collagen, acellular dermis, fascia, Teflon, silicone, and other materials. The largest proportion of papers described the use of fat injection.[150] Direct comparison across injectable materials occurs less commonly, but a recent (nonrandomized)

TABLE 10.1
Examples of Vocal Fold Injection Materials

Material	Sample Trade Names	Length of Effect	Amount Injected	Needle Gauge	FDA Approval	Comments	Estimated Cost
Autologous fat	NA	? years; variable	Overinject	18–22	NA	Requires harvest	NA
Cadaveric micronized dermis	Cymetra (LifeCell, Branchburg NJ)	2–4 months; some >1 year	Overinject	18–25	Yes	Requires preparation	$448
Calcium hydroxyl-apatite (CaHA)	Prolaryn Plus, previously called Radiesse Voice (Merz Aesthetics, San Mateo, CA); Renu Voice (RegenScientific)	>1 year	Slightly overinject	25	Yes	Place lateral to ligament; poor rheologic properties	$210–625
Carboxymethyl-cellulose	Prolaryn Gel, previously called Radiesse Voice Gel (Merz Aesthetics); Renu Gel (Regen-Scientific)	2–3 months	Slightly overinject	27	Yes		$190–625
Hyaluronic acid gels	Restylane, Perlane, Juvederm (Medicis Aesthetics, Scotts-dale, AZ)	6–9 months	Slightly overinject	27	No	Good compliance, rheologic properties	~$680

Several collagen preparations, including Zyplast, Cosmoplast, and Cosmoderm, and the hyaluronic acid preparations Hylaform and Hylaform Plus (Allergan, Irvine, CA) have been discontinued. Information presented in this table was acquired from multiple sources, including relevant papers in the literature[156–163] and vendor/manufacturer information where available, as well as trade organization information as needed.[164]
FDA, U.S. Food and Drug Administration.

comparison of autologous fat versus calcium hydroxyl-apatite demonstrated comparable treatment results with both substances.[151]

A multi-institutional retrospective review by Sulica et al. gave a sense of current practice patterns, with methylcellulose (35%), bovine collagen (28%), and calcium hydroxylapatite (26%) used most commonly for awake injections and calcium hydroxylapatite (36%) and methylcellulose (35%) used most commonly in the operating room.[147] Although Teflon had previously enjoyed popularity because of its long duration and easy injectability, Teflon injection is associated with giant cell granulomas that persist decades after injection[152] and are challenging to address surgically.[153] Some problems may have been related to technique,[154,155] and some authors describe vocal rehabilitation with multiple surgical procedures, but the potential disadvantages render Teflon difficult to support, particularly when other alternatives exist.

Individual surgeon preferences for use of a given injectable may also depend upon characteristics of each material, including duration, ease of use, cost, and rheologic properties. Several of the commonly used injectable materials are summarized in Table 10.1. The physical setting of the injection may be another consideration. Screening criteria for identifying the small proportion of patients who would benefit from having their injections performed in a monitored setting rather than an unmonitored office setting have been proposed.[165] In addition, injections performed in endoscopy suites cost less than those performed in operating rooms.[166]

Although there is an estimated duration of effect quoted for each injectable, the literature reveals a wide range of reported durations. For example, some studies have described a greater than 1 year effect in patients with uvfp who underwent injections with micronized dermis.[160,161] The assessment of duration of effect for injection medialization may be complex because of the possibility of partial improvement in neurologic function, which may improve the tone of the paralyzed vocal fold without restoring motion.

That there remain numerous injectables in active use suggests that no single injectable is definitively superior to the others, and nuanced decision making with respect to selection of injectable may be appropriate. Systematic review of the literature has not identified any definite best substances for injection.[167] Further investigation, perhaps with more randomized head-to-head comparisons, may clarify the potential utility of different substances.

As described earlier, complications are relatively rare. Reported risks include prolonged stridor, need for intubation, and postinjection dysphonia[168] secondary to subepithelial injection and/or overinjection.[147] Particular caution is important to avoid superficial injection, as the injectate can persist for years.[169] Rare but serious risks include immediate or delayed injection site inflammation requiring management with steroids,[170,171] intralaryngeal migration of injectate,[172] abscess at the site of injection[173] or extralaryngeally,[174] and severe laryngeal inflammation leading to decreased vocal fold mobility, and laryngeal web.[175] Injections can be accomplished at bedside in recent postoperative patients, including those on anticoagulation.[176] Although this chapter is not intended to cover technical detail in depth, there is also a growing literature on techniques that facilitate successful vocal fold injections in awake patients,[177–183] as well as pitfalls to avoid.[184]

It remains controversial whether the timing of injection medialization affects longer-term outcomes, largely because the probability of recovery changes over time. In all comers, the overall need for permanent medialization (e.g., medialization thyroplasty) is approximately 20%–30% after injection.[161,185] Early medialization (1–4 days) after the onset of uvfp after thoracic surgery has been associated with significantly fewer cases of pneumonia and a shorter length of stay when compared with late medialization (>5 days after onset).[186] Some studies have suggested that early injection medialization may be associated with a lower rate of eventual need for permanent medialization thyroplasty,[187–189] but others have not found this to be the case.[190] A small randomized study of hyaluronic acid injection showed no differences in voice-related measures compared with conservative management at 6 months but did suggest better mental health-related quality of life in the injection group, suggesting a valuable benefit from injection even if long-term voice outcomes are unchanged.[190a] Taken together, these data do suggest that *early injection medialization* is helpful;

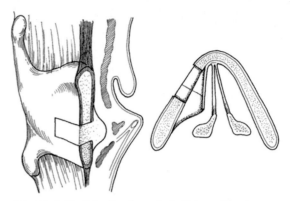

FIG. 10.2 Medialization thyroplasty. Schematic representation of a polymer implant used in a medialization thyroplasty to permanently medially displace the vocal fold. This allows adjustment of the position of the vocal fold in three dimensions. On the left is an oblique coronal view; on the right is an axial view. (From Fried MP, ed. *The Larynx*. 2nd ed. St. Louis, MO (Mosby): Elsevier; 1996:213, with permission.)

further studies are necessary to determine whether early injection influences longer-term outcomes. The use of a nomogram to help identify patients who may benefit from early thyroplasty has also been proposed.[191]

Future frontiers include different materials and technology for injected agents in uvfp treatment. The use of novel materials has been reported in the world literature, including different augmentation materials, such as polydimethylsiloxane[192] and auricular cartilage,[193] as well as bioactive molecules, such as basic fibroblast-derived growth factor, that are used with the goal to promote muscle regeneration.[194]

Medialization thyroplasty (level 2–4). A more long-lasting approach to medialization of the paralyzed true vocal fold was originally described by Payr in 1915, who used a cartilage flap pressed inward from a thyroid cartilage window to reposition the paralyzed vocal fold.[195] This technique was later modified by Isshiki, who described the use of mobilized thyroid cartilage inserted through the window[196] and further adapted it with the use of alloplastic material (Fig. 10.2).[197] As with injection medialization, early medialization thyroplasty has been associated with fewer diagnoses of pneumonia and shorter lengths of stay after thoracic surgeries, as mentioned earlier.[186] The procedure has commonly necessitated overnight observation, but some have moved toward risk stratification,[198] suggesting that in patients with few risk factors for complications, day surgery could be considered.[199]

As with injection medialization, a variety of implant types is available, although the current literature most commonly presents data for patients undergoing medialization with a carved Silastic (polymeric silicone, Dow Corning, Midland, MI) implant. In a 2008 comprehensive evidence-based review by Paniello, 52 papers describing the impact of open implant medialization on subjective and objective voice outcomes were summarized. There was no level 1 evidence; there was some level 2 evidence for Silastic, Montgomery (Boston Medical Products, Westborough, MA), GORE-Tex (W.L. Gore and Associates, Elkton, MD), and other types of implants. The majority reported improvement in voice outcomes using auditory-perceptual and aerodynamic/acoustic measures.[150] A large 2010 survey of US otolaryngologists indicated that the most commonly used materials were Silastic, Montgomery, and Gore-tex implants.[200] Some direct comparisons between titanium implants and other materials have also been published, with some suggestion that titanium may be superior for restoration of voice quality,[201,202] but additional work is necessary before a definitive conclusion, particularly given the report of a low rate of explants necessitated by granulation.[203] Thyroplasty with nasal septal cartilage may be another option,[204] potentially especially useful in cost-limited settings.

Although the specifics of the procedure may be somewhat surgeon-specific, it has been shown that intraoperative measurement of acoustic and aerodynamic measurements such as *maximum phonation time* may be useful in predicting postoperative outcomes. Although the maximum phonation time is typically lower when the patient is supine and may be lower under sedation, the relative improvement in maximum phonation time at the time of medialization seems to be informative.[205]

Adjunct procedures at the time of medialization thyroplasty may include arytenoid adduction,[206] arytenopexy,[207] or even cricothyroid approximation.[208] It is important to be aware that endoscopy alone does not necessarily provide a definitive way to assess the need for arytenoid adduction and arytenoid adduction does not necessarily change the laryngoscopic appearance in a predictable way.[209] Some data suggest that arytenopexy may also lead to improved phonatory results[210]; a cadaver study suggests improved harmonic profile with arytenopexy as compared with arytenoid adduction.[211] To our knowledge there are no studies that directly compare results of the two techniques in vivo.

For medialization thyroplasty there is an 8% estimated rate of complications requiring medical or surgical intervention,[212] including edema, wound complications, extrusion, and/or need for tracheotomy. A higher risk of complications has been observed in patients on anticoagulation, with atrophic/absent tissue, and/or undergoing revision surgery.[199] Although a history of neck radiation has also been considered to be a contraindication to medialization, reports indicate that medialization can safely be performed in this patient population.[213,214] Rare reported thyroplasty complications include the creation of a window in cricoid cartilage, leading to airway obstruction when the implant was placed[215] and saccular cyst development caused by gland obstruction,[216] as well as implant extrusion in 2.1% and implant malpositioning in 1.3%.[150] Common indications for revision surgery include persistent glottic insufficiency, overclosure, implant malposition, decreased vocal fold pliability, and implant extrusion[217,218]; it has also been noted that sheet medialization is associated with a higher prevalence of undercorrection than silicone block medialization.[219] Airway complications are more commonly reported after arytenoid adduction than after medialization laryngoplasty.[220] Although medialization is often described as reversible because the implant may be removed, placement of the implant has been associated with permanent changes in joint mobility and/or fibrosis in an experimental animal model.[221]

The long-term effect of medialization thyroplasty on voice seems to be very good overall. Although some have raised the question of late-onset vocal fold atrophy and whether that renders implant medialization less effective over time,[217] most authors demonstrate excellent persistence of vocal improvement at 3 months post procedure, with stable or greater improvement at the 1-year time point.[222–226] Longer-term data are scant, but Leder and Sasaki demonstrated long-term improvement in maximum phonation time and other characteristics that persisted over 3 years after medialization thryoplasty,[223] and Ryu et al. have observed that outcomes at 1 year were generally predictive of outcomes at 5 years.[227] Thus, although there may be some variability over the first several months after medialization, overall the *vocal improvement seems to be robust and long-lasting.*

Although medialization thyroplasty is clearly effective, there may yet be room for improvement. Gray et al. assessed vocal function in 15 patients 1 year after type I thyroplasty with cartilage, Silastic, or GORE-Tex and variable etiology of vocal fold paralysis. Some voice characteristics (pitch, intonation, loudness) were not statistically different from normal; others (strain, breathiness, hoarseness, harshness, unsteadiness) were different. When surveyed, 92% patients reported that surgery helped with their voice and 73%

were generally or extremely satisfied. However, 87% felt their voices were still abnormal and 25% had adjusted their employment to accommodate voice.[228] This information is very important to keep in mind when counseling patients regarding postoperative expectations.

Comparing injection medialization with medialization thyroplasty (level 3)

Voice. A number of studies have compared the results of injection medialization and medialization thyroplasty. Many have not demonstrated a meaningful difference between the two techniques,[229-231] but several reported a trend toward greater improvement after medialization thyroplasty over the long term.[232-234] As noted by Paniello in a systematic review of a subset of these papers, a challenge to the interpretation of these data is the variable length of follow-up time and small sample sizes. Studies with longer follow-up time tended to favor results of medialization thyroplasty,[150] although a few studies with at least 1-year follow-up have suggested that long-acting injectables, such as fat and calcium hydroxylapatite, can provide comparable or superior voice outcomes compared with thyroplasty.[235,236] Different injection and thyroplasty materials across studies and, in some cases, incomplete data render overall comparisons difficult to make. In addition, randomization to injection medialization versus medialization thyroplasty may not be acceptable to patients. The available data suggest that *in the short term, injection medialization and medialization thyroplasty are likely comparable with respect to voice outcomes but that in the long term, medialization thyroplasty may provide better voice results.* A recent cost analysis based on a decision analytic model suggested that in-clinic medialization injection laryngoplasty with calcium hydroxylapatite is more cost-effective than medialization thyroplasty (Montgomery implant), factoring an assumption that injection would need to be repeated annually.[237] Patient preferences and the psychosocial impact of needing and awaiting multiple injections would likely also play a role in decision making. More investigation is needed to clarify and compare longer-term outcomes across these treatment types.

Swallowing. Fewer studies have compared the impact of injection medialization with that of medialization thyroplasty on swallowing, but *no significant difference* has been detected in the improvement of swallowing between patients who underwent injection medialization and those who underwent medialization thyroplasty.[238,239]

Medialization thyroplasty versus medialization thyroplasty with arytenoid adduction (levels 3–4). Another oft-debated topic is the consideration of arytenoid adduction when medialization thyroplasty is performed. In excised canine larynges, studies suggested differences between injection, thyroplasty, and thyroplasty with arytenoid adduction; injection reduced mucosal wave amplitude, but medialization thyroplasty with or without arytenoid adduction increased amplitude. Overall, medialization with arytenoid adduction resulted in the greatest improvement in phonatory measurements, including phonation threshold flow, phonation threshold power, and signal to noise ratio.[240]

A small number of studies have undertaken this comparison in patients, with some demonstrating no difference between the two groups[212] and others demonstrating greater improvement or a trend in that direction after medialization thyroplasty with arytenoid adduction.[212,241-243] Formal summary evaluation of these studies is difficult because of heterogeneous patient groups, implant types, and measurement of pre- and postoperative outcomes. There is little evidence on whether these techniques have a differential impact on swallowing.

Laryngeal reinnervation (levels 1–4)

Another approach to the management of uvfp has been laryngeal reinnervation, which takes advantage of the presence of other functioning nerves in the anatomic vicinity to improve tone and/or mobility of the paralyzed side (Figs. 10.3 and 10.4).[244] Options for laryngeal reinnervation include ansa,[144] phrenic,[144] hypoglossal,[245] and nerve-muscle pedicles.[246-248] Approaches have included selective innervation of different muscles in the same setting (e.g., adductor and abductor)[144] or targeted reinnervation of a selected muscle (e.g., lateral cricoarytenoid or thyroarytenoid).[248] Some studies have described the use of various laryngeal reinnervation techniques in combination with arytenoid adduction.[249-251]

In a systematic review of the literature, Paniello identified 11 studies, levels 3–4, with either a trend toward or statistically significant improvement of voice parameters as assessed by auditory-perceptual evaluation, acoustic/aerodynamic measures, and/or laryngoscopy or stroboscopy. The complication rate was low, with one delayed tracheostomy tube placement reported (2%).[150] As he noted, there is great clinical variability in the evidence currently in the literature—depending upon the study, there are different reinnervation techniques, possible concomitant procedures, different timing of reinnervation, patient ages, and length of follow-up.[150] A varying degree of synkinesis from

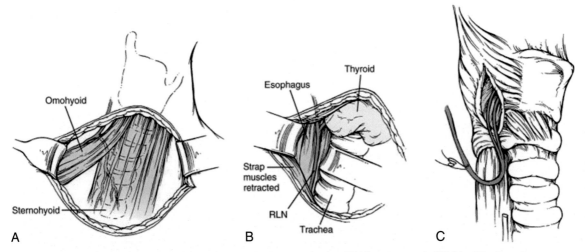

FIG. 10.3 Illustrations of direct ansa–recurrent laryngeal nerve (RLN) anastomosis (**(A)** identification of ansa cervicalis branch to sternohyoid muscle; **(B)** identification of recurrent laryngeal nerve; **(C)** anastomosis of the two nerves). (From *Cummings Otolaryngology*. 5th ed. Mosby: Elsevier, Figs. 68-2 and 68-1.)

misdirected reinnervation of laryngeal abductors and/or adductors can also complicate the picture,[129,252–254] as can the use of voice therapy.

Medialization thyroplasty versus laryngeal reinnervation (levels 1–3). Tucker compared nerve-muscle pedicle with medialization thyroplasty with medialization thyroplasty alone; expert listeners rated voice outcomes better after combined reinnervation and medialization thyroplasty.[255] This study was not randomized but helped to lay the groundwork for a major trial.

Paniello et al. performed a *multicenter randomized clinical trial comparing medialization thyroplasty with reinnervation using the ansa cervicalis nerve*.[256] The trial included 24 patients, 12 in each arm. Pre- and postoperative voice were evaluated using perceptual rating by untrained listeners, blinded speech pathologists' GRBAS ratings, the VRQOL Scale, and secondarily, maximum phonation time, cepstral analysis, and EMG. At 12 months postoperatively, both groups had significant improvement in perceptual ratings, GRBAS, and VRQOL and there was *no significant difference* between the groups. However, a more detailed analysis revealed that *patient age* seemed to be an important variable.

Patients under the age of 52 years who underwent reinnervation had better postoperative auditory-perceptual ratings than those in the same age group who underwent medialization. Furthermore, patients under the age of 52 years who underwent reinnervation had better voice results than those over the age of 52 years who underwent reinnervation. In the over-52-year age group, voice results were better after medialization thyroplasty than after reinnervation.

As in prior studies of surgical intervention for uvfp, most of the voice results did not reach "normal" as measured by GRBAS and VRQOL. However, cepstral analysis demonstrated better voicing in the reinnervated group and patients under the age of 52 years who underwent reinnervation approached normal values. At the conclusion of study, several additional surgeries were planned for study patients, including injection augmentation in two of the patients who underwent medialization and thyroplasties in two of the patients who underwent reinnervation, suggesting that some patients may benefit from multiple procedures.

In addition to a new nuanced picture of tailored surgical approaches for patients of different ages who present with uvfp, this trial provided some valuable insight into the challenges of performing this type of study. The authors described difficulty with both accrual and randomization, noting that both patients and surgeons had difficulty accepting randomization. A study examining patient perceptions reported that patients expressed greater interest in reinnervation than in thyroplasty, suggesting that phraseology may also be an important component in trials in this area.[257] Nonetheless, Paniello et al.'s thyroplasty versus reinnervation study is an inspiring example of a well-conducted study that addressed a focused and meaningful clinical question.

A 2016 systematic review comparing medialization thyroplasty, injection augmentation, arytenoid adduction, and reinnervation reported positive comparable outcomes for patients with uvfp,[258] although studies reported varying outcomes and follow-up times, clearly demonstrating that further work is needed. Thus at present, evidence supports surgical intervention when recovery and/or conservative treatment do not lead to adequate vocal function but does not identify a single best surgical approach to management.

FUTURE HORIZONS

Multiple investigators have developed animal (both in and ex vivo), human (ex vivo larynges), and computational models that will lead to a better understanding of the effects and treatment of uvfp. These

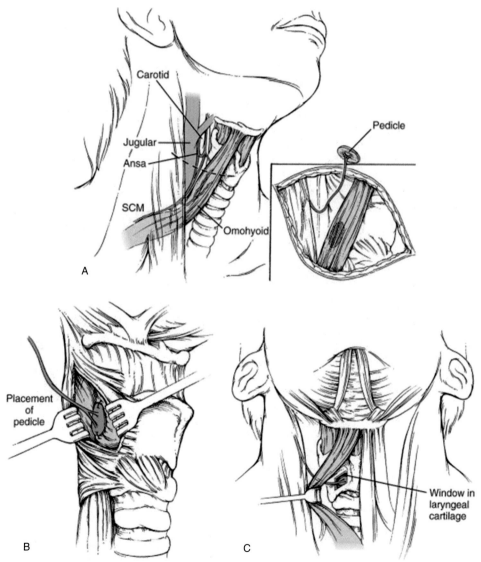

FIG. 10.4 Illustrations of the use of neuromuscular pedicle ((**A**) neuromuscular pedicle harvest using ansa cervicalis branch to omohyoid muscle; (**B**) neuromuscular pedicle placement into lateral cricoarytenoid muscle via (**C**) laryngeal cartilage window). *SCM*, sternocleidomastoid muscle. (From *Cummings Otolaryngology*. 5th ed. Mosby: Elsevier, Figs. 68-2 and 68-1.)

types of models allow the examination of factors such as the role of synkinesis and how tissue and geometric properties of the true vocal folds affect voice production.[259-262] They also facilitate investigations into improving treatments, such as the size and shape of vocal fold implants for thyroplasty,[263,264] less invasive approaches for arytenoid repositioning,[265] and/or characteristics of injectable materials.[266] Studies are also ongoing into potential adjunct treatments, such as chemotherapeutics to decrease synkinesis following denervation[267,268] and nimodipine to improve nerve regeneration and subsequent recovery of mobility.[269]

BOTTOM LINE: WHAT DOES THE EVIDENCE TELL US?

- PRESENTATION (Evidence Grade C): A wide variety of etiologies can lead to uvfp; the distribution of these etiologies has evolved over time. Postsurgical uvfp, neoplasm-related uvfp, and idiopathic uvfp remain common.
- EVALUATION (Evidence Grade C): In the workup of uvfp, imaging may be reasonable (CXR not sufficient, CT more informative, ultrasonography may be useful), but the routine use of serology is not well supported. LEMG with fibrillations, positive sharp waves, and/or absent or reduced voluntary motor unit potentials predicts a lack of functionally meaningful recovery, but the ideal timing of LEMG after symptom onset remains to be defined.
- MANAGEMENT (Evidence Grade B): Data on voice therapy suggest a positive impact, but further studies are needed. Injection medialization is widely used, and there is a variety of injectables that may be considered. The current evidence suggests that short-term voice outcomes after injection medialization are similar to those after medialization thyroplasty, but longer-term results may favor the latter. Finally, laryngeal reinnervation has been shown to have comparable vocal impact to that of medialization thyroplasty, and surgical decision making should take patient age into account. Some patients may benefit from multiple procedures.
- There is a need for ongoing systematic reviews of the literature and more randomized controlled trials.

ACKNOWLEDGMENTS

S.M. was supported by the National Institute on Deafness and other Communication Disorders of the National Institutes of Health, award number K23DC016335. The content is solely the responsibility of the authors and does not necessarily represent the official views of the National Institutes of Health.

REFERENCES

1. Lee KE, Koo do H, Kim SJ, et al. Outcomes of 109 patients with papillary thyroid carcinoma who underwent robotic total thyroidectomy with central node dissection via the bilateral axillo-breast approach. *Surgery.* 2010;148:1207–1213.
2. Chandrasekhar SS, Randolph GW, Seidman MD, et al. Clinical practice guideline: improving voice outcomes after thyroid surgery. *Otolaryngol Head Neck Surg.* 2013; 148(6 suppl):S1–S37.
3. Jeannon JP, Orabi AA, Bruch GA, Abdalsalam HA, Simo R. Diagnosis of recurrent laryngeal nerve palsy after thyroidectomy: a systematic review. *Int J Clin Pract.* 2009;63:624–629.
4. Bhattacharyya N, Fried MP. Assessment of the morbidity and complications of total thyroidectomy. *Arch Otolaryngol Head Neck Surg.* 2002;128:389–392.
5. Papaleontiou M, Hughes DT, Guo C, Banerjee M, Haymart MR. Population-based assessment of complications following surgery for thyroid cancer. *J Clin Endocrinol Metab.* 2017. http://dx.doi.org/10.1210/jc.2017-00255.
6. Francis DO, Pearce EC, Ni S, Garrett CG, Penson DF. Epidemiology of vocal fold paralyses after total thyroidectomy for well-differentiated thyroid cancer in a medicare population. *Otolaryngol Head Neck Surg.* 2014;150(4):548–557.
7. Netterville JL, Koriwchak MJ, Winkle M, Courey MS, Ossoff RH. Vocal fold paralysis following the anterior approach to the cervical spine. *Ann Otol Rhinol Laryngol.* 1996;105:85–91.
8. Heeneman H. Vocal cord paralysis following approaches to the anterior cervical spine. *Laryngoscope.* 1973;83:17–21.
9. Merati AL, Shemirani N, Smith TL, Toohill RJ. Changing trends in the nature of vocal fold motion impairment. *Am J Otolaryngol.* 2006;27:106–108.
10. Tan TP, Govindarajulu AP, Massicotte EM, Venkatraghavan L. Vocal cord palsy after anterior cervical spine surgery: a qualitative systematic review. *Spine J.* 2014;14(7):1332–1342.
11. Kriskovich MD, Apfelbaum RI, Haller JR. Vocal fold paralysis after anterior cervical spine surgery: incidence, mechanism, and prevention of injury. *Laryngoscope.* 2000;110:1467–1473.
11a. Pertl L, Zacherl J, Mancusi G, et al. High risk of unilateral recurrent laryngeal nerve paralysis after esophagectomy using cervical anastomosis. *Eur Arch Otorhinolaryngol.* 2011. http://dx.doi.org/10.1007/s00405-011-1679-7.
11b. Loochtan MJ, Balcarcel D, Carroll E, Foecking EM, Thorpe EJ, Charous SJ. Vocal Fold Paralysis after Esophagectomy for Carcinoma. *Otolaryngol Head Neck Surg.* 2016;155(1):122–126.

12. Itagaki T, Kikura M, Sato S. Incidence and risk factors of postoperative vocal cord paralysis in 987 patients after cardiovascular surgery. *Ann Thorac Surg.* 2007;83:2147–2152.

13. Widstrom A. Palsy of the recurrent nerve following mediastinoscopy. *Chest.* 1975;67:365–366.

14. Roberts JR, Wadsworth J. Recurrent laryngeal nerve monitoring during mediastinoscopy: predictors of injury. *Ann Thorac Surg.* 2007;83:388–391. Discussion 391–392.

15. Bando H, Nishio T, Bamba H, Uno T, Hisa Y. Vocal fold paralysis as a sign of chest diseases: a 15-year retrospective study. *World J Surg.* 2006;30:293–298.

16. Hardy JD, Webb WR, Timmis H, Watson DG, Blake TM. Patent ductus arteriosus: operative treatment of 100 consecutive patients with isolated lesions without mortality. *Ann Surg.* 1966;164:877–882.

17. Robinson LC, Winston KR. Relationship of vocal cord paralysis to the coil diameter of vagus nerve stimulator leads. *J Neurosurg.* 2015;122(3):532–535.

18. Sheahan P, O'Connor A, Murphy MS. Risk factors for recurrent laryngeal nerve neuropraxia postthyroidectomy. *Otolaryngol Head Neck Surg.* 2012;146(6):900–905.

19. Kandil E, Abdel Khalek M, Aslam R, Friedlander P, Bellows CF, Slakey D. Recurrent laryngeal nerve: significance of the anterior extralaryngeal branch. *Surgery.* 2011;149(6):820–824.

20. Franch-Arcas G, González-Sánchez C, Aguilera-Molina YY, Rozo-Coronel O, Estévez-Alonso JS, Muñoz-Herrera Á. Is there a case for selective, rather than routine, preoperative laryngoscopy in thyroid surgery? *Gland Surg.* 2015;4(1):8–18.

21. Kadakia S, Mourad M, Hu S, Brown R, Lee T, Ducic Y. Utility of intraoperative nerve monitoring in thyroid surgery: 20-year experience with 1418 cases. *Oral Maxillofac Surg.* 2017. http://dx.doi.org/10.1007/s10006-017-0637-y.

22. Bergenfelz A, Salem AF, Jacobsson H, Nordenström E, Almquist M, Steering Committee for the Scandinavian Quality Register for Thyroid, Parathyroid and Adrenal Surgery (SQRTPA). Risk of recurrent laryngeal nerve palsy in patients undergoing thyroidectomy with and without intraoperative nerve monitoring. *Br J Surg.* 2016;103(13):1828–1838.

23. Yang S, Zhou L, Lu Z, Ma B, Ji Q, Wang Y. Systematic review with meta-analysis of intraoperative neuromonitoring during thyroidectomy. *Int J Surg.* 2017; 39:104–113.

24. Yoshioka K, Miyauchi A, Fukushima M, Kobayashi K, Kihara M, Miya A. Surgical methods and experiences of surgeons did not significantly affect the recovery in phonation following reconstruction of the recurrent laryngeal nerve. *World J Surg.* 2016;40(12):2948–2955.

25. Kikura M, Suzuki K, Itagaki T, Takada T, Sato S. Age and comorbidity as risk factors for vocal cord paralysis associated with tracheal intubation. *Br J Anaesth.* 2007;98:524–530.

26. Lowinger D, Benjamin B, Gadd L. Recurrent laryngeal nerve injury caused by a laryngeal mask airway. *Anaesth Intensiv Care.* 1999;27:202–205.

27. Fang TJ, Tam YY, Courey MS, Li HY, Chiang HC. Unilateral high vagal paralysis: relationship of the severity of swallowing disturbance and types of injuries. *Laryngoscope.* 2011;121:245–249.

28. Norris BK, Schweinfurth JM. Arytenoid dislocation: an analysis of the contemporary literature. *Laryngoscope.* 2011;121:142–146.

29. Leonetti JP, Collins SL, Jablokow V, Lewy R. Laryngeal chondrosarcoma as a late-appearing cause of "idiopathic" vocal cord paralysis. *Otolaryngol Head Neck Surg.* 1987; 97:391–395.

30. McCaffrey TV, Lipton RJ. Thyroid carcinoma invading the upper aerodigestive system. *Laryngoscope.* 1990;100: 824–830.

31. Coover LR. Permanent iatrogenic vocal cord paralysis after I-131 therapy: a case report and literature review. *Clin Nucl Med.* 2000;25:508–510.

32. Snyder S. Vocal cord paralysis after radioiodine therapy. *J Nucl Med.* 1978;19:975–976.

33. Stern Y, Marshak G, Shpitzer T, Segal K, Feinmesser R. Vocal cord palsy: possible late complication of radiotherapy for head and neck cancer. *Ann Otol Rhinol Laryngol.* 1995;104:294–296.

34. Westbrook KC, Ballantyne AJ, Eckles NE, Brown GR. Breast cancer and vocal cord paralysis. *South Med J.* 1974;67:805–807.

35. Crawley BK, Sulica L. Vocal fold paralysis as a delayed consequence of neck and chest radiotherapy. *Otolaryngol Head Neck Surg.* 2015;153(2):239–243.

36. Lau DP, Lo YL, Wee J, Tan NG, Low WK. Vocal fold paralysis following radiotherapy for nasopharyngeal carcinoma: laryngeal electromyography findings. *J Voice.* 2003;17:82–87.

37. Steele NP, Myssiorek D. West Nile virus induced vocal fold paralysis. *Laryngoscope.* 2006;116:494–496.

38. Chitose SI, Umeno H, Hamakawa S, Nakashima T, Shoji H. Unilateral associated laryngeal paralysis due to varicella-zoster virus: virus antibody testing and videofluoroscopic findings. *J Laryngol Otol.* 2008;122:170–176.

39. Schroeter V, Belz GG, Blenk H. Paralysis of recurrent laryngeal nerve in Lyme disease. *Lancet.* 1988;2:1245.

40. Gayathri Devi HJ, Mohan Rao KN, Prathima KM, Moideen R. Pulmonary mucormycosis presenting with vocal cord paralysis. *Respir Med Case Rep.* 2013;9:15–17.

41. Allen JE, Belafsky PC. Laryngeal coccidioidomycosis with vocal fold paralysis. *Ear Nose Throat J.* 2011;90(5):E1–E5.

42. Rabkin R. Paralysis of the larynx due to central nervous system syphilis. *Eye Ear Nose Throat Mon.* 1963;42:53.

43. Chijimatsu Y, Tajima J, Washizaki M, Homma H. Hoarseness as an initial manifestation of sarcoidosis. *Chest.* 1980;78:779–781.

44. Kraus A, Guerra-Bautista G. Laryngeal involvement as a presenting symptom of systemic lupus erythematosus. *Ann Rheum Dis.* 1990;49:421.

45. Flores-Suárez LF, Alba MA, Tona G. Severe microscopic polyangiitis with unilateral vocal cord paralysis as initial manifestation. *Colomb Med.* 2017;48(1):32–34.

46. Carpenter 3rd RJ, McDonald TJ, Howard Jr FM. The otolaryngologic presentation of myasthenia gravis. *Laryngoscope.* 1979;89:922–928.

47. Yoskovitch A, Kantor S. Cervical osteophytes presenting as unilateral vocal fold paralysis and dysphagia. *J Laryngol Otol.* 2001;115:422–424.

48. Kapoor J, Trinidade A, Mochloulis G, Mohamid W. Plasmacytoma of the atlas presenting as hoarseness: a rare cause of unilateral vocal fold palsy. *J Laryngol Otol.* 2012;126(8):870–872.

49. Rontal E, Rontal M, Wald J, Rontal D. Botulinum toxin injection in the treatment of vocal fold paralysis associated with multiple sclerosis: a case report. *J Voice.* 1999;13:274–279.

50. Naunheim MR, Plotkin SR, Franco RA, Song PC. Laryngeal manifestations of neurofibromatosis. *Otolaryngol Head Neck Surg.* 2016;154(3):494–497.

51. Polkey MI, Lyall RA, Green M, Nigel Leigh P, Moxham J. Expiratory muscle function in amyotrophic lateral sclerosis. *Am J Respir Crit Care Med.* 1998;158:734–741.

52. Holinger LD, Holinger PC, Holinger PH. Etiology of bilateral abductor vocal cord paralysis: a review of 389 cases. *Ann Otol Rhinol Laryngol.* 1976;85:428–436.

53. Plasse HM, Lieberman AN. Bilateral vocal cord paralysis in Parkinson's disease. *Arch Otolaryngol.* 1981;107:252–253.

54. Schechter GL, Kostianovsky M. Vocal cord paralysis in diabetes mellitus. *Trans Am Acad Ophthalmol Otolaryngol.* 1972;76:729–740.

55. Ahn TB, Cho JW, Jeon BS. Unusual neurological presentations of vitamin B(12) deficiency. *Eur J Neurol.* 2004;11:339–341.

56. Lerat J, Lacoste M, Prechoux J-M, et al. An uncommon case of dyspnea with unilateral laryngeal paralysis in acromegaly. *Auris Nasus Larynx.* 2016;43(1):105–107.

57. Burns BV, Shotton JC. Vocal fold palsy following vinca alkaloid treatment. *J Laryngol Otol.* 1998;112:485–487.

58. Kwon OJ, Park JJ, Kim JP, Woo SH. Vocal cord paralysis caused by stingray. *Eur Arch Otorhinolaryngol.* 2013; 270(12):3191–3194.

59. Titche LL. Causes of recurrent laryngeal nerve paralysis. *Arch Otolaryngol.* 1976;102:259–261.

60. Parnell FW, Brandenburg JH. Vocal cord paralysis. A review of 100 cases. *Laryngoscope.* 1970;80:1036–1045.

61. Maisel RH, Ogura JH. Evaluation and treatment of vocal cord paralysis. *Laryngoscope.* 1974;84:302–316.

62. Ramadan HH, Wax MK, Avery S. Outcome and changing cause of unilateral vocal cord paralysis. *Otolaryngol Head Neck Surg.* 1998;118:199–202.

63. Rosenthal LH, Benninger MS, Deeb RH. Vocal fold immobility: a longitudinal analysis of etiology over 20 years. *Laryngoscope.* 2007;117:1864–1870.

64. Spataro EA, Grindler DJ, Paniello RC. Etiology and time to presentation of unilateral vocal fold paralysis. *Otolaryngol Head Neck Surg.* 2014;151(2):286–293.

65. Takano S, Nito T, Tamaruya N, Kimura M, Tayama N. Single institutional analysis of trends over 45 years in etiology of vocal fold paralysis. *Auris Nasus Larynx.* 2012;39(6):597–600.

66. Cantarella G, Dejonckere P, Galli A, et al. A retrospective evaluation of the etiology of unilateral vocal fold paralysis over the last 25 years. *Eur Arch Otorhinolaryngol.* 2017;274(1):347–353.

67. El Badawey MR, Punekar S, Zammit-Maempel I. Prospective study to assess vocal cord palsy investigations. *Otolaryngol Head Neck Surg.* 2008;138:788–790.

68. Chen HC, Jen YM, Wang CH, Lee JC, Lin YS. Etiology of vocal cord paralysis. *ORL J Otorhinolaryngol Relat Spec.* 2007;69:167–171.

69. Furukawa M, Furukawa MK, Ooishi K. Statistical analysis of malignant tumors detected as the cause of vocal cord paralysis. *ORL J Otorhinolaryngol Relat Spec.* 1994;56:161–165.

70. Behkam R, Roberts KE, Bierhals AJ, et al. Aortic arch compliance and idiopathic unilateral vocal fold paralysis. *J Appl Physiol.* 2017. http://dx.doi.org/10.1152/japplphysiol.00239.2017.

71. Pei Y-C, Li H-Y, Chen C-L, Wong AMK, Huang P-C, Fang T-J. Disease characteristics and electromyographic findings of nonsurgery-related unilateral vocal fold paralysis. *Laryngoscope.* 2017;127(6):1381–1387.

72. Huppler EG, Schmidt HW, Devine KD, Gage RP. Ultimate outcome of patients with vocal-cord paralysis of undetermined cause. *Am Rev Tuberc.* 1956;73:52–60.

73. Sulica L. The natural history of idiopathic unilateral vocal fold paralysis: evidence and problems. *Laryngoscope.* 2008;118:1303–1307.

74. Brunner E, Friedrich G, Kiesler K, Chibidziura-Priesching J, Gugatschka M. Subjective breathing impairment in unilateral vocal fold paralysis. *Folia Phoniatr Logop.* 2011;63:142–146.

75. Francis DO, McKiever ME, Garrett CG, Jacobson B, Penson DF. Assessment of patient experience with unilateral vocal fold immobility: a preliminary study. *J Voice.* 2014;28(5):636–643.

76. Leder SB, Ross DA. Incidence of vocal fold immobility in patients with dysphagia. *Dysphagia.* 2005;20:163–167. Discussion 168–169.

77. Bhattacharyya N, Kotz T, Shapiro J. The effect of bolus consistency on dysphagia in unilateral vocal cord paralysis. *Otolaryngol Head Neck Surg.* 2003;129:632–636.

78. Domer AS, Leonard R, Belafsky PC. Pharyngeal weakness and upper esophageal sphincter opening in patients with unilateral vocal fold immobility. *Laryngoscope.* 2014;124(10):2371–2374.

79. McHorney CA, Ware Jr JE, Raczek AE. The MOS 36-item short-form health survey (SF-36): II. Psychometric and clinical tests of validity in measuring physical and mental health constructs. *Med Care.* 1993;31:247–263.

80. Jacobson BH, Johnson A, Grywalski C, et al. The voice handicap index (VHI): development and validation. *Am J Speech Lang Pathol.* 1997;6:66–70.

81. Gliklich RE, Glovsky RM, Montgomery WW. Validation of a vKoice outcome survey for unilateral vocal cord paralysis. *Otolaryngol Head Neck Surg.* 1999;120: 153–158.

82. Spector BC, Netterville JL, Billante C, Clary J, Reinisch L, Smith TL. Quality-of-life assessment in patients with unilateral vocal cord paralysis. *Otolaryngol Head Neck Surg.* 2001;125:176–182.

83. Hogikyan ND, Wodchis WP, Terrell JE, Bradford CR, Esclamado RM. Voice-related quality of life (V-RQOL) following type I thyroplasty for unilateral vocal fold paralysis. *J Voice.* 2000;14:378–386.

84. Billante CR, Spector B, Hudson M, Burkard K, Netterville JL. Voice outcome following thyroplasty in patients with cancer-related vocal fold paralysis. *Auris Nasus Larynx.* 2001;28:315–321.

85. Wang W, Chen D, Chen S, et al. Laryngeal reinnervation using ansa cervicalis for thyroid surgery-related unilateral vocal fold paralysis: a long-term outcome analysis of 237 cases. *PLoS One.* 2011;6:e19128.

86. Stojadinovic A, Henry LR, Howard RS, et al. Prospective trial of voice outcomes after thyroidectomy: evaluation of patient-reported and clinician-determined voice assessments in identifying postthyroidectomy dysphonia. *Surgery.* 2008;143:732–742.

87. Kreiman J, Gerratt BR, Ito M. When and why listeners disagree in voice quality assessment tasks. *J Acoust Soc Am.* 2007;122:2354–2364.

88. Kreiman J, Gerratt BR. Sources of listener disagreement in voice quality assessment. *J Acoust Soc Am.* 2000;108:1867–1876.

89. Kreiman J, Gerratt BR, Precoda K. Listener experience and perception of voice quality. *J Speech Hear Res.* 1990;33:103–115.

90. Eadie T, Sroka A, Wright DR, Merati A. Does knowledge of medical diagnosis bias auditory-perceptual judgments of dysphonia? *J Voice.* 2011;25:420–429.

91. Eadie TL, Kapsner M, Rosenzweig J, Waugh P, Hillel A, Merati A. The role of experience on judgments of dysphonia. *J Voice.* 2010;24:564–573.

92. Karnell MP, Melton SD, Childes JM, Coleman TC, Dailey SA, Hoffman HT. Reliability of clinician-based (GRBAS and CAPE-V) and patient-based (V-RQOL and IPVI) documentation of voice disorders. *J Voice.* 2007;21:576–590.

93. Behrman A. Evidence-based treatment of paralytic dysphonia: making sense of outcomes and efficacy data. *Otolaryngol Clin North Am.* 2004;37:75–104, vi.

94. Little MA, Costello DA, Harries ML. Objective dysphonia quantification in vocal fold paralysis: comparing nonlinear with classical measures. *J Voice.* 2011;25:21–31.

95. Colton RH, Paseman A, Kelley RT, Stepp D, Casper JK. Spectral moment analysis of unilateral vocal fold paralysis. *J Voice.* 2011;25:330–336.

96. Balasubramanium RK, Bhat JS, Fahim 3rd S, Raju 3rd R. Cepstral analysis of voice in unilateral adductor vocal fold palsy. *J Voice.* 2011;25:326–329.

97. Peterson EA, Roy N, Awan SN, Merrill RM, Banks R, Tanner K. Toward validation of the cepstral spectral index of dysphonia (CSID) as an objective treatment outcomes measure. *J Voice.* 2013;27(4):401–410.

98. Dastolfo C, Gartner-Schmidt J, Yu L, Carnes O, Gillespie AI. Aerodynamic outcomes of four common voice disorders: moving toward disorder-specific assessment. *J Voice.* 2015. http://dx.doi.org/10.1016/j.jvoice.2015.03.017.

99. Sinclair CF, Bumpous JM, Haugen BR, et al. Laryngeal examination in thyroid and parathyroid surgery: an American Head and Neck Society consensus statement: AHNS consensus statement. *Head Neck.* 2016;38(6):811–819.

100. Madden LL, Rosen CA. Evaluation of vocal fold motion abnormalities: are we all seeing the same thing? *J Voice.* 2017;31(1):72–77.

101. Rosen CA, Mau T, Remacle M, et al. Nomenclature proposal to describe vocal fold motion impairment. *Eur Arch Otorhinolaryngol.* 2016;273(8):1995–1999.

102. Woodson GE. Configuration of the glottis in laryngeal paralysis. I: clinical study. *Laryngoscope.* 1993;103:1227–1234.

103. Menon JKR, Nair RM, Priyanka S. Unilateral vocal fold paralysis: can laryngoscopy predict recovery? A prospective study. *J Laryngol Otol.* 2014;128(12): 1095–1104.

104. Hiramatsu H, Tokashiki R, Nakamura M, Motohashi R, Yoshida T, Suzuki M. Characterization of arytenoid vertical displacement in unilateral vocal fold paralysis by three-dimensional computed tomography. *Eur Arch Otorhinolaryngol.* 2009;266:97–104.

105. Steffen N, Vieira VP, Yazaki RK, Pontes P. Modifications of vestibular fold shape from respiration to phonation in unilateral vocal fold paralysis. *J Voice.* 2011;25:111–113.

106. Harries ML, Morrison M. The role of stroboscopy in the management of a patient with a unilateral vocal fold paralysis. *J Laryngol Otol.* 1996;110:141–143.

107. de Miguel M, Peláez EM, Caubet E, González Ó, Velasco M, Rigual L. Accuracy of transcutaneous laryngeal ultrasound for detecting vocal cord paralysis in the immediate postoperative period after total thyroidectomy. *Minerva Anestesiol.* june 2017. http://dx.doi.org/10.23736/S0375-9393.17.11755-4.

108. Kandil E, Deniwar A, Noureldine SI, et al. Assessment of vocal fold function using transcutaneous laryngeal ultrasonography and flexible laryngoscopy. *JAMA Otolaryngol Head Neck Surg.* 2016;142(1):74–78.

109. Woo J-W, Suh H, Song R-Y, et al. A novel lateral-approach laryngeal ultrasonography for vocal cord evaluation. *Surgery.* 2016;159(1):52–56.

110. Carneiro-Pla D, Miller BS, Wilhelm SM, et al. Feasibility of surgeon-performed transcutaneous vocal cord ultrasonography in identifying vocal cord mobility: a multi-institutional experience. *Surgery.* 2014;156(6):1597–1602. Discussion 1602–1604.

111. Merati AL, Halum SL, Smith TL. Diagnostic testing for vocal fold paralysis: survey of practice and evidence-based medicine review. *Laryngoscope.* 2006;116:1539–1552.

112. Song SW, Jun BC, Cho KJ, Lee S, Kim YJ, Park SH. CT evaluation of vocal cord paralysis due to thoracic diseases: a 10-year retrospective study. *Yonsei Med J.* 2011;52:831–837.

113. Glazer HS, Aronberg DJ, Lee JK, Sagel SS. Extralaryngeal causes of vocal cord paralysis: CT evaluation. *Am J Roentgenol.* 1983;141:527–531.

114. Liu AY, Yousem DM, Chalian AA, Langlotz CP. Economic consequences of diagnostic imaging for vocal cord paralysis. *Acad Radiol.* 2001;8:137–148.

115. Altman JS, Benninger MS. The evaluation of unilateral vocal fold immobility: is chest X-ray enough? *J Voice.* 1997;11:364–367.

116. Hojjat H, Svider PF, Folbe AJ, et al. Cost-effectiveness of routine computed tomography in the evaluation of idiopathic unilateral vocal fold paralysis. *Laryngoscope.* 2017;127(2):440–444.

117. Noel JE, Jeffery CC, Damrose E. Repeat imaging in idiopathic unilateral vocal fold paralysis: is it necessary? *Ann Otol Rhinol Laryngol.* 2016;125(12):1010–1014.

118. Tsikoudas A, Paleri V, El-Badawey MR, Zammit-Maempel I. Recommendations on follow-up strategies for idiopathic vocal fold paralysis: evidence-based review. *J Laryngol Otol.* 2012;126(6):570–573.

119. Chen DW, Young A, Donovan DT, Ongkasuwan J. Routine computed tomography in the evaluation of vocal fold movement impairment without an apparent cause. *Otolaryngol Head Neck Surg.* 2015;152(2):308–313.

120. Wang CP, Chen TC, Lou PJ, et al. Neck ultrasonography for the evaluation of the etiology of adult unilateral vocal fold paralysis. *Head Neck.* 2011. http://dx.doi.org/10.1002/hed.21794.

121. Heller MT, Meltzer CC, Fukui MB, et al. Superphysiologic FDG uptake in the non-paralyzed vocal cord. Resolution of a false-positive PET result with combined PET-CT imaging. *Clin Positron Imaging.* 2000;3:207–211.

122. Kamel EM, Goerres GW, Burger C, von Schulthess GK, Steinert HC. Recurrent laryngeal nerve palsy in patients with lung cancer: detection with PET-CT image fusion – report of six cases. *Radiology.* 2002;224:153–156.

123. Yeretsian RA, Blodgett TM, Branstetter 4th BF, Roberts MM, Meltzer CC. Teflon-induced granuloma: a false-positive finding with PET resolved with combined PET and CT. *Am J Neuroradiol.* 2003;24:1164–1166.

124. Tessonnier L, Fakhry N, Taieb D, Giovanni A, Mundler O. False-positive finding on FDG-PET/CT after injectable elastomere implant (Vox implant) for vocal cord paralysis. *Otolaryngol Head Neck Surg.* 2008;139:738–739.

125. Hall EJ, Brenner DJ. Cancer risks from diagnostic radiology. *Br J Radiol.* 2008;81:362–378.

126. White M, Meenan K, Patel T, Jaworek A, Sataloff RT. Laboratory evaluation of vocal fold paralysis and paresis. *J Voice.* 2017;31(2):168–174.

127. Rickert SM, Childs LF, Carey BT, Murry T, Sulica L. Laryngeal electromyography for prognosis of vocal fold palsy: a meta-analysis. *Laryngoscope.* 2012;122:158–161.

128. Statham MM, Rosen CA, Nandedkar SD, Munin MC. Quantitative laryngeal electromyography: turns and amplitude analysis. *Laryngoscope.* 2010;120:2036–2041.

129. Statham MM, Rosen CA, Smith LJ, Munin MC. Electromyographic laryngeal synkinesis alters prognosis in vocal fold paralysis. *Laryngoscope.* 2010;120:285–290.

130. Munin MC, Heman-Ackah YD, Rosen CA, et al. Consensus statement: using laryngeal electromyography for the diagnosis and treatment of vocal cord paralysis. *Muscle Nerve.* 2016;53(6):850–855.

131. Young VN, Smith LJ, Rosen C. Voice outcome following acute unilateral vocal fold paralysis. *Ann Otol Rhinol Laryngol.* 2013;122(3):197–204.

132. Mau T, Pan H-M, Childs LF. The natural history of recoverable vocal fold paralysis: implications for kinetics of reinnervation. *Laryngoscope.* 2017. http://dx.doi.org/10.1002/lary.26734.

133. Peterson KL, Fenn J. Treatment of dysphagia and dysphonia following skull base surgery. *Otolaryngol Clin North Am.* 2005;38. 809–817, xi.

134. D'Alatri L, Galla S, Rigante M, Antonelli O, Buldrini S, Marchese MR. Role of early voice therapy in patients affected by unilateral vocal fold paralysis. *J Laryngol Otol.* 2008;122:936–941.

135. Heuer RJ, Thayer Sataloff R, Emerich K, et al. Unilateral recurrent laryngeal nerve paralysis: the importance of "preoperative" voice therapy. *J Voice.* 1997;11:88–94.

136. Busto-Crespo O, Uzcanga-Lacabe M, Abad-Marco A, et al. Longitudinal voice outcomes after voice therapy in unilateral vocal fold paralysis. *J Voice.* 2016;30(6):767. e9-e767.e15.

137. Kao Y-C, Chen S-H, Wang Y-T, Chu P-Y, Tan C-T, Chang W-ZD. Efficacy of voice therapy for patients with early unilateral adductor vocal fold paralysis. *J Voice.* 2017. http://dx.doi.org/10.1016/j.jvoice.2017.01.007.

138. Mattioli F, Bergamini G, Alicandri-Ciufelli M, et al. The role of early voice therapy in the incidence of motility recovery in unilateral vocal fold paralysis. *Logop Phoniatr Vocal.* 2011;36:40–47.

139. Kelchner LN, Stemple JC, Gerdeman E, Le Borgne W, Adam S. Etiology, pathophysiology, treatment choices, and voice results for unilateral adductor vocal fold paralysis: a 3-year retrospective. *J Voice.* 1999;13:592–601.

140. Schindler A, Bottero A, Capaccio P, Ginocchio D, Adorni F, Ottaviani F. Vocal improvement after voice therapy in unilateral vocal fold paralysis. *J Voice.* 2008;22:113–118.

141. Walton C, Conway E, Blackshaw H, Carding P. Unilateral vocal fold paralysis: a systematic review of speech-language pathology management. *J Voice.* 2017;31(4): 509.e7–e509.e22.

142. Cates DJ, Venkatesan NN, Strong B, Kuhn MA, Belafsky PC. Effect of vocal fold medialization on dysphagia in patients with unilateral vocal fold immobility. *Otolaryngol Head Neck Surg.* 2016;155(3):454–457.

143. Kupfer RA, Merati AL, Sulica L. Medialization laryngoplasty for odynophonia. *JAMA Otolaryngol Head Neck Surg.* 2015;141(6):556–561.

144. Crumley RL. Selective reinnervation of vocal cord adductors in unilateral vocal cord paralysis. *Ann Otol Rhinol Laryngol.* 1984;93:351–356.

145. Gacek M, Gacek RR. Cricoarytenoid joint mobility after chronic vocal cord paralysis. *Laryngoscope.* 1996;106:1528–1530.

146. Colman MF, Schwartz I. The effect of vocal cord paralysis on the cricoarytenoid joint. *Otolaryngol Head Neck Surg.* 1981;89:419–422.

147. Sulica L, Rosen CA, Postma GN, et al. Current practice in injection augmentation of the vocal folds: indications, treatment principles, techniques, and complications. *Laryngoscope.* 2010;120:319–325.

148. Rosow DE. Trends in utilization of vocal fold injection procedures. *Otolaryngol Head Neck Surg.* 2015;153(5):812–814.

149. Mau T, Weinheimer KT. Three-dimensional arytenoid movement induced by vocal fold injections. *Laryngoscope.* 2010;120:1563–1568.

150. Shin JL, Hartnick CJ, Randolph GW. *Evidence-Based Otolaryngology.* New York, NY: Springer; 2008.

151. Zeleník K, Walderová R, Kučová H, Jančatová D, Komínek P. Comparison of long-term voice outcomes after vocal fold augmentation using autologous fat injection by direct microlaryngoscopy versus office-based calcium hydroxylapatite injection. *Eur Arch Otorhinolaryngol.* 2017;274(8):3147–3151.

152. Dedo HH, Carlsoo B. Histologic evaluation of Teflon granulomas of human vocal cords. A light and electron microscopic study. *Acta Otolaryngol.* 1982;93:475–484.

153. Ossoff RH, Koriwchak MJ, Netterville JL, Duncavage JA. Difficulties in endoscopic removal of Teflon granulomas of the vocal fold. *Ann Otol Rhinol Laryngol.* 1993;102:405–412.

154. Nakayama M, Ford CN, Bless DM. Teflon vocal fold augmentation: failures and management in 28 cases. *Otolaryngol Head Neck Surg.* 1993;109:493–498.

155. Kasperbauer JL, Slavit DH, Maragos NE. Teflon granulomas and overinjection of Teflon: a therapeutic challenge for the otorhinolaryngologist. *Ann Otol Rhinol Laryngol.* 1993;102:748–751.

156. O'Leary MA, Grillone GA. Injection laryngoplasty. *Otolaryngol Clin North Am.* 2006;39:43–54.

157. Lau DP, Lee GA, Wong SM, et al. Injection laryngoplasty with hyaluronic acid for unilateral vocal cord paralysis. Randomized controlled trial comparing two different particle sizes. *J Voice.* 2010;24:113–118.

158. Rosen CA, Gartner-Schmidt J, Casiano R, et al. Vocal fold augmentation with calcium hydroxylapatite: twelve-month report. *Laryngoscope.* 2009;119:1033–1041.

159. Kwon TK, Rosen CA, Gartner-Schmidt J. Preliminary results of a new temporary vocal fold injection material. *J Voice.* 2005;19:668–673.

160. Milstein CF, Akst LM, Hicks MD, Abelson TI, Strome M. Long-term effects of micronized Alloderm injection for unilateral vocal fold paralysis. *Laryngoscope.* 2005;115:1691–1696.

161. Tan M, Woo P. Injection laryngoplasty with micronized dermis: a 10-year experience with 381 injections in 344 patients. *Laryngoscope.* 2010;120:2460–2466.

162. Mikaelian DO, Lowry LD, Sataloff RT. Lipoinjection for unilateral vocal cord paralysis. *Laryngoscope.* 1991;101:465–468.

163. McCulloch TM, Andrews BT, Hoffman HT, Graham SM, Karnell MP, Minnick C. Long-term follow-up of fat injection laryngoplasty for unilateral vocal cord paralysis. *Laryngoscope.* 2002;112:1235–1238.

164. Dermal Fillers Cost. American Society of Plastic Surgeons. https://www.plasticsurgery.org/cosmetic-procedures/dermal-fillers/cost.

165. Madden LL, Ward J, Ward A, et al. A cardiovascular prescreening protocol for unmonitored in-office laryngology procedures. *Laryngoscope.* 2017;127(8):1845–1849.

166. Hillel AT, Ochsner MC, Johns 3rd MM, Klein AM. A cost and time analysis of laryngology procedures in the endoscopy suite versus the operating room. *Laryngoscope.* 2016;126(6):1385–1389.

167. Lakhani R, Fishman JM, Bleach N, Costello D, Birchall M. Alternative injectable materials for vocal fold medialisation in unilateral vocal fold paralysis. *Cochrane Database Syst Rev.* 2012;10:CD009239.

168. Anderson TD, Sataloff RT. Complications of collagen injection of the vocal fold: report of several unusual cases and review of the literature. *J Voice.* 2004;18:392–397.

169. Ford CN, Bless DM. Clinical experience with injectable collagen for vocal fold augmentation. *Laryngoscope.* 1986;96:863–869.

170. Cohen JC, Reisacher W, Malone M, Sulica L. Severe systemic reaction from calcium hydroxylapatite vocal fold filler. *Laryngoscope.* 2013;123(9):2237–2239.

171. Upton DC, Johnson M, Zelazny SK, Dailey SH. Prospective evaluation of office-based injection laryngoplasty with hyaluronic acid gel. *Ann Otol Rhinol Laryngol.* 2013;122(9):541–546.

172. Bock JM, Lee JH, Robinson RA, Hoffman HT. Migration of Cymetra after vocal fold injection for laryngeal paralysis. *Laryngoscope.* 2007;117:2251–2254.

173. Zapanta PE, Bielamowicz SA. Laryngeal abscess after injection laryngoplasty with micronized AlloDerm. *Laryngoscope.* 2004;114:1522–1524.

174. Young VN, Wijewickrama RC, Pizzuto MA, Rosen CA. An unusual complication of vocal fold lipoinjection: case report and review of the literature. *Arch Otolaryngol Head Neck Surg.* 2012;138(4):418–420.

175. Shamanna SG, Bosch JD. Injection laryngoplasty: a serious reaction to hyaluronic acid. *J Otolaryngol Head Neck Surg.* 2011;40(5):E39–E42.

176. Barbu AM, Gniady JP, Vivero RJ, Friedman AD, Burns JA. Bedside injection medialization laryngoplasty in immediate postoperative patients. *Otolaryngol Head Neck Surg.* 2015;153(6):1007–1012.

177. Gadkaree SK, Best SRA, Walker C, Akst LM, Hillel AT. Patient tolerance of transoral versus percutaneous thyrohyoid office-based injection laryngoplasty: a case-controlled study of forty-one patients. *Clin Otolaryngol.* 2015;40(6):717–721.

178. Jayaram SC, Costello D. Technical tip for difficult injection laryngoplasty: the use of a hypodermic needle as a retractor. *Laryngoscope.* 2015;125(9):2157–2158.

179. Clary MS, Milam BM, Courey MS. Office-based vocal fold injection with the laryngeal introducer technique. *Laryngoscope.* 2014;124(9):2114–2117.

180. Chhetri DK, Jamal N. Percutaneous injection laryngoplasty. *Laryngoscope.* 2014;124(3):742–745.

181. Achkar J, Song P, Andrus J, Franco Jr R. Double-bend needle modification for transthyrohyoid vocal fold injection. *Laryngoscope.* 2012;122(4):865–867.

182. Amin MR. Thyrohyoid approach for vocal fold augmentation. *Ann Otol Rhinol Laryngol.* 2006;115: 699–702.

183. Mayerhoff RM, Kuo C, Meyer T. A novel approach to the challenging injection laryngoplasty. *Ann Otol Rhinol Laryngol.* 2016;125(5):415–420.

184. Jamal N, Mundi J, Chhetri DK. Higher risk of superficial injection during injection laryngoplasty in women. *Am J Otolaryngol.* 2014;35(2):159–163.

185. Arviso LC, Johns 3rd MM, Mathison CC, Klein AM. Long-term outcomes of injection laryngoplasty in patients with potentially recoverable vocal fold paralysis. *Laryngoscope.* 2010;120:2237–2240.

186. Bhattacharyya N, Batirel H, Swanson SJ. Improved outcomes with early vocal fold medialization for vocal fold paralysis after thoracic surgery. *Auris Nasus Larynx.* 2003;30:71–75.

187. Friedman AD, Burns JA, Heaton JT, Zeitels SM. Early versus late injection medialization for unilateral vocal cord paralysis. *Laryngoscope.* 2010;120:2042–2046.

188. Alghonaim Y, Roskies M, Kost K, Young J. Evaluating the timing of injection laryngoplasty for vocal fold paralysis in an attempt to avoid future type 1 thyroplasty. *J Otolaryngol Head Neck Surg.* 2013;42:24.

189. Yung KC, Likhterov I, Courey MS. Effect of temporary vocal fold injection medialization on the rate of permanent medialization laryngoplasty in unilateral vocal fold paralysis patients. *Laryngoscope.* 2011;121:2191–2194.

190. Francis DO, Williamson K, Hovis K, et al. Effect of injection augmentation on need for framework surgery in unilateral vocal fold paralysis. *Laryngoscope.* 2015. http://dx.doi.org/10.1002/lary.25431.

190a. Pei Y-C, Fang T-J, Hsin L-J, Li H-Y, Wong AM. Early hyaluronate injection improves quality of life but not neural recovery in unilateral vocal fold paralysis: an open-label randomized controlled study. *Restor Neurol Neurosci.* 2015;33(2):121–130.

191. Mor N, Wu G, Aylward A, Christos PJ, Sulica L. Predictors for permanent medialization laryngoplasty in unilateral vocal fold paralysis. *Otolaryngol Head Neck Surg.* 2016;155(3):443–453.

192. Mattioli F, Bettini M, Botti C, et al. Polydimethylsiloxane injection laryngoplasty for unilateral vocal fold paralysis: long-term results. *J Voice.* 2017;31(4):517. e1-e517.e7.

193. Lim Y-S, Lee YS, Lee J-C, et al. Intracordal auricular cartilage injection for unilateral vocal fold paralysis. *J Biomed Mater Res B Appl Biomater.* 2015;103(1):47–51.

194. Kanazawa T, Kurakami K, Kashima K, et al. Injection of basic fibroblast growth factor for unilateral vocal cord paralysis. *Acta Otolaryngol.* 2017;137(9):962–967.

195. Payr E. Plastik am Schildknorpel zur Behebung der Folgen einseitiger Stimmbanclahmung. *Dtsch Med Wochenschr.* 1915;43:1265–1270.

196. Isshiki N, Okamura H, Ishikawa T. Thyroplasty type I (lateral compression) for dysphonia due to vocal cord paralysis or atrophy. *Acta Otolaryngol.* 1975;80:465–473.

197. Isshiki N, Taira T, Kojima H, Shoji K. Recent modifications in thyroplasty type I. *Ann Otol Rhinol Laryngol.* 1989;98:777–779.

198. Zhao X, Roth K, Fung K. Type I thyroplasty: risk stratification approach to inpatient versus outpatient postoperative management. *J Otolaryngol Head Neck Surg.* 2010;39:757–761.

199. Bray D, Young JP, Harries ML. Complications after type one thyroplasty: is day-case surgery feasible? *J Laryngol Otol.* 2008;122:715–718.

200. Young VN, Zullo TG, Rosen CA. Analysis of laryngeal framework surgery: 10-year follow-up to a national survey. *Laryngoscope.* 2010;120:1602–1608.

201. van Ardenne N, Vanderwegen J, Van Nuffelen G, De Bodt M, Van de Heyning P. Medialization thyroplasty: vocal outcome of silicone and titanium implant. *Eur Arch Otorhinolaryngol.* 2011;268:101–107.

202. Storck C, Fischer C, Cecon M, et al. Hydroxyapatite versus titanium implant: comparison of the functional outcome after vocal fold medialization in unilateral recurrent nerve paralysis. *Head Neck.* 2010;32:1605–1612.

203. Schneider-Stickler B, Gaechter J, Bigenzahn W. Long-term results after external vocal fold medialization thyroplasty with titanium vocal fold medialization implant (TVFMI). *Eur Arch Otorhinolaryngol.* 2013;270(5):1689–1694.

204. Mesallam TA, Khalil YA, Malki KH, Farahat M. Medialization thyroplasty using autologous nasal septal cartilage for treating unilateral vocal fold paralysis. *Clin Exp Otorhinolaryngol.* 2011;4(3):142–148.

205. Lundy DS, Casiano RR, Xue JW. Can maximum phonation time predict voice outcome after thyroplasty type I? *Laryngoscope.* 2004;114:1447–1454.

206. Isshiki N, Tanabe M, Sawada M. Arytenoid adduction for unilateral vocal cord paralysis. *Arch Otolaryngol.* 1978;104:555–558.

207. Zeitels SM, Hochman I, Hillman RE. Adduction aryten-opexy: a new procedure for paralytic dysphonia with implications for implant medialization. *Ann Otol Rhinol Laryngol Suppl.* 1998;173:2–24.
208. Thakar A, Sikka K, Verma R, Preetam C. Cricothyroid approximation for voice and swallowing rehabilitation of high vagal paralysis secondary to skull base neo-plasms. *Eur Arch Otorhinolaryngol.* 2011. http://dx.doi.org/10.1007/s00405-011-1614-y.
209. Li AJ, Johns MM, Jackson-Menaldi C, et al. Glottic clo-sure patterns: type I thyroplasty versus type I thyroplasty with arytenoid adduction. *J Voice.* 2011;25:259–264.
210. Franco RA, Andrus JG. Aerodynamic and acoustic char-acteristics of voice before and after adduction aryten-opexy and medialization laryngoplasty with GORE-TEX in patients with unilateral vocal fold immobility. *J Voice.* 2009;23:261–267.
211. McNamar J, Montequin DW, Welham NV, Dailey SH. Aerodynamic, acoustic, and vibratory comparison of ar-ytenoid adduction and adduction arytenopexy. *Laryngo-scope.* 2008;118:552–558.
212. Abraham MT, Gonen M, Kraus DH. Complications of type I thyroplasty and arytenoid adduction. *Laryngoscope.* 2001;111:1322–1329.
213. Rosow DE, Al-Bar MH. Type I thyroplasty in previously irradiated patients: assessing safety and efficacy. *Otolar-yngol Head Neck Surg.* 2015;153(4):582–585.
214. White JR, Orbelo DM, Noel DB, Pittelko RL, Maragos NE, Ekbom DC. Thyroplasty in the previously irradiated neck: a case series and short-term outcomes. *Laryngo-scope.* 2016;126(8):1849–1853.
215. Senkal HA, Yilmaz T. Type I thyroplasty revision 1 year after a window was mistakenly created on the cricoid cartilage. *Ear Nose Throat J.* 2010;89:E14–E16.
216. Benscoter BJ, Akst LM. Saccular cyst as a complication of medialization laryngoplasty: a case report. *Ear Nose Throat J.* 2014;93(8):E1–E3.
217. Woo P, Pearl AW, Hsiung MW, Som P. Failed mediali-zation laryngoplasty: management by revision surgery. *Otolaryngol Head Neck Surg.* 2001;124:615–621.
218. Parker NP, Barbu AM, Hillman RE, Zeitels SM, Burns JA. Revision transcervical medialization laryngoplasty for unilateral vocal fold paralysis. *Otolaryngol Head Neck Surg.* 2015;153(4):593–598.
219. Iwahashi T, Ogawa M, Hosokawa K, Mochizuki R, Inohara H. Computed tomographic assessment of the causal factors of unsuccessful medialization thyroplasty. *Acta Otolaryngol.* 2015;135(3):283–289.
220. Rosen CA. Complications of phonosurgery: results of a national survey. *Laryngoscope.* 1998;108:1697–1703.
221. Paniello RC, Dahm JD. Reversibility of medialization laryngoplasty. An experimental study. *Ann Otol Rhinol Laryngol.* 1997;106:902–908.
222. Sasaki CT, Leder SB, Petcu L, Friedman CD. Longitudi-nal voice quality changes following Isshiki thyroplasty type I: the Yale experience. *Laryngoscope.* 1990;100:849–852.
223. Leder SB, Sasaki CT. Long-term changes in vocal qual-ity following Isshiki thyroplasty type I. *Laryngoscope.* 1994;104:275–277.
224. Netterville JL, Stone RE, Luken ES, Civantos FJ, Os-soff RH. Silastic medialization and arytenoid ad-duction: the Vanderbilt experience. A review of 116 phonosurgical procedures. *Ann Otol Rhinol Laryngol.* 1993;102:413–424.
225. Billante CR, Clary J, Childs P, Netterville JL. Voice gains following thyroplasty may improve over time. *Clin Oto-laryngol Allied Sci.* 2002;27:89–94.
226. Lundy DS, Casiano RR, Xue JW, Lu FL. Thyroplasty type I: short- versus long-term results. *Otolaryngol Head Neck Surg.* 2000;122:533–536.
227. Ryu IS, Nam SY, Han MW, Choi S-H, Kim SY, Roh J-L. Long-term voice outcomes after thyroplasty for unilat-eral vocal fold paralysis. *Arch Otolaryngol Head Neck Surg.* 2012;138(4):347–351.
228. Gray SD, Barkmeier J, Jones D, Titze I, Druker D. Vo-cal evaluation of thyroplastic surgery in the treat-ment of unilateral vocal fold paralysis. *Laryngoscope.* 1992;102:415–421.
229. Dejonckere PH. Teflon injection and thyroplasty: objec-tive and subjective outcomes. *Rev Laryngol Otol Rhinol.* 1998;119:265–269.
230. Lundy DS, Casiano RR, McClinton ME, Xue JW. Early results of transcutaneous injection laryngoplasty with micronized acellular dermis versus type-I thyroplasty for glottic incompetence dysphonia due to unilateral vocal fold paralysis. *J Voice.* 2003;17:589–595.
231. Morgan JE, Zraick RI, Griffin AW, Bowen TL, Johnson FL. Injection versus medialization laryngoplasty for the treatment of unilateral vocal fold paralysis. *Laryngoscope.* 2007;117:2068–2074.
232. Tsuzuki T, Fukuda H, Fujioka T, Takayama E, Kawaida M. Voice prognosis after liquid and solid silicone injection. *Am J Otolaryngol.* 1991;12:165–169.
233. D'Antonio LL, Wigley TL, Zimmerman GJ. Quan-titative measures of laryngeal function following Teflon injection or thyroplasty type I. *Laryngoscope.* 1995;105:256–262.
234. Vinson KN, Zraick RI, Ragland FJ. Injection versus me-dialization laryngoplasty for the treatment of unilateral vocal fold paralysis: follow-up at six months. *Laryngo-scope.* 2010;120:1802–1807.
235. Shen T, Damrose EJ, Morzaria S. A meta-analysis of voice outcome comparing calcium hydroxylapatite injection laryngoplasty to silicone thyroplasty. *Otolaryngol Head Neck Surg.* 2013;148(2):197–208.
236. Umeno H, Chitose S-I, Sato K, Ueda Y, Nakashima T. Long-term postoperative vocal function after thyroplasty type I and fat injection laryngoplasty. *Ann Otol Rhinol Laryngol.* 2012;121(3):185–191.
237. Tam S, Sun H, Sarma S, Siu J, Fung K, Sowerby L. Me-dialization thyroplasty versus injection laryngoplasty: a cost minimization analysis. *J Otolaryngol Head Neck Surg.* 2017;46(1):14.

238. Bhattacharyya N, Kotz T, Shapiro J. Dysphagia and aspiration with unilateral vocal cord immobility: incidence, characterization, and response to surgical treatment. *Ann Otol Rhinol Laryngol.* 2002;111:672–679.

239. Nayak VK, Bhattacharyya N, Kotz T, Shapiro J. Patterns of swallowing failure following medialization in unilateral vocal fold immobility. *Laryngoscope.* 2002;112: 1840–1844.

240. Hoffman MR, Witt RE, Chapin WJ, McCulloch TM, Jiang JJ. Multiparameter comparison of injection laryngoplasty, medialization laryngoplasty, and arytenoid adduction in an excised larynx model. *Laryngoscope.* 2010;120:769–776.

241. McCulloch TM, Hoffman HT, Andrews BT, Karnell MP. Arytenoid adduction combined with Gore-Tex medialization thyroplasty. *Laryngoscope.* 2000;110:1306–1311.

242. Thompson DM, Maragos NE, Edwards BW. The study of vocal fold vibratory patterns in patients with unilateral vocal fold paralysis before and after type I thyroplasty with or without arytenoid adduction. *Laryngoscope.* 1995;105:481–486.

243. Mortensen M, Carroll L, Woo P. Arytenoid adduction with medialization laryngoplasty versus injection or medialization laryngoplasty: the role of the arytenoidopexy. *Laryngoscope.* 2009;119:827–831.

244. Tucker HM. Reinnervation of the paralyzed larynx: a review. *Head Neck Surg.* 1979;1:235–242.

245. Paniello RC, Lee P, Dahm JD. Hypoglossal nerve transfer for laryngeal reinnervation: a preliminary study. *Ann Otol Rhinol Laryngol.* 1999;108:239–244.

246. Tucker HM, Rusnov M. Laryngeal reinnervation for unilateral vocal cord paralysis: long-term results. *Ann Otol Rhinol Laryngol.* 1981;90:457–459.

247. Tucker HM. Long-term results of nerve-muscle pedicle reinnervation for laryngeal paralysis. *Ann Otol Rhinol Laryngol.* 1989;98:674–676.

248. Goding Jr GS. Nerve-muscle pedicle reinnervation of the paralyzed vocal cord. *Otolaryngol Clin North Am.* 1991;24:1239–1252.

249. Hassan MM, Yumoto E, Baraka MA, Sanuki T, Kodama N. Arytenoid rotation and nerve-muscle pedicle transfer in paralytic dysphonia. *Laryngoscope.* 2011;121:1018–1022.

250. Yumoto E, Sanuki T, Toya Y, Kodama N, Kumai Y. Nerve-muscle pedicle flap implantation combined with arytenoid adduction. *Arch Otolaryngol Head Neck Surg.* 2010;136:965–969.

251. Chhetri DK, Gerratt BR, Kreiman J, Berke GS. Combined arytenoid adduction and laryngeal reinnervation in the treatment of vocal fold paralysis. *Laryngoscope.* 1999;109:1928–1936.

252. Woo P, Mangaro M. Aberrant recurrent laryngeal nerve reinnervation as a cause of stridor and laryngospasm. *Ann Otol Rhinol Laryngol.* 2004;113:805–808.

253. Maronian NC, Robinson L, Waugh P, Hillel AD. A new electromyographic definition of laryngeal synkinesis. *Ann Otol Rhinol Laryngol.* 2004;113:877–886.

254. Crumley RL. Laryngeal synkinesis revisited. *Ann Otol Rhinol Laryngol.* 2000;109:365–371.

255. Tucker HM. Long-term preservation of voice improvement following surgical medialization and reinnervation for unilateral vocal fold paralysis. *J Voice.* 1999;13:251–256.

256. Paniello RC, Edgar JD, Kallogjeri D, Piccirillo JF. Medialization versus reinnervation for unilateral vocal fold paralysis: a multicenter randomized clinical trial. *Laryngoscope.* 2011;121:2172–2179.

257. Mat Baki M, Yu R, Rubin JS, Chevretton E, Sandhu G, Birchall MA. Patient perception of a randomised, controlled trial of laryngeal reinnervation versus thyroplasty for unilateral vocal fold paralysis. *J Laryngol Otol.* 2015;129(7):693–701.

258. Siu J, Tam S, Fung K. A comparison of outcomes in interventions for unilateral vocal fold paralysis: a systematic review. *Laryngoscope.* 2016;126(7):1616–1624.

259. Jiang W, Zheng X, Xue Q. Computational modeling of fluid-structure-acoustics interaction during voice production. *Front Bioeng Biotechnol.* 2017;5:7.

260. Samlan RA, Story BH. Influence of left-right asymmetries on voice quality in simulated paramedian vocal fold paralysis. *J Speech Lang Hear Res.* 2017;60(2):306–321.

261. Paniello RC. Synkinesis following recurrent laryngeal nerve injury: a computer simulation. *Laryngoscope.* 2016;126(7):1600–1605.

262. Oren L, Khosla S, Gutmark E. Effect of vocal fold asymmetries on glottal flow. *Laryngoscope.* 2016;126(11): 2534–2538.

263. Mittal R, Zheng X, Bhardwaj R, Seo JH, Xue Q, Bielamowicz S. Toward a simulation-based tool for the treatment of vocal fold paralysis. *Front Physiol.* 2011;2:19.

264. Zhang Z, Chhetri DK, Bergeron JL. Effects of implant stiffness, shape, and medialization depth on the acoustic outcomes of medialization laryngoplasty. *J Voice.* 2015;29(2):230–235.

265. Hoffman HT, Heaford AC, Dailey SH, et al. Arytenoid repositioning device. *Ann Otol Rhinol Laryngol.* 2014;123(3):195–205.

266. Kim YS, Choi JW, Park J-K, et al. Efficiency and durability of hyaluronic acid of different particle sizes as an injectable material for VF augmentation. *Acta Otolaryngol.* 2015;135(12):1311–1318.

267. Park AM, Bhatt NK, Paniello RC. Paclitaxel inhibits post-traumatic recurrent laryngeal nerve regeneration into the posterior cricoarytenoid muscle in a canine model. *Laryngoscope.* 2017;127(3):651–655.

268. Paniello RC, Park A. Effect on laryngeal adductor function of vincristine block of posterior cricoarytenoid muscle 3 to 5 months after recurrent laryngeal nerve injury. *Ann Otol Rhinol Laryngol.* 2015;124(6):484–489.

269. Rosen CA, Smith L, Young V, Krishna P, Muldoon MF, Munin MC. Prospective investigation of nimodipine for acute vocal fold paralysis. *Muscle Nerve.* 2014;50(1):114–118.

Evidence-Based Practice: Management of Hoarseness/ Dysphonia

DANIEL J. CATES, MD • DERRICK R. RANDALL, MD, MSC, FRCSC

KEY POINTS

The following points list the level of evidence as based on Oxford Center for Evidence-Based Medicine. Additional critical points are provided and points here are expanded at the conclusion of the chapter.

- Antibiotics should not be used for acute laryngitis unless a bacterial infection is identified (Level 1a).
- Antireflux medications, in particular proton pump inhibitors (PPIs), improve symptoms of laryngopharyngeal reflux (LPR), such as globus, dysphagia, and cough (Level 1a-), but they are not proven in the treatment of dysphonia or as empiric therapy.
- Medialization thyroplasty and injection laryngoplasty seem to be equivalent in short-term voice outcomes (Level 2a-).
- Laryngeal electromyography (LEMG) provides diagnostic and prognostic information for vocal fold paralysis and vocal fold paresis (Level 3a).
- Phonomicrosurgery, potassium titanyl phosphate (KTP), and pulsed-dye laser (PDL) therapy provide similar outcomes for vocal fold polyps (Level 3b) but have not been compared with voice therapy.
- Laryngostroboscopy improves diagnostic accuracy and can be delivered through a flexible or rigid laryngoscope with equivalent diagnostic accuracy (Level 4).
- The otolaryngologist must rule out malignancy in patients with persistent dysphonia (Level 5).

OVERVIEW

Hoarseness is a symptom described by a patient, whereas dysphonia refers to the medical definition of producing voice with impairment in social or professional communication.[1] Hoarseness is a common complaint with a lifetime prevalence of 29%–47%; it has a point prevalence of 7% in the adult population and may be as common as 29.1% in the elderly.[2,3] High-vocal-demand occupations, such as teachers, exercise instructors, priests, and telemarketers, have a higher rate of dysphonia.[2,4–8] Voice disorders are associated with decreased quality of life, poor work productivity, difficulty obtaining employment, and $2.5 billion in lost wages.[9–13]

Many people with acute dysphonia do not present to a physician, but they are more likely to do so if it persists or steadily worsens. Assessment by an otolaryngologist–head and neck surgeon mandates exclusion of life-threatening disease, such as malignancy, severe infection, or airway obstruction. Secondary to this is recognition of the degree of impairment to quality of life or limitation in work capacity. Appropriate treatment of patients with dysphonia can be immensely beneficial to the patient and gratifying to the voice practitioner.

The objective of this article is to present and review the evidence for diagnosis and management of patients with dysphonia. It does not aim to provide a clinical practice guideline, as this has been produced by the American Academy of Otolaryngology–Head and Neck Surgery and is undergoing revision with an update slated for release shortly. Extensive review of all conditions causing dysphonia is beyond the reach of this article, and so select topics and interventions for benign conditions causing dysphonia are addressed.

EVIDENCE-BASED CLINICAL ASSESSMENT

A thorough history and head and neck examination is a critical first step in the assessment of all patients presenting with unexplained hoarseness. This allows the clinician to assess potential etiologies, evaluate the degree of morbidity, and plan further investigations. However, expert survey suggests a low diagnostic accuracy of history and physical examination alone.[14] Although recently published clinical practice guidelines suggest that laryngeal visualization may be delayed for 3 months in the absence of serious underlying conditions,[15] several retrospective reviews and expert surveys advocate for a much shorter duration between symptom onset and diagnostic laryngoscopy.[16–18] The ideal timing of visualizing the larynx in acute-onset dysphonia deserves further study. This section reviews the evidence-based literature regarding techniques for (1) visualization of the larynx, (2) assessment of vocal fold vibration, (3) diagnostic testing, and (4) measurement of the degree of dysphonia.

Visualization of the Larynx
Laryngoscopy
Following a thorough history and head and neck examination, including subjective evaluation of the voice, visualization of the larynx in the dysphonic patient is of paramount importance. Classically this has been accomplished with an angled laryngeal mirror and light directed by a semispherical reflector, which has been the standard of laryngeal examination for over 100 years.[19] Although mirror laryngoscopy remains an important part of the head and neck examination, modern comprehensive evaluation of the larynx and interventions demand greater resolution, a larger field of view, and the ability to record and play back logged examinations. Advances in optics led to the development of an array of rigid telescopes, flexible fiberoptic endoscopes, and flexible distal chip endoscopes that provide high resolution and magnification and can be attached to video recording devices for examination storage and review. Two studies prospectively compared the use of laryngeal mirror and rigid endoscopy with regard to patient tolerance and accuracy of diagnosis. Barker and Dort successfully performed rigid endoscopy using a 90-degree telescope in 83% of patients compared with only 52% with laryngeal mirror examination; direct laryngoscopy confirmed no false-negative rigid endoscopy evaluations.[20] In 2009, Dunkelbarger et al. found rigid laryngoscopy using a 30-degree endoscope to be more comfortable and preferred by a majority of patients (80%) when compared with mirror examination, provided greater detail to the clinician, and was helpful to 84% of patients to see the examinations on the monitor.[21] Direct comparison of mirror examination and flexible laryngoscopy has not

been reported. Studies comparing flexible and rigid laryngoscopy are varied with regard to patient demographics, study design, and outcome measures. Overall, flexible transnasal laryngoscopy is well tolerated by the majority of adult patients with minimal morbidity.[22] However, although flexible laryngoscopy was tolerated by all participants in a study of 35 pediatric patients, 80% of children preferred rigid transoral examinations because of less perceived pain and irritation.[23]

With regard to image quality, flexible fiberoptic and distal chip endoscopes have been criticized for distortion and "barreling effect" that is not present in rigid telescopes. Two 2008 studies comparing the diagnostic capabilities of flexible fiberoptic, flexible distal chip, and rigid endoscopes in a controlled, single-blinded fashion reported that the rigid examination provided more information in one-third of patients and changed diagnosis in 10% of patients with benign vocal fold lesions.[24,25] However, in more recent single-blinded studies comparing rigid and flexible distal chip laryngoscopy, there was no statistical difference between the two techniques when evaluating stroboscopic vibratory amplitude[26] and early glottic cancer,[27] with high interrater and intrarater agreement. Thus, although certain advantages are intrinsic to rigid per oral endoscopy (no "barreling effect," less painful) and transnasal flexible endoscopy (evaluation of dynamic voice tasks, avoidance of gag reflex), ongoing advancements in optics, video-capture devices, and imaging processors will likely make the difference in image quality between the two technologies less perceptible.

Narrow-band imaging
Narrow-band imaging (NBI) is a relatively new and widely available technology that uses filtered light to highlight the superficial vasculature of the laryngeal mucosa. Only blue and green light are used, corresponding to the peak absorption of hemoglobin, which penetrates the laryngeal mucosa and enhances small vessels just under the surface.[28] The principle for using NBI to detect cancer or precancerous changes is based on its ability to identify specific patterns of neoangiogenesis caused by neoplastic lesions that would otherwise be overlooked with typical full-spectrum light imaging.[29] In a series of 34 patients, Watanabe et al. first used NBI to evaluate laryngeal lesions suspicious for malignancy by comparing final histopathology to NBI-based predictions, yielding a sensitivity and specificity of 91% and 92%, respectively.[30] Two larger studies of prospectively enrolled patients undergoing microlaryngoscopic biopsy demonstrated that the use of NBI on screening endoscopy was more sensitive than

white light alone in detecting malignant or premalignant lesions, with a significantly higher negative predictive value (98%–99%).[31,32] Positive predictive values, however, were equivalent in both studies.[31,32]

Assessment of Vocal Fold Vibration

Vocal folds oscillate at frequencies of 100–250 Hz during normal phonation, so mucosal vibration cannot be seen under constant illumination in real time and requires special methods to evaluate. This has traditionally been accomplished with stroboscopic techniques, although advances in high-speed photography make continuous evaluation of the vibratory cycle possible.

Laryngostroboscopy

The concept of stroboscopy was first applied to laryngoscopy in the late 19th century in the form of interrupted illumination through a rotating disc.[33] Since that time, laryngostroboscopy has become the leading method of evaluating the vocal fold mucosal wave. Modern stroboscopy uses a strobe light source that is synchronized to the vibratory frequency of the patient's vocal folds using a microphone placed on the neck. The standard strobe rate is 1.5 Hz above the fundamental frequency, which produces the illusion of visualizing the vibratory cycle in slow motion. This allows the clinician to evaluate any alterations in the vibratory cycle or mucosal wave.

Laryngostroboscopy has been demonstrated to improve diagnostic accuracy of voice disorders when compared with laryngoscopy alone in multiple retrospective and observational studies. In 1991, Sataloff et al. reported a series of 1900 consecutive patients undergoing laryngostroboscopy, representing the largest single-institution study of its kind.[34] Prestroboscopy diagnoses were found to be incorrect in 18% of patients, and nearly half of all patients had their incoming diagnoses modified.[34] Two subsequent observational studies of single-institution tertiary laryngology practices including 438 patients reported diagnostic changes in 10%–14% of cases.[35,36] A recent large retrospective study reported results of 4000 patients extracted from a national US claims database who underwent specialty voice evaluation with laryngostroboscopy within 90 days of a previous laryngoscopy.[37] The final diagnosis was changed in 48% of patients, resulting in frequent changes in treatment, with acute laryngitis and vocal fold paresis being the most likely diagnoses to be changed and laryngeal cancer and nonspecific dysphonia the least likely.[37] As interest in new technology and clearer images develops, high definition and 4K recording have entered the laryngeal examination. Two studies

examining diagnostic accuracy and anatomic clarity found diagnosis changed following 4K examination in 4% compared with conventional charge-coupled device (CCD) digital imaging, but CCD may provide a better assessment of color and vascularity.[38,39] Using high-definition cameras with a small viewing monitor (10-inch) did not provide any benefit; however, a larger monitor (42-inch) required high definition to appreciate examination subtleties.[38]

High-speed digital imaging

Although laryngostroboscopy remains the contemporary standard of assessment of laryngeal function, advances in high-speed digital imaging (HSDI) permit entire vibratory cycle evaluation and avoid the shortcomings of stroboscopy. High-speed cameras are capable of recording between 2000 and 5000 frames per second, well above the frequency of vocal fold vibration, thus allowing image capture even in the case of aperiodicity of the vibratory cycle.[40] Patel et al. reported outcomes of 252 patients examined with either HSDI or laryngostroboscopy divided into three groups including those with neuromuscular, epithelial, and subepithelial abnormalities.[41] Stroboscopic data were unsatisfactory because of severity of dysphonia in 63% of patients, whereas HSDI recordings could be evaluated in 100% of patients, with those having neuromuscular disorders the most likely to benefit from HSDI.[41] Although high-speed imaging is becoming more widely available with decreasing costs, the video output remains cumbersome to review in that a 2-s recording can take up to 7 min to play back at normal frame rates and is largely limited to specialized voice laboratories.[42]

Direct laryngoscopy

Operative direct microlaryngoscopy remains the gold standard for the assessment of the laryngeal epithelium and can be an invaluable tool in the assessment of certain voice disorders. Operative laryngoscopy allows for examination of the larynx through palpation of the laryngeal epithelium and the cricoarytenoid joint as well as offers the opportunity to perform diagnostic biopsy or phonomicrosurgery. Difficult laryngeal exposure may limit the utility of direct laryngoscopy in certain patients, especially in the population with head and neck cancer, although angled telescopes and curved or flexible instrumentation may help overcome these challenges.[43]

Multiple retrospective studies suggest that operative direct laryngoscopy affords a greater degree of diagnostic accuracy in the evaluation of benign vocal fold lesions as compared with rigid stroboscopy, despite the relative lack of dynamic vibratory data afforded intraoperatively. A study of 221 patients in 2003 found the diagnosis changed in 36% of cases and additional lesions were discovered in 31% of patients undergoing microlaryngoscopy following preoperative stroboscopic examinations in a general otolaryngology clinic.[44] Lesions missed during stroboscopy were predominantly intracordal.[44] In another review of 100 patients by Dailey and colleagues, an additional 16 lesions were identified in 9 patients at the time of microlaryngoscopy, with alteration of the surgical plan in nearly half of those patients.[45] A more recent review of 85 prospectively enrolled patients at a single tertiary center reported that additional lesions were found in half of patients and 18% of patients had their diagnosis changed.[46]

Other Techniques to Assess Vocal Fold Motion

Beyond direct and indirect endoscopic visualization of the laryngeal surface, other techniques have emerged that allow static and dynamic visualization of the vocal folds. These imaging modalities traditionally require direct tissue contact or near-contact to function, although potential endoscopic applications are emerging.[47]

Ultrasonography

Ultrasonography is a ubiquitous tool that is readily available in countless medical centers, but its use in laryngeal evaluation is relatively new.[48] Although its adoption was initially slow because of perceived difficulty and a steep learning curve, a recent study of eight surgical residents found that 95% of vocal cords could be assessed accurately after seven examinations, suggesting that surgical trainees could successfully measure vocal fold mobility after a brief formal training period.[49,50] In one single-surgeon experience, 204 pre- and postthyroidectomy patients were evaluated with both laryngeal ultrasonography and flexible laryngoscopy, yielding a sensitivity and specificity of 93% and 98%, respectively.[51] Similar results were reported in the pediatric population in a 2016 case-control study by Ongkasuwan and colleagues, who demonstrated 84% sensitivity and 95% specificity for identifying vocal fold immobility in a pediatric cardiovascular intensive care unit.[52] Further investigations have demonstrated that lower-frequency ultrasound and a lateral neck placement of the transducer increase diagnostic yield.[53,54] Laryngeal ultrasound imaging has been applied toward the identification and echogenic characterization of vocal fold lesions, with early work suggesting it is most useful in identifying lesions greater than 2 mm.[55] A 2016 case-control study of 46 pediatric patients who had previously been evaluated with flexible laryngostroboscopy demonstrated a sensitivity and specificity of 100% and 87%, respectively, with a high interrater agreement ($\kappa = 0.70$) for detecting vocal fold nodules with ultrasound by blinded radiologists.[56]

Optical coherence tomography

Optical coherence tomography (OCT) is an imaging technique analogous to ultrasonography that uses near-infrared light instead of sound to create cross-sectional images of target tissues. Substantial work has been done to assess the appearance of static OCT images of the human larynx with direct comparison with microscopic histology demonstrating excellent fidelity.[57–60] However, these studies have necessarily been performed with patients under general anesthesia because of the need for direct tissue contact with the OCT probe. Technological advances in the last several years allow a reduction in image acquisition time and motion artifact, opening the doors to real-time endoscopic assessment in awake patients. Coughlan and colleagues demonstrated the use of long-range OCT via transoral rigid endoscopy in the clinic, producing high-speed panoramic cross-sectional imaging of the vocal folds during phonation.[61]

Ancillary Diagnostic Testing for Dysphonia

A thorough history, physical examination, and laryngoscopy often comprise an adequate workup in the dysphonic patient. However, further diagnostic testing is warranted in selected patients, particularly in those with unilateral vocal fold paralysis (UVFP).

Laryngeal electromyography

LEMG assesses function and electrical activity of targeted laryngeal muscles in an effort to generate diagnostic and prognostic information. LEMG has been used to evaluate a wide variety of laryngeal neuromuscular disorders and dystonias, with the most prevalent use in the evaluation of vocal fold immobility. In the first evidence-based review on the topic in 2003, Sataloff et al. concluded that LEMG was "probably useful" in guiding botulinum toxin injections, but evidence for other uses was lacking.[62] A survey of members of the American Broncho-Esophagological Association (ABEA) found that 75% of respondents used LEMG to evaluate UVFP, typically in an unblinded fashion.[63]

The Neurolaryngology Study Group convened a multidisciplinary panel to generate recommendations for the use of LEMG based on the available literature and expert opinion.[64] One of the largest studies reviewed from Koufman and colleagues reported that LEMG altered the clinical management in 40% of patients and reclassified vocal fold paralysis as fixation in 12%.[65] However, the Neurolaryngology Study Group posited that LEMG is primarily qualitative and further studies are needed to help standardize techniques, analysis, and outcome measures.[64] In 2012, Rickert et al. published a meta-analysis analyzing the utility of LEMG in cases of UVFP across 503 patients in 10 studies.[66] The meta-analysis determined that 91% of those with poor prognostic findings, including fibrillations, positive sharp waves, and absent or reduced voluntary motor unit potentials, had no recovery of vocal fold motion, with positive predictive values ranging from 0.714 to 1.0.[66] A quantitative approach to LEMG interpretation has been described using interference pattern analysis to describe motor unit recruitment by measuring the number of turns per second during phonation, termed "turns analysis."[67] In a study of 23 patients with acute-onset vocal fold paralysis, addition of turns analysis to conventional LEMG techniques improved prognostic accuracy, yielding positive and negative predictive values of 100% and 90%, respectively.[68]

Radiographic imaging

Although evaluation of patients with dysphonia does not often warrant ancillary imaging studies, specific findings on history, physical examination, or laryngoscopy may deserve further radiographic investigation. In the case of suspected laryngeal malignancy, CT or MRI of the neck should be obtained for locoregional staging purposes.[69] If UVFP is identified, imaging may be warranted as part of the initial workup, although practice is varied among voice experts. In a survey of ABEA members, 72% of respondents felt CT is "always" or "often" necessary and chest X-ray is "always" or "often" necessary in the case of idiopathic UVFP.[70] MRI was felt to be necessary by 31%. Several authors have sought to quantify the diagnostic yield of CT imaging in unexplained UVFP.[71–73] One prospective cohort study of 86 patients with UVFP but otherwise normal head and neck examination identified responsible lesions on CT of the neck and chest in 36% of patients, mostly intrathoracic.[71] In a larger retrospective single-institution study, causative lesions were identified on CT imaging in 24% of 153 patients with idiopathic UVFP.[72] Cost analysis data indicate that CT of the neck and chest in patients with unexplained UVFP is cost-effective.[74] Noel and colleagues reported a cohort of 207 patients with idiopathic UVFP where 8 developed an alternative diagnosis with a mean time to detection of 27 months, leading the authors to recommend consideration of repeat CT imaging 2 years following initial presentation; repeat imaging had little utility after 5 years.[75] Similar studies investigating the utility of CT imaging in vocal fold paresis demonstrated low yield (0%–3%) for identifying causative lesions.[76,77]

Measurement of Degree of Dysphonia

The task of quantifying the degree and quality of dysphonia is both critical and complex. The available measures of dysphonia continue to evolve and incorporate perceptual and acoustic analysis, aerodynamic analysis, and tools to assess psychosocial patient impact.

Patient-reported outcome measures

Patient-reported outcome measures (PROMs) are increasingly used instruments to quantify patients' views of their symptoms. Evidence is emerging that routine use of such outcome measures may help to both guide treatments and improve health outcomes.[78] One of the original voice symptom-specific PROMs is the Voice Handicap Index (VHI), consisting of 30 items comprising three domains: functional, emotional, and physical.[79] The VHI subsequently underwent item reduction and factor analysis to produce the streamlined VHI-10, and both instruments have been translated into more than 20 languages.[80,81] The Voice-Related Quality of Life (V-RQOL) is another widely used 10-item PROM with high correlation to the VHI and the VHI-10 in a variety of voice complaints.[82–84] To target specific populations, specialized versions of the VHI have been developed, including the pediatric VHI[85] and the singing VHI.[86] Interestingly, despite a high burden of voice complaints in the elderly, no instrument specifically targeting the geriatric population has been developed.

Across all areas of medicine, there is growing emphasis on determining the degree of PROM score change that represents a clinically meaningful change in disease state.[87] Such values have yet to be identified for the voice PROMs. Several studies comparing both the VHI and V-RQOL to perceptual and acoustic analysis suggest that patient-reported voice handicap is weakly to moderately correlated with clinician-rated measures of dysphonia severity.[88–91] In a survey of experienced voice therapists, 94% of respondents reported that voice-related quality of life instruments are important for the assessment of treatment outcomes.[92] The VHI has been used to compare pre- and posttreatment effects in many voice disorders, including spasmodic dysphonia[93,94] and vocal fold paralysis,[95,96] and is capable of demonstrating statistically significant changes. Furthermore, in a group of 45 patients undergoing medialization laryngoplasty, the reductions in VHI were significantly correlated with the widely used measure of general health-related quality of life Short Form-36 (SF-36).[97]

Clinician-rated measures

Auditory-perceptual measures are frequently used in both research and clinical practice and rely heavily on clinician expertise. Proposed by Hirano in 1981, GRBAS (Grade, Roughness, Breathiness, Asthenia, and Strain) is a 0–3 point scale across five domains that subjectively assesses the degree of perceived voice disorder severity.[98] In 2009 the Consensus Auditory Perceptual Evaluation of Voice (CAPE-V) was developed by the American Speech-Language Hearing Association in an attempt to standardize the perceptual analysis and improve consistency of measurements.[99] Although the CAPE-V demonstrated slightly better interrater reliability compared with GRBAS,[100] the instruments are subject to bias as a result of clinician experience and prior knowledge of the patient's diagnosis or history.[101–103] These tools may be useful to follow individual patients over time, although as mentioned earlier do not correlate well with patient-reported measures.[88,89,91]

Measures of vocal physiology most commonly include acoustic and aerodynamic analyses, with more than 80 different acoustic markers of voice quality identified in a recent meta-analysis.[104] Although often thought of as objective, bias may be introduced into such measures due to the need for behavioral investment by both patient and clinician during testing.[105] In addition, the classically used perturbation measures, including jitter, shimmer, and noise-to-harmonic ratio, rely on linear cycle analysis, which holds uncertain validity in the case of irregular vocal fold vibration or incomplete glottal closure.[105,106]

EVIDENCE-BASED MANAGEMENT OF DYSPHONIA

Selection of an appropriate therapy for dysphonia depends on an accurate diagnosis. Treatment may be single- or multimodal, depending on the primary disease process and if there are secondary lesions or compensatory changes incorporated by the patient. Above all, life-threatening conditions such as cancer and airway compromise cannot be neglected. Description of management of these topics, as well as other subjects including laryngotracheal trauma, cough, vocal process granuloma, spasmodic dysphonia, and postoperative voice change are not covered in this paper. This chapter focuses on the utility of voice, medical, and surgical therapies in the treatment of functional voice disorders, inflammatory lesions of the vocal folds, benign vocal fold lesions, and glottic incompetence. Sensibly, the therapeutic objective of these techniques varies. Voice therapy aims to optimize voice production techniques with the existing anatomy and physiology, improve voice hygiene by avoiding injurious behaviors, and target abnormal phonation in dysphonic voice.[107] Medical therapy directs efforts at the underlying medical disease as it manifests in the vocal folds, whereas surgical therapy aims to correct abnormal anatomy or physiology through removing abnormal tissue or augmenting inadequate tissue.

Functional Voice Disorders

Functional voice disorders develop from psychological and personality characteristics, vocal misuse, and compensation for underlying disease.[107,108] Functional voice disorders are generally assumed to be dysphonia in the presence of a normal laryngeal examination, commonly termed primary muscle tension dysphonia, and can be hyperfunctional or hypofunctional. However, organic disease can lead to a secondary functional dysphonia, for example, false vocal fold phonation in patients with glottic incompetence, where adaptive behaviors attempting to compensate for the primary issue lead to a degree of dysphonia excessive for the apparent laryngeal deficiency.

Voice therapy

A systematic review of voice therapy techniques found good evidence for benefit in physiologic treatments, with some support for patient education to address vocal hygiene, and observational data supporting symptomatic approaches.[107] Therapy with a speech language pathologist with expertise in voice is the mainstay of treatment to assist these patients by emphasizing healthy vocal hygiene through patient education, voice therapy, and circumlaryngeal therapy and eliminating phonotraumatic behaviors.[108] In patients with secondary muscle tension dysphonia, the underlying disease process should be addressed—or at least considered in the context of the particular patient's needs—with voice therapy used as an adjunct to refine voice outcomes. For patients who undergo laryngeal surgery, voice therapy can be beneficial to reduce factors that contributed to the organic disease.[109,110]

Medical therapy

Medical interventions have little role in primary functional voice disorders; however, consideration of underlying medical conditions or mental health disorders and their treatment is important. Studies evaluating the prevalence of depression and severity of anxiety found greater rates in patients with functional voice disorders than in controls.[111,112] Inclusion of a psychologist in a voice team may help stratify these patients better and improve selection for appropriate treatment.[113] As yet, there are no clinical trials or reviews of voice symptoms in patients with functional voice disorders who undergo therapy for coincident mental health concerns.

Surgical therapy

Under the premise that muscle tension dysphonia represents laryngeal hyperfunction as compensation in select patients, surgical therapy can be directed at the primary etiology. In some instances, there may not be an underlying etiology. Case reports and small series exist of patients with ventricular dysphonia that responded favorably to botulinum toxin injection or CO_2 laser resection of the redundant false vocal fold mucosa.[114-117] These are extreme measures and should only be considered in a very limited population with no other underlying cause of disease leading to the hyperfunction and failed extensive voice therapy.[118] There is consideration that vocal fold augmentation may be useful to reduce the apparent strain in the case of glottic insufficiency, and a parallel outcome has been shown in chronic cough where injection laryngoplasty decreased cough severity, potentially through decreased hyperfunction with speech.[119]

Inflammatory Laryngeal Pathology

Inflammation can affect any of the laryngeal subsites: supraglottis, glottis, or subglottis. Voice disorder develops from irregular or stiffened vocal fold vibration when the glottis is involved, whereas decreased airflow can alter voice if there is significant subglottic inflammation or restriction of vocal fold mobility. When inflammation involves the supraglottis, dysphonia can arise from altered resonance of the pharynx or from decreased mobility of the structures because of pain, as in the classic "hot potato" voice of a peritonsillar abscess. Etiologies for inflammation include infection, allergy, LPR, and phonotrauma. When an agent causing laryngeal inflammation is identified, medical therapy is a key component to managing the initial insult and preventing disease recurrence.

Voice therapy

The primary objective for voice therapy in the setting of laryngeal inflammation is reducing phonotrauma

and correcting poor compensatory hyperfunction behaviors, which can expedite recovery and prevent recurrence.[107]

Medical therapy

Laryngitis. A 2015 update to the Cochrane review on antibiotics in the presentation of acute laryngitis reports a paucity of good quality data, finding only three randomized controlled trials (RCTs) involving 351 participants with one of the most common clinical conditions in primary care.[120] The authors admit they cannot be definitive given the low-quality, biased data but report no benefit to antibiotics in objective improvement to voice. There may be improvements in cough, as a secondary outcome, but these benefits do not outweigh the costs and risks of population-level excessive antibiotic use. Culture-directed antibiotic therapy is an appropriate course when patients have a bacterial infection, but most acute laryngitis are not cultured.

Chronic laryngitis is generally considered noninfectious and results from failure of the body to mount adequate response to a noxious agent or continuous exposure to an injurious agent.[121] A small study found that mucous secretions from the larynges of patients with chronic laryngitis have abundant bacteria but few neutrophils, indicating bacteria are colonizers rather than contributors to the inflammation.[122] Although empiric treatment with antibiotics is commonly employed, it leads to modest improvement with regular relapse after treatment cessation.[123] Bacterial biofilms are an emerging topic in otolaryngology disease, and Kinnari et al. found bacterial biofilms in 62% of a small sample of patients with chronic laryngitis.[124] Nonetheless, there is no literature evaluating antibiotic types or regimen efficacy in treating chronic laryngitis. Similarly, fungal infection can cause chronic laryngitis, but there is no level of evidence higher than expert opinion and case reports describing effective treatment. One prospective, nonrandomized study analyzing posterior commissural thickening found 67% of patients responded to PPI therapy,[125] but there has not yet been a study investigating the efficacy or safety of empiric PPI therapy in chronic laryngitis or dysphonia or appropriate treatment duration.

Another intriguing consideration in managing inflammatory vocal fold lesions is acupuncture. Following a randomized, placebo-controlled trial of acupuncture versus sham acupuncture that demonstrated improved quality of life, acoustics, and perceptual voice measures,[126] a prospective RCT with patients affected by chronic laryngitis, vocal fold nodules, or polyps found improved quality of life, vocal function, and reduced lesion size following genuine acupuncture to nine voice-related acupoints.[127] More investigation is required to validate these findings.

Laryngopharyngeal reflux. Since Koufman described a correlation between laryngeal symptoms and pH monitor abnormalities in the lower and upper esophagus,[128] gastroesophageal reflux affecting the larynx, most commonly referred to as LPR, blossomed into a contentious topic within otolaryngology. Two recent meta-analyses on the use of PPI therapy for dysphonia found good response to treatment in reflux symptom index (RSI) scores but no benefit to reflux finding score (RFS).[129,130] An earlier systematic review of several of the same studies included in the meta-analyses concluded that the existing literature is too inconsistent in defining LPR and used inconsistent outcome measures to support or refute the use of PPI therapy in dysphonia.[131] The 2006 Cochrane review on the effectiveness of PPI therapy for dysphonia did not find any studies adequate for inclusion, and the 2015 update was withdrawn, as it was deemed to be out of date.[132] A major limitation of the studies investigating PPI use in dysphonia, despite gastroesophageal reflux disease (GERD) affecting 10% of the adult population, is small enrollment numbers. The highest quality studies that have been randomized, placebo-controlled studies did not use a validated symptom score for voice outcomes[133-138]; had controls with normal pretreatment symptom scores[137]; did not find a change in endoscopic appearance or acoustic measures[133-137]; relied on nonvoice laryngeal symptoms such as globus, throat clearing, cough, and dysphagia to demonstrate therapeutic benefit[134,138-140]; or did not find a benefit of treatment.[133,135,137,141] In essence, many of the higher quality studies used to support the use of PPI therapy for dysphonia did not explicitly measure dysphonia. One single-center study also found PPIs do not affect VHI, GRBAS, or acoustic outcomes following phonomicrosurgery.[142]

In contrast, the use of Nissen fundoplication for professional voice users with dysphonia refractory to high-dose PPI therapy and 24-h pH monitor-proven GERD found that 86% of patients required less medication, postoperative pH monitor testing improved, and 76% were satisfied with their decision to undergo surgery, although RFS had not changed.[143] A small retrospective study of patients with multichannel impedance monitor-proven LPR found improvements of typical GERD symptoms following Nissen fundoplication and 100% reported their primary complaint resolved; however, it should be noted that all patients presented with nonvoice primary complaints, such as globus, cough, throat clearing, and dysphagia.[144]

The questions of whether empiric PPI therapy is useful for dysphonia in suspected LPR or how long treatment should be continued are also unknown. A 2011 prospective, double-blind trial by Masaany et al. testing empiric PPI therapy for presumed LPR—23% presented with hoarseness—found improved RSI and RFS measures after 2 months of therapy and further improvements up to 4 months but did not measure dysphonia.[138] There are no studies rigorously evaluating appropriate treatment duration or cessation protocols.

A 2016 Italian position paper on the use of PPIs states they are invaluable drugs for acid-related disease and outweigh the risks of harm but indicates use outside of evidence-based indications exposes people to risk.[145] It is worthwhile to note that hoarseness, dysphonia, and LPR are not referred to in this publication, although benefit is listed as uncertain for all forms of extradigestive GERD.[145] It is all too common that a patient presents with dysphonia and has been on empiric PPI therapy for several years but does not recall any benefit to the medication. Several studies have found alternative diagnoses for dysphonia in patients who do not respond to PPI therapy.[146-148] Anecdotally and according to expert opinion there are patients with dysphonia who improve with PPI therapy. Attempts to improve patient selection may be under way with oropharyngeal pH monitoring, but addressing the progress and limitations of the diagnostics, development, and validation of this test are outside the scope of this chapter.

Steroids. Steroid treatment for laryngeal disease is commonplace in patients with airway obstruction and in professional voice users, but there are no data available to demonstrate efficacy. Theoretically, laryngeal inflammation stiffens and impairs mucosal vibration; ergo employing steroids to reduce this inflammation should be beneficial. Phonotraumatic stress creates an inflammatory milieu in laryngeal secretions, and a very small, randomized proof-of-principle trial treating patients with 100 mg oral hydrocortisone caused a reduction of inflammatory markers versus placebo.[149,150] Croup is the best studied condition affecting the larynx that is responsive to steroid, with a Cochrane review finding resolution within hours and decreased readmissions, repeat visits, and hospital length of stay.[151] Multiple case reports and case series of systemic inflammatory diseases, localized inflammation (lichen planus), and autoimmune disorders showing improvement with corticosteroids exist, but these conditions are too infrequent to produce large series.[152-158]

Allergy. Increasing suspicion has developed that allergy is a cause of laryngeal inflammation, which is plausible under the premise of the unified airway hypothesis.[159] A retrospective review of patients with refractory laryngeal symptoms, including hoarseness, globus, phlegm, cough, or throat clearing, demonstrated a similar rate of positive in vitro allergy testing to patients with allergic rhinitis, sinusitis, and otitis media.[160] In patients with documented birch allergy, VHI scores, visual analog dysphonia scores, and perceptual voice assessments by an SLP were found to be worse during the pollen season compared with controls without voice concerns.[161] Forty-nine patients with allergic rhinitis undergoing immunotherapy had higher vocal symptom scores on an established Finnish voice questionnaire than controls.[162] In contrast, 30 patients with allergic rhinitis reported higher VHI scores but did not have differences in stroboscopic appearance or other acoustic measures compared with nonallergic controls.[163] A prospective, pseudocontrolled study of patients with allergic rhinitis in Turkey found reduced nasal symptom and VHI scores, along with improved acoustic measures, following nasal corticosteroid and systemic antihistamine treatment.[164] These measures approached those of controls who did not undergo therapy.

Benign Laryngeal Lesions

Dysphonia develops from benign lesions in the larynx by mass effect, interrupting smooth glottic closure, and asynchronous or tethered mucosal wave. Treatment for a benign lesion should be considered when patient's voice is bothersome or unsatisfactory to him or her, which is a subjective assessment and depends on a patient's perceived disability or dysfunction. Certainly there are many people with dysphonia who are not affected by their voice; although this may register as dysphonic to a voice professional, the patient will not necessarily be happy with the resultant voice if some form of therapy is undertaken. In these instances, confirmation that a lesion does not have a worrisome appearance, often through reevaluation to ensure no interval change, or biopsy may be necessary to ensure no interval worsening occurred. The door should always be left open to these patients should they decide later that their voice affects them.

For those patients appropriate for intervention, lesion type and location are key factors in vocal outcome, and efforts to categorize benign vocal fold lesions with structured nomenclature and their likelihood for surgical success are under way.[165,166] As shown by do Amaral Catani et al. in a large series of

vocal performers, those with superficial lesions had improved acoustic parameters 1 month after phonomicrosurgery,[167] whereas deep lesions responded after 3 months. Similarly, the University of Pittsburgh group found VHI-10 improvement with phonomicrosurgery for superficial and deep lesions, but less improvement occurred with lesions involving the vocal ligament.[166] These results can be used to counsel patients in regards to potential surgical outcomes, but there is no similar trial to provide prognosis to patients undergoing voice or medical therapy based on lesion location.

Voice therapy

Voice therapy is targeted at educating patients about general behaviors and practices that traumatize the midmembranous region, reducing compensatory maladaptive behaviors that serve to worsen the trauma, and addressing patient-specific factors that worsen the injury.[168] Voice therapy is the established treatment for vocal fold nodules and is traditionally listed as a first-line therapy for benign vocal fold lesions, with surgical excision reserved for treatment failure[109,168–170]; a survey of American Academy of Otolaryngology–Head and Neck Surgery members with 1208 respondents found 91% use voice therapy as the primary treatment for nodules.[171] Although voice therapy has been well studied, most of the investigations supporting voice therapy for nodules are retrospective, do not compare alternative treatments, or do not find a difference in outcomes between methods.[169,172–174] Moreover, a Cochrane review comparing voice therapy versus surgery for managing vocal fold nodules found no randomized trials suitable for inclusion.[175] Nonetheless, with the likelihood for equivalent outcomes between voice therapy and surgery,[169] avoiding risk for complication swings the balance in favor of voice therapy.

There is renewed interest in voice therapy as the primary treatment modality for benign midmembranous lesions. De Vasconcelos et al. offer a small series with selection bias comparing lip and tongue trill exercises in comparison with phonomicrosurgery for the management of polyps that found improvements in several voice parameters; however, they exceeded the statistical capability to evaluate the number of outcomes, plus there was a noticeable absence of benefit in the "control" surgical group.[176] Voice therapy seems to be successful in treating 20%–56% of vocal fold polyps,[177–181] indicating a need to determine features to aid in patient selection. Retrospective studies evaluating predictors of successful voice therapy for polyps are female sex; nonhemorrhagic, white polyps; small polyps less than one-quarter the length of the vocal fold; and sessile polyps;

smoking did not seem to affect the likelihood for success.[180,182] A randomized controlled study involving unilateral vocal fold polyps (hemorrhagic, gelatinous, and fibrous) investigated phonomicrosurgery versus a strict and prolonged "Voice Therapy Expulsion" protocol, which purports to cause progressive thinning of a polyp's stalk until it can be coughed out. The authors found excellent improvements between GRBAS, VHI, and VRQOL scores before and after treatment, with no significant difference between groups.[183]

Medical therapy

As office-based procedures become more common in laryngology, techniques that decrease operating room utilization gain steady support. A systematic review and meta-analysis of percutaneous steroid injections (PSIs) for benign vocal fold lesions was published in 2013 and reported statistically significant improvements in VHI and MPT.[184] These data were uncontrolled and heterogeneous, with vocal fold scarring included. An update on the results of a prospective, uncontrolled, nonrandomized study of percutaneous triamcinolone injections for nodules, polyps, and Reinke edema after 2 years was provided by Lee and Park, which found 70.2% of all patients had improvement in endoscopic appearance and 44% of all patients had complete lesion resolution, defined as >80% reduction in size.[185] There was no statistically significant difference in the result based on lesion type. Of the remaining patients, 6% had no effect and 24% showed recurrence of the lesion, generally within 1 year. More current prospective studies lacking control groups or randomization also show short-term improvements in acoustic and VHI data.[186,187] Steroid injection into the subepithelial space following phonomicrosurgery was associated with reduced lesion recurrence in one retrospective cohort study.[188]

A retrospective review of nonrandomized patients receiving either PSI or vocal hygiene instructions (without SLP direction) found equivalent lesion size reduction for vocal fold nodules between groups at 2 months, whereas vocal fold polyps showed a greater size reduction with PSI.[189] The authors argue patients with high vocal demand occupations showed a better response with PSI based on relative size reduction, but the patients in this subgroup analysis receiving vocal hygiene instruction started with a smaller mean lesion size.[189]

Surgical therapy

Numerous uncontrolled retrospective reviews report improved voice and glottal function parameters following laryngeal microsurgery using cold steel or CO_2 laser,[109,190–193] and it is accepted that this is the standard treatment if voice therapy fails. Benninger provided the first prospective RCT comparing phonomicrosurgery and CO_2 excision of benign vocal fold lesions and found no difference in perceptual measures or recovery time between groups.[194] Several publications appeared demonstrating the beneficial effect of other surgical and nonsurgical techniques, but as yet there is no well-designed, randomized prospective study comparing the developing techniques.[195]

Laser treatment

The tools of greatest interest and increased adoption into clinical practice have been fiber-based lasers that can be used in the operating room or on unsedated, awake patients in the outpatient setting. Retrospective reviews of single-center experiences with KTP or PDL treatment of benign lesions found improvement or restoration of normal VHI scores, regression of lesion size, and improved acoustic parameters among patients with vocal fold polyps, with or without concurrent polypectomy; similar outcomes result for procedures performed in the office or with the patient under general anesthesia.[196–202] A multicenter review of laser experience found excellent lesion regression, although often incomplete, for numerous types of lesions with KTP treatment.[203] There is heterogeneity in lesion response within each study, but polyps and vascular ectasias consistently show good results. Reinke edema also shows subjective and objective improvement with KTP treatment, but response is less successful than with other lesions.[198,202–204] There has not been a direct comparison between the two laser types to determine whether one modality is more effective or safer.

There are no modern prospective data with appropriate randomization comparing different surgical treatment modalities. A retrospective review of patients who underwent KTP versus microflap treatment of vocal fold polyps found equivalent postoperative acoustic and aerodynamic parameters between groups, but 15% of patients treated with KTP required more than one treatment.[205] One prospective, nonrandomized study comparing diode laser with cold steel excision of vocal fold polyps found no differences in VHI or acoustic measures at 8 weeks postoperatively, although no description of polyp size or type was provided.[206]

Glottic Insufficiency

Glottic insufficiency encompasses UVFP, vocal fold paresis, presbyphonia, and vocal fold scar, with the ultimate effect being inadequate glottic closure, poor-quality vibratory character, and dysphonia. The most common causes of vocal fold hypomobility include iatrogenic, idiopathic, postinfectious, neurologic, malignancy, and internal or external trauma, with relative proportions varying by practice referral pattern.[207] Voice therapy is typically the first treatment employed, but in patients who do not realize adequate improvement, surgical therapy to medialize the vocal fold (or vocal folds) and facilitate glottic closure is undertaken.

Voice therapy

Uncontrolled retrospective and prospective studies on the utility of early voice therapy (2–4 weeks post onset) for UVFP found improved glottic closure, vocal fold motion, subjective, perceptual, and acoustic measures in patients with various causes of UVFP.[208–210] Many of these patients had iatrogenic injuries following thyroidectomy, and a high rate of return of vocal fold motion suggests these were temporary injuries with spontaneous recovery. This highlights the limitation of these uncontrolled studies since it is difficult to attribute voice outcomes to the voice therapy rather than the return of mobility. Nonetheless, it is suggested that two-thirds of patients with UVFP do not need medialization surgery with good voice therapy.[211] In a larger study of 171 patients with UVFP of various causes (mostly iatrogenic), the authors assert early (less than 4 weeks) or intermediate (4–8 weeks) voice therapy is necessary to promote improved voice outcomes and return of mobility, with better results in these groups compared with patients who started voice therapy more than 8 weeks after UVFP onset.[212] In a population where 62% of patients regained vocal fold motion, it is again difficult to attribute the recovery to voice therapy, although in those in whom function returned, late voice therapy may have poorer acoustic outcomes.[212] Similarly, emerging data in animal models suggest early nerve stimulation following nerve crush injury results in earlier return of laryngeal nerve function, although all groups eventually reach similar results.[213] However, Busto-Crespo et al. found improvements in voice parameters among all patients who underwent voice therapy for UVFP, regardless of duration until commencing treatment, although a greater effect was seen for those who started treatment within 1 year of onset.[214]

A systematic review on SLP management of UVFP was written in 2016, which highlighted the variety in treatment modalities and intensities, duration of time from symptom onset to beginning treatment, etiology of UVFP, different outcome measures, lack of control groups, and other key parameters that limit the ability to estimate the effectiveness of voice therapy on UVFP outcomes.[215] A more recent but inadequately powered prospective, controlled study assessing voice therapy following early (less than 6 months) UVFP among patients with a mixture of idiopathic and iatrogenic etiologies found aerodynamic, acoustic, and perceptual improvements in voice for those who underwent a structured voice therapy program using resonant voice therapy, vocal function exercise, and hard glottal attack.[216]

In those patients with vocal fold paresis or presbylaryngis, voice therapy is commonly used as the primary treatment modality, with aims to strengthen respiratory support for phonation, decrease maladaptive hyperfunction, and improve resonance.[217] As the population ages and presbylaryngis prevalence increases, it should be kept in mind that a large series of patients found the majority did not pursue any treatment.[218] This tendency away from treatment may reflect patient disinterest following reassurance that no pathology is identified or practitioner bias. Expert opinion dictates that presbylaryngis is difficult to treat by any modality, and existing data agree in its inconsistency. A small retrospective series of patients with presbylaryngis who followed a voice therapy regimen found improved VRQOL, whereas those who elected no treatment found no change.[219] Interestingly, a separate small uncontrolled study of geriatric patients with presbylaryngis undergoing weekly voice therapy sessions for 6 weeks reported decreased effort and improved voice, despite no statistical difference between pre- and posttreatment perceptual, stroboscopic, and acoustic parameters.[220] Acoustic parameters were also shown to improve with regular voice therapy, although vocal assessments were not included.[221] A larger retrospective study found 81% of patients with presbylaryngis felt improved with voice therapy, but the magnitude of improvement was small.[218] Voice therapy was associated with improved voice among patients with presbylaryngis in 85% of patients, and patients with larger glottic gaps are less likely to experience benefit.[222]

Medical therapy

One prospective, open-label, nonrandomized trial using nimodipine in 28 patients with 30 vocal folds affected by acute vocal fold paralysis (89% postsurgical, 11% idiopathic or intubation related, 7% bilateral) found 60% of paralyzed vocal folds regained purposeful motion.[223] This was reportedly higher than their institution's typical expected spontaneous recovery rate but is similar to a recovery rate reported in the use of voice therapy for UVFP.[212] A follow-up study with larger patient numbers found timing of medication implementation was not a factor.[224] These data are interesting but require well-designed, controlled studies to verify potential utility.

Surgical therapy

Present surgical options for glottic incompetence are directed at medializing the immobile or atrophic vocal fold to provide better contact with the contralateral vocal fold. There are no techniques available to produce purposeful movement of a paralyzed vocal fold. Surgical therapy for glottic incompetence over the last few decades has relied primarily on medialization thyroplasty, but the increasing popularity of injection laryngoplasty has made it a common tool in the management of glottic incompetence. The injection material selected depends on the clinical context, desired duration of effect, and rheologic properties. No study has comprehensively compared all available injection materials, but a multiinstitutional review of tertiary laryngology centers found no preference for any particular material.[225] Vocal fold injections can be performed in the clinic with a patient who is awake or under general anesthesia, with no differences in vocal outcomes found between locations.[226] The popularity of office-based injections is increasing because of convenience, comfort with the procedure, equivalent complication rates, and institutional costs, among other factors.[225] A systematic review of 10 retrospective studies comparing subjective and perceptual voice outcomes, acoustic measures, and stroboscopy parameters in patients with UVFP who received injection laryngoplasty versus medialization thyroplasty (with or without arytenoid adduction) generally found no difference between groups, with occasional outliers between individual studies.[227] A cost analysis (reported in Canadian dollars) by the same group found a mean cost savings of $1556 per patient, with forecasting to 5 years post initial treatment.[228]

Despite the temporary nature, injection laryngoplasty can provide a durable effect beyond the expected lifetime. One retrospective study found a decreased proportion of patients required permanent medialization following injection with short-term injectable material (26%) compared with those who underwent observation or voice therapy (66%) at least 9 months post diagnosis.[229] Another retrospective study followed up 28 patients who underwent short-term injectable material laryngoplasty but had no recovery of vocal fold motion at 10 months: 57% compensated well enough to need no further treatment, with the remainder undergoing medialization thyroplasty.[230]

Medialization thyroplasty is a well-established technique for glottic incompetence with durable results. Arytenoid adduction, which aims to rotate the vocal process medially and provide better vertical height match between vocal folds is more controversial in terms of voice outcomes or improvement. A limited number of studies compared medialization thyroplasty plus arytenoid adduction with thyroplasty alone. One study found improved acoustic measures and posterior glottic closure with arytenoid adduction at 3 months,[231] whereas others

did not find any differences and noted an increased hospitalization time with risk of edema and tracheotomy.[232,233]

Laryngeal reinnervation was originally described before medialization procedures and involves reanastomosis of an injured recurrent laryngeal nerve (RLN) (generally at the time of injury or shortly afterward); nerve cable grafting between proximal and distal RLN; anastomosis of a branch of the ansa cervicalis, transverse cervical, or supraclavicular nerve to the distal recurrent laryngeal nerve; or neuromuscular pedicle implant.[234,235] These techniques cannot provide vocal fold motion but instead rely on a degree of synkinesis supporting muscle bulk and minimizing atrophy resulting from peripheral neuropathy. Neuromuscular pedicle implants have largely fallen out of favor for the other techniques, and the optimal individual techniques depend on the degree of gap between nerve stumps.[235] One multicenter prospective trial to compare reinnervation with thyroplasty was attempted, but it had to be terminated early because of slow recruitment with only 24 patients enrolled.[236] No significant difference was found between reinnervation or static medialization. A subgroup analysis suggested patients over the age of 52 years had poorer outcomes with laryngeal reinnervation, but this age was selected on the basis of median age and for convenient group size rather than any physiologic feature.

Despite the seemingly simple deficiency of inadequate closure and prolonged open phase, and in contrast to the generally reliable and predictable results of medialization in UVFP, presbylaryngis and bilateral hypomobility have proven challenging to treat with acceptable patient satisfaction.[237,238] In the largest studies of patients with presbylaryngis, 5%–6% of patients presenting to tertiary laryngology practices with isolated presbylaryngis underwent surgical treatment, underscoring the need for appropriate patient selection and how patients feel about their voice.[218,239] Single-center retrospective series in patients with glottic incompetence found thyroplasty or injection laryngoplasty to be inconsistent in providing positive vocal outcomes.[218,239–242] Patient selection is likely a factor in producing successful outcomes for vocal fold medialization in presbylaryngis, and trial vocal fold injection was suggested as a method to address this.[243] Two retrospective studies found mixed predictability of thyroplasty success based on trial vocal fold injection with carboxymethylcellulose.[244,245] Further work may develop this understanding to improve selection.

Vocal fold scar has been equally, or perhaps more, difficult to successfully treat. Various methods including mucosal slicing, microflap scar excision, thyroplasty, injection laryngoplasty, Gray minithyrotomy, and grafting techniques have been inconsistent and less successful in producing good voice outcomes compared with the degree of success for other vocal fold surgeries.[242,246–254] The infrequency of these procedures and inability to determine good patient selection again challenges the development of an effective, consistent technique.

Regenerative medicine, the next great frontier, offers some hope for glottic incompetence, with a case report and clinical trial showing reduced VHI-10, improved mucosal wave, and reduced glottic gap up to 1 year after basic fibroblast growth factor injection, but multiple injections were required for most patients.[255–257] Although this is intriguing, it will require extensive replication and validation.

WHAT THE EVIDENCE TELLS US (THE BOTTOM LINE)

Clinical studies in the management of dysphonia are generally of low-quality evidence, and improving this through multicenter prospective trials would be valuable. Patients presenting to an otolaryngologist with dysphonia need complete evaluation to ensure there is no life-threatening disease process at hand. This is accomplished by history and examination of the larynx, which can be accomplished by either rigid or flexible laryngoscopy. Malignant or other life-threatening disease is recognized by either technique accurately, but refined evaluation of the mucosal wave requires stroboscopy and certain diagnoses can be missed otherwise. High-definition imaging provides better optics but does not alter diagnosis as frequently as stroboscopy. Diagnostic imaging is useful in some instances, such as identifying a malignant lesion in the skull base, neck, or chest, but it is not likely to provide a diagnosis for hoarseness without laryngoscopy. CT scans are cost-effective for UVFP with no apparent cause following head and neck examination with laryngoscopy, but they do not seem to be helpful for vocal fold paresis. Most diagnoses can be made in the clinic, and operative laryngoscopy should be reserved for select cases or when biopsies or procedures are necessary. LEMG can provide prognosis for vocal fold paralysis but is not useful for the primary workup of dysphonia.

Once a diagnosis for dysphonia is identified, various treatment options may be available. Full discussion of all treatment options for all conditions is not possible in this chapter. Voice therapy is an excellent primary treatment for many causes of dysphonia, with surgical intervention useful in the event of treatment failure or incomplete response. There is no evidence to strongly support the use of antibiotics, antifungals, or steroids for dysphonia, although expert opinion suggests certain clinical conditions may benefit. PPIs provide effective treatment of nonvoice symptoms associated with LPR, but endoscopic appearance of the larynx may not change following treatment. Likewise, empiric therapy of dysphonia with PPIs has not been proven efficacious. Surgical therapy is a good option for benign vocal fold lesions and UVFP but has not produced reliable success in other causes of glottic insufficiency. Phonomicrosurgery and laser treatment for benign laryngeal lesions seem to be equivalent.

CRITICAL POINTS
- Antibiotics should not be used for acute laryngitis unless a bacterial infection is identified (Level 1a).
- Antireflux medications, in particular PPIs, improve symptoms of LPR, such as globus, dysphagia, and cough (Level 1a-), but they are not proven in the treatment of dysphonia or as empiric therapy.
- Medialization thyroplasty and injection laryngoplasty seem to be equivalent in short-term voice outcomes (Level 2a-).
- LEMG provides diagnostic and prognostic information for vocal fold paralysis and vocal fold paresis (Level 3a).
- Laryngeal surgery improves vocal outcomes for benign vocal fold lesions and glottic insufficiency (Level 3a).
- Voice therapy can be effective therapy for some benign vocal fold lesions, including nodules, polyps, and inflammation (Level 3b).
- Phonomicrosurgery, KTP, and PDL therapy provide similar outcomes for vocal fold polyps (Level 3b) but have not been compared with voice therapy.
- Oral steroids have a limited role in managing dysphonia in a select patient population (Level 4).
- Angled rigid laryngoscopy with normal light may provide additional information over flexible laryngoscopy (Level 4).
- PSI may improve some benign vocal fold lesions (Level 4).
- Stroboscopy improves diagnostic accuracy and can be delivered through a flexible or rigid laryngoscope with equivalent diagnostic accuracy (Level 4).
- Patient-related outcome measures should be used to evaluate dysphonia and monitor treatment progress (Level 5).
- The otolaryngologist must rule out malignancy in patients with persistent dysphonia (Level 5).

REFERENCES

1. Chang JI, Bevans SE, Schwartz SR. Otolaryngology clinic of North America: evidence-based practice. Management of hoarseness/dysphonia. *Otolaryngol Clin North Am.* 2012;45(5):1109–1126. http://dx.doi.org/10.1016/j.otc.2012.06.012.

2. Roy N, Merrill RM, Thibeault S, Parsa RA, Gray SD, Smith EM. Prevalence of voice disorders in teachers and the general population. *J Speech Lang Hear Res.* 2004;47(2):281. http://dx.doi.org/10.1044/1092-4388(2004/023).

3. Roy N, Stemple J, Merrill RM, Thomas L. Epidemiology of voice disorders in the elderly: preliminary findings. *Laryngoscope.* 2007;117(4):628–633. http://dx.doi.org/10.1097/MLG.0b013e3180306da1.

4. Heidel SE, Torgerson JK. Vocal problems among aerobic instructors and aerobic participants. *J Commun Disord.* 1993;26(3):179–191. http://www.ncbi.nlm.nih.gov/pubmed/8227503.

5. Jones K, Sigmon J, Hock L, Nelson E, Sullivan M, Ogren F. Prevalence and risk factors for voice problems among telemarketers. *Arch Otolaryngol Head Neck Surg.* 2002;128(5):571–577. http://www.ncbi.nlm.nih.gov/pubmed/12003590.

6. Angelillo M, Di Maio G, Costa G, Angelillo N, Barillari U. Prevalence of occupational voice disorders in teachers. *J Prev Med Hyg.* 2009;50(1):26–32. http://www.ncbi.nlm.nih.gov/pubmed/19771757.

7. Hočevar-Boltežar I. Prevalence and risk factors for voice problems in priests. *Wien Klin Wochenschr.* 2009;121(7–8):276–281. http://dx.doi.org/10.1007/s00508-009-1163-1.

8. Rumbach AF. Vocal problems of group fitness instructors: prevalence of self-reported sensory and auditory-perceptual voice symptoms and the need for preventative education and training. *J Voice.* 2013;27(4):524.e11–524.e21. http://dx.doi.org/10.1016/j.jvoice.2013.01.016.

9. Ramig LO, Verdolini K. Treatment efficacy: voice disorders. *J Speech Lang Hear Res.* 1998;41(1):S101–S116. http://www.ncbi.nlm.nih.gov/pubmed/9493749.

10. Mirza N, Ruiz C, Baum ED, Staab JP. The prevalence of major psychiatric pathologies in patients with voice disorders. *Ear Nose Throat J.* 2003;82(10):808–810, 812, 814 http://www.ncbi.nlm.nih.gov/pubmed/14606179.

11. Cohen SM, Dupont WD, Courey MS. Quality-of-life impact of non-neoplastic voice disorders: a meta-analysis. *Ann Otol Rhinol Laryngol.* 2006;115(2):128–134. http://dx.doi.org/10.1177/000348940611500209.

12. Dietrich M, Verdolini Abbott K, Gartner-Schmidt J, Rosen CA. The frequency of perceived stress, anxiety, and depression in patients with common pathologies affecting voice. *J Voice.* 2008;22(4):472–488. http://dx.doi.org/10.1016/j.jvoice.2006.08.007.

13. Isetti DD, Baylor CR, Burns MI, Eadie TL. Employer reactions to adductor spasmodic dysphonia: exploring the influence of symptom severity and disclosure of diagnosis during a simulated telephone interview. *Am J Speech Lang Pathol.* 2017:1. http://dx.doi.org/10.1044/2016_AJSLP-16-0040.

14. Paul BC, Chen S, Sridharan S, Fang Y, Amin MR, Branski RC. Diagnostic accuracy of history, laryngoscopy, and stroboscopy. *Laryngoscope.* 2013;123(1):215–219. http://dx.doi.org/10.1002/lary.23630.

15. Schwartz SR, Cohen SM, Dailey SH, et al. Clinical practice guideline: hoarseness (dysphonia). *Otolaryngol Neck Surg.* 2009;141(3 suppl):1–31. http://dx.doi.org/10.1016/j.otohns.2009.06.744.

16. Keesecker SE, Murry T, Sulica L. Patterns in the evaluation of hoarseness: time to presentation, laryngeal visualization, and diagnostic accuracy. *Laryngoscope.* 2015;125(3):667–673. http://dx.doi.org/10.1002/lary.24955.

17. Sadoughi B, Fried MP, Sulica L, Blitzer A. Hoarseness evaluation: a transatlantic survey of laryngeal experts. *Laryngoscope.* 2014;124:221–226. http://dx.doi.org/10.1002/lary.24178.

18. Paul BC, Branski RC, Amin MR. Diagnosis and management of new-onset hoarseness: a survey of the American Broncho-Esophagological Association. *Ann Otol Rhinol Laryngol.* 2012;121(10):629–634. http://dx.doi.org/10.1177/000348941212101001.

19. Peter WA. The history of laryngology: a centennial celebration. *Otolaryngol Head Neck Surg.* 1996;114(3):345–354. http://dx.doi.org/10.1016/S0194-59989670202-4.

20. Barker M, Dort JC. Laryngeal examination: a comparison of mirror examination with a rigid lens system. *J Otolaryngol.* 1991;20(2):100–103. http://www.ncbi.nlm.nih.gov/pubmed/2041058.

21. Dunklebarger J, Rhee D, Kim S, Ferguson B. Video rigid laryngeal endoscopy compared to laryngeal mirror examination: an assessment of patient comfort and clinical visualization. *Laryngoscope.* 2009;119(2):269–271. http://dx.doi.org/10.1002/lary.20020.

22. Paul BC, Rafii B, Achlatis S, Amin MR, Branski RC. Morbidity and patient perception of flexible laryngoscopy. *Ann Otol Rhinol Laryngol.* 2012;121(11):708–713. http://dx.doi.org/10.1177/000348941212101102.

23. Demirci S, Tuzuner A, Callioglu EE, Akkoca O, Aktar G, Arslan N. Rigid or flexible laryngoscope: the preference of children. *Int J Pediatr Otorhinolaryngol.* 2015;79(8):1330–1332. http://dx.doi.org/10.1016/j.ijporl.2015.06.004.

24. Eller R, Ginsburg M, Lurie D, Heman-Ackah Y, Lyons K, Sataloff R. Flexible laryngoscopy: a comparision of fiber optic and distal chip technologies. Part 1: vocal fold masses. *J Voice.* 2008;22(6):746–750. http://dx.doi.org/10.1016/j.jvoice.2007.04.003.

25. Eller R, Ginsburg M, Lurie D, Heman-Ackah Y, Lyons K, Sataloff R. Flexible laryngoscopy: a comparison of fiber optic and distal chip technologies-part 2: laryngopharyngeal reflux. *J Voice.* 2009;23(3):389–395. http://dx.doi.org/10.1016/j.jvoice.2007.10.007.

26. Hosbach-Cannon CJ, Lowell SY, Kelley RT, Colton RH. A preliminary quantitative comparison of vibratory amplitude using rigid and flexible stroboscopic assessment. *J Voice.* 2016;30(4):485–492. http://dx.doi.org/10.1016/j.jvoice.2015.05.018.

27. Makki FM, Hilal A, Fung E, Hart R, Taylor SM, Brown T. Accuracy of flexible versus rigid laryngoscopic photo-documentation in the diagnosis of early glottic cancer. *J Laryngol Otol.* 2013;127(9):890–896. http://dx.doi.org/10.1017/S0022215113001825.

28. Piazza C, Del Bon F, Peretti G, Nicolai P. Narrow band imaging in endoscopic evaluation of the larynx. *Curr Opin Otolaryngol Head Neck Surg.* 2012;20(6):1. http://dx.doi.org/10.1097/MOO.0b013e32835908ac.

29. Lin YC, Wang WH, Lee KF, Tsai WC, Weng HH. Value of narrow band imaging endoscopy in early mucosal head and neck cancer. *Head Neck.* 2012;34(11):1574–1579. http://dx.doi.org/10.1002/hed.21964.

30. Watanabe A, Taniguchi M, Tsujie H, Hosokawa M, Fujita M, Sasaki S. The value of narrow band imaging for early detection of laryngeal cancer. *Eur Arch Otorhinolaryngol.* 2009;266(7):1017–1023. http://dx.doi.org/10.1007/s00405-008-0835-1.

31. Piazza C, Cocco D, Del Bon F, Mangili S, Nicolai P, Peretti G. Narrow band imaging and high definition television in the endoscopic evaluation of upper aero-digestive tract cancer. *Acta Otorhinolaryngol Ital.* 2011;31(2):70–75. http://www.ncbi.nlm.nih.gov/pubmed/22065027.

32. Kraft M, Fostiropoulos K, Gürtler N, Arnoux AE, Davaris N, Arens C. Value of narrow band imaging in the early diagnosis of laryngeal cancer. *Head Neck.* 2015;38(1):15–20. http://dx.doi.org/10.1002/hed.23838.

33. Moore P. A short history of laryngeal investigation. *Q J Speech.* 1937;23(4):531–564. http://dx.doi.org/10.1080/00335633709380306.

34. Spiegel JR, Sataloff RT, Hawkshaw MJ. Strobovideolaryngoscopy: results and clinical value. *Ann Otol Rhinol Laryngol.* 1991;100(9):725–727. http://dx.doi.org/10.1177/000348949110000907.

35. Woo P, Colton R, Casper J, Brewer D. Diagnostic value of stroboscopic examination in hoarse patients. *J Voice.* 1991;5(3):231–238. http://dx.doi.org/10.1016/S0892-1997(05)80191-2.

36. Casiano RR, Zaveri V, Lundy DS. Efficacy of videostroboscopy in the diagnosis of voice disorders. *Otolaryngol Head Neck Surg.* 1992;107(1):95–100. http://dx.doi.org/10.1177/019459989210700115.

37. Cohen SM, Kim J, Roy N, Wilk A, Thomas S, Courey M. Change in diagnosis and treatment following specialty voice evaluation: a national database analysis. *Laryngoscope.* 2015;125(7):1660–1666. http://dx.doi.org/10.1002/lary.25192.

38. Otto KJ, Hapner ER, Baker M, Johns MM. Blinded evaluation of the effects of high definition and magnification on perceived image quality in laryngeal imaging. *Ann Otol Rhinol Laryngol.* 2006;115(2):110–113. http://dx.doi.org/10.1177/000348940611500205.

39. Woo P. 4K video-laryngoscopy and video-stroboscopy: preliminary findings. *Ann Otol Rhinol Laryngol.* 2016;125(1):77–81. http://dx.doi.org/10.1177/0003489415595639.

40. Krausert CR, Olszewski AE, Taylor LN, McMurray JS, Dailey SH, Jiang JJ. Mucosal wave measurement and visualization techniques. *J Voice.* 2011;25(4):395–405. http://dx.doi.org/10.1016/j.jvoice.2010.02.001.

41. Patel R, Dailey S, Bless D. Comparison of high-speed digital imaging with stroboscopy for laryngeal imaging of glottal disorders. *Ann Otol Rhinol Laryngol.* 2008;117(6):413–424. http://dx.doi.org/10.1177/000348940811700603.

42. Woo P. Objective measures of laryngeal imaging: what have we learned since Dr. Paul Moore. *J Voice.* 2014;28(1):69–81. http://dx.doi.org/10.1016/j.jvoice.2013.02.001.

43. Kawaida M, Fukuda H, Kohno N. Video-assisted rigid endoscopic laryngosurgery: application to cases with difficult laryngeal exposure. *J Voice.* 2001;15(2):305–312. http://dx.doi.org/10.1016/S0892-1997(01)00032-7.

44. Poels PJP, De Jong FI, Schutte HK. Consistency of the preoperative and intraoperative diagnosis of benign vocal fold lesions. *J Voice.* 2003;17(3):425–433. http://dx.doi.org/10.1067/S0892-1997(03)00010-9.

45. Dailey SH, Spanou K, Zeitels SM. The evaluation of benign glottic lesions: rigid telescopic stroboscopy versus suspension microlaryngoscopy. *J Voice.* 2007;21(1):112–118. http://dx.doi.org/10.1016/j.jvoice.2005.09.006.

46. Akbulut S, Altintas H, Oguz H. Videolaryngostroboscopy versus microlaryngoscopy for the diagnosis of benign vocal cord lesions: a prospective clinical study. *Eur Arch Otorhinolaryngol.* 2015;272(1):131–136. http://dx.doi.org/10.1007/s00405-014-3181-5.

47. Deliyski DD, Hillman RE. State of the art laryngeal imaging: research and clinical implications. *Curr Opin Otolaryngol Head Neck Surg.* 2010;18(3):147–152. http://dx.doi.org/10.1097/MOO.0b013e3283395dd4.

48. Parangi S. Editorial: translaryngeal vocal cord ultrasound: ready for prime time. *Surgery (United States).* 2016;159(1):67–69. http://dx.doi.org/10.1016/j.surg.2015.10.014.

49. Sidhu S, Stanton R, Shahidi S, Chu J, Chew S, Campbell P. Initial experience of vocal cord evaluation using grey-scale, real-time, b-mode ultrasound. *ANZ J Surg.* 2001;71(12):737–739. http://dx.doi.org/10.1046/j.1445-1433.2001.02257.x.

50. Wong KP, Lang BHH, Lam S, Au KP, Chan DTY, Kotewall NC. Determining the learning curve of transcutaneous laryngeal ultrasound in vocal cord assessment by CUSUM analysis of eight surgical residents: when to abandon laryngoscopy. *World J Surg.* 2016;40:659–664. http://dx.doi.org/10.1007/s00268-015-3348-2.

51. Wong KP, Lang BHH, Ng SH, Cheung CY, Chan CTY, Lo CY. A prospective, assessor-blind evaluation of surgeon-performed transcutaneous laryngeal ultrasonography in vocal cord examination before and after thyroidectomy. *Surgery (United States).* 2013;154(6):1158–1165. http://dx.doi.org/10.1016/j.surg.2013.04.063.

52. Ongkasuwan J, Ocampo E, Tran B. Laryngeal ultrasound and vocal fold movement in the pediatric cardiovascular intensive care unit. *Laryngoscope.* 2016;127(1):167–172. http://dx.doi.org/10.1002/lary.26051.

53. Woo J-W, Park I, Choe JH, Kim J-H, Kim JS. Comparison of ultrasound frequency in laryngeal ultrasound for vocal cord evaluation. *Surgery.* 2017;161(4):1108–1112. http://dx.doi.org/10.1016/j.surg.2016.10.013.

54. Woo JW, Suh H, Song RY, et al. A novel lateral-approach laryngeal ultrasonography for vocal cord evaluation. *Surgery (United States).* 2016;159:52–56. http://dx.doi.org/10.1016/j.surg.2015.07.043.

55. Sirikci A, Karatas E, Durucu C, et al. Noninvasive assessment of benign lesions of vocal folds by means of ultrasonography. *Ann Otol Rhinol Laryngol.* 2007;116(11):827–831. http://dx.doi.org/10.1177/000348940711601106.

56. Ongkasuwan J, Devore D, Hollas S, Jones J, Tran B. Laryngeal ultrasound and pediatric vocal fold nodules. *Laryngoscope.* 2016;127(3):1–3. http://dx.doi.org/10.1002/lary.26209.

57. Maturo S, Benboujja F, Boudoux C, Hartnick C. Quantitative distinction of unique vocal fold subepithelial architectures using optical coherence tomography. *Ann Otol Rhinol Laryngol.* 2012;121(11):754–760. http://dx.doi.org/10.1177/000348941212101109.

58. Klein AM, Pierce MC, Zeitels SM, et al. Imaging the human vocal folds in vivo with optical coherence tomography: a preliminary experience. *Ann Otol Rhinol Laryngol.* 2006;115(4):277–284. http://dx.doi.org/10.1177/000348940611500405.

59. Kaiser ML, Rubinstein M, Vokes DE, et al. Laryngeal epithelial thickness: a comparison between optical coherence tomography and histology. *Clin Otolaryngol.* 2009;34(5):460–466. http://dx.doi.org/10.1111/j.1749-4486.2009.02005.x.

60. Burns JA, Zeitels SM, Anderson RR, Kobler JB, Pierce MC, de Boer JF. Imaging the mucosa of the human vocal fold with optical coherence tomography. *Ann Otol Rhinol Laryngol.* 2005;114(9):671–676. http://dx.doi.org/10.1177/000348940511400903.

61. Coughlan CA, Chou L-D, Jing JC, et al. In vivo cross-sectional imaging of the phonating larynx using long-range Doppler optical coherence tomography. *Sci Rep.* 2016;6(October 2015):22792. http://dx.doi.org/10.1038/srep22792.

62. Sataloff RT, Mandel S, Mann EA, Ludlow CL. AAEM Laryngeal Task Force. Laryngeal electromyography: an evidence-based review. *Muscle Nerve.* 2003;28(6):767–772. http://dx.doi.org/10.1002/mus.10503.

63. Halum SL, Patel N, Smith TL, Jaradeh S, Toohill RJ, Merati AL. Laryngeal electromyography for adult unilateral vocal fold immobility: a survey of the American Broncho-Esophagological Association. *Ann Otol Rhinol Laryngol.* 2005;114(6):425–428. http://dx.doi.org/10.1177/000348940511400602.

64. Blitzer A, Crumley RL, Dailey SH, et al. Recommendations of the Neurolaryngology Study Group on laryngeal electromyography. *Otolaryngol Head Neck Surg.* 2009;140(6):782–793. http://dx.doi.org/10.1016/j.otohns.2009.01.026.

65. Koufman JA, Postma GN, Whang CS, et al. Diagnostic laryngeal electromyography: the Wake Forest experience 1995-1999. *Otolaryngol Head Neck Surg.* 2001;124(6):603–606. http://dx.doi.org/10.1067/mhn.2001.115856.

66. Rickert SM, Childs LF, Carey BT, Murry T, Sulica L. Laryngeal electromyography for prognosis of vocal fold palsy: a meta-analysis. *Laryngoscope.* 2012;122(1):158–161. http://dx.doi.org/10.1002/lary.22354.

67. Statham MM, Rosen CA, Nandedkar SD, Munin MC. Quantitative laryngeal electromyography: turns and amplitude analysis. *Laryngoscope.* 2010;120(10):2036–2041. http://dx.doi.org/10.1002/lary.21046.

68. Smith LJ, Rosen CA, Niyonkuru C, Munin MC. Quantitative electromyography improves prediction in vocal fold paralysis. *Laryngoscope.* 2012;122(4):854–859. http://dx.doi.org/10.1002/lary.21884.

69. Pretorius PM, Milford CA. Investigating the hoarse voice. *BMJ.* 2008;337(337):1726. http://www.bmj.com/content/337/bmj.a1726.

70. Merati AL, Halum SL, Smith TL. Diagnostic testing for vocal fold paralysis: survey of practice and evidence-based medicine review. *Laryngoscope.* 2006;116(9):1539–1552. http://dx.doi.org/10.1097/01.mlg.0000234937.46306.c2.

71. El Badawey MR, Punekar S, Zammit-Maempel I. Prospective study to assess vocal cord palsy investigations. *Otolaryngol Head Neck Surg.* 2008;138(6):788–790. http://dx.doi.org/10.1016/j.otohns.2008.03.004.

72. Kang BC, Roh J-L, Lee JH, et al. Usefulness of computed tomography in the etiologic evaluation of adult unilateral vocal fold paralysis. *World J Surg.* 2013;37(6):1236–1240. http://dx.doi.org/10.1007/s00268-013-1991-z.

73. Chin SC, Edelstein S, Chen CY, Som PM. Using CT to localize side and level of vocal cord paralysis. *Am J Roentgenol.* 2003;180(4):1165–1170. http://dx.doi.org/10.2214/ajr.180.4.1801165.

74. Hojjat H, Svider PF, Folbe AJ, et al. Cost-effectiveness of routine computed tomography in the evaluation of idiopathic unilateral vocal fold paralysis. *Laryngoscope.* 2017;127(2):440–444. http://dx.doi.org/10.1002/lary.26152.

75. Noel JE, Jeffery CC, Damrose E. Repeat imaging in idiopathic unilateral vocal fold paralysis: is it necessary? *Ann Otol Rhinol Laryngol.* 2016;125(12):1010–1014. http://dx.doi.org/10.1177/0003489416670654.

76. Paddle PM, Mansor MB, Song PC, Franco RA. Diagnostic yield of computed tomography in the evaluation of idiopathic vocal fold paresis. *Otolaryngol Head Neck Surg (United States).* 2015;153(3):414–419. http://dx.doi.org/10.1177/0194599815593268.

77. Badia PI, Hillel AT, Shah MD, Johns MM, Klein AM. Computed tomography has low yield in the evaluation of idiopathic unilateral true vocal fold paresis. *Laryngoscope.* 2013;123(1):204–207. http://dx.doi.org/10.1002/lary.23538.

78. Black N. Patient reported outcome measures may transform healthcare. *Br Med J.* 2013;346(7896):19–21. http://www.bmj.com/content/346/bmj.f167.full.

79. Jacobson BH, Johnson A, Grywalski C, et al. The voice handicap index (VHI): development and validation. *Am J Speech Lang Pathol.* 1997;6(3):66–69. http://dx.doi.org/10.1044/1058-0360.0603.66.

80. Rosen CA, Lee AS, Osborne J, Zullo T, Murry T. Development and validation of the voice handicap index-10. *Laryngoscope.* 2004;114(9):1549–1556. http://dx.doi.org/10.1097/00005537-200409000-00009.

81. Gilbert MR, Gartner-Schmidt JL, Rosen CA. The VHI-10 and VHI item reduction translations—are we all speaking the same language? *J Voice.* 2016;31(2):250.e1–250.e7. http://dx.doi.org/10.1016/j.jvoice.2016.07.016.

82. Hogikyan ND, Sethuraman G. Validation of an instrument to measure voice-related quality of life (V-RQOL). *J Voice.* 1999;13(4):557–569. http://dx.doi.org/10.1016/s0892-1997(99)80010-1.

83. Portone CR, Hapner ER, McGregor L, Otto K, Johns MM. Correlation of the voice handicap index (VHI) and the voice-related quality of life measure (V-RQOL). *J Voice.* 2007;21(6):723–727. http://dx.doi.org/10.1016/j.jvoice.2006.06.001.

84. Romak JJ, Orbelo DM, Maragos NE, Ekbom DC. Correlation of the voice handicap index-10 (VHI-10) and voice-related quality of life (V-RQOL) in patients with dysphonia. *J Voice.* 2014;28(2):237–240. http://dx.doi.org/10.1016/j.jvoice.2013.07.015.

85. Zur KB, Cotton S, Kelchner L, Baker S, Weinrich B, Lee L. Pediatric voice handicap index (pVHI): a new tool for evaluating pediatric dysphonia. *Int J Pediatr Otorhinolaryngol.* 2007;71(1):77–82. http://dx.doi.org/10.1016/j.ijporl.2006.09.004.

86. Cohen SM, Jacobson BH, Garrett CG, et al. Creation and validation of the singing voice handicap index. *Ann Otol Rhinol Laryngol.* 2007;116(6):402–406. http://dx.doi.org/10.1177/000348940711600602.

87. McGlothlin AE, Lewis RJ. Minimal clinically important difference. *JAMA.* 2014;312(13):1342. http://dx.doi.org/10.1001/jama.2014.13128.

88. Bauer V, Aleric Z, Jancic E. Comparing voice self-assessment with auditory perceptual analysis in patients with multiple sclerosis. *Int Arch Otorhinolaryngol.* 2015;19(2):100–105. http://dx.doi.org/10.1055/s-0034-1397332.

89. Murry T, Medrado R, Hogikyan ND, Aviv JE. The relationship between ratings of voice quality and quality of life measures. *J Voice.* 2004;18(2):183–192. http://dx.doi.org/10.1016/j.jvoice.2003.11.003.

90. Karnell MP, Melton SD, Childes JM, Coleman TC, Dailey SA, Hoffman HT. Reliability of clinician-based (GRBAS and CAPE-V) and patient-based (V-RQOL and IPVI) documentation of voice disorders. *J Voice.* 2007;21(5):576–590. http://dx.doi.org/10.1016/j.jvoice.2006.05.001.

91. Rojas GVE, Ricz H, Tumas V, Rodrigues GR, Toscano P, Aguiar-Ricz L. Vocal parameters and self-perception in individuals with adductor spasmodic dysphonia. *J Voice.* 2017;31(3):391.e7–391.e18. http://dx.doi.org/10.1016/j.jvoice.2016.09.029.

92. Behrman A. Common practices of voice therapists in the evaluation of patients. *J Voice.* 2005;19(3):454–469. http://dx.doi.org/10.1016/j.jvoice.2004.08.004.

93. Mendelsohn AH, Berke GS. Surgery or botulinum toxin for adductor spasmodic dysphonia: a comparative study. *Ann Otol Rhinol Laryngol.* 2012;121(4):231–238. http://dx.doi.org/10.1177/000348941212100408.

94. Morzaria S, Damrose EJ. A comparison of the VHI, VHI-10, and V-RQOL for measuring the effect of botox therapy in adductor spasmodic dysphonia. *J Voice.* 2012;26(3):378–380. http://dx.doi.org/10.1016/j.jvoice.2010.07.011.

95. Young VN, Smith LJ, Rosen C. Voice outcome following acute unilateral vocal fold paralysis. *Ann Otol Rhinol Laryngol.* 2013;122(3):197–204. http://dx.doi.org/10.1177/000348941312200309.

96. Cates DJ, Venkatesan NN, Strong B, Kuhn MA, Belafsky PC. Effect of vocal fold medialization on dysphagia in patients with unilateral vocal fold immobility. *Otolaryngol Head Neck Surg.* 2016;155(3):454–457. http://dx.doi.org/10.1177/0194599816645765.

97. Spector B, Netterville JL, Billante C, Clary J, Reinisch L, Smith TL. Quality-of-life assessment in patients with unilateral vocal cord paralysis. *Otolaryngol Head Neck Surg.* 2001;125(3):176–182. http://dx.doi.org/10.1067/mhn.2001.117714.

98. Hirano M. *Clinical Examination of Voice.* Springer-Verlag; 1981. https://openlibrary.org/books/OL4272267M/Clinical_examination_of_voice.

99. Kempster GB, Gerratt BR, Verdolini Abbott K, et al. Consensus auditory-perceptual evaluation of voice: development of a standardized clinical protocol. *Am J Speech Lang Pathol.* 2009;18(2):124. http://dx.doi.org/10.1044/1058-0360(2008/08-0017).

100. Zraick RI, Kempster GB, Connor NP, et al. Establishing validity of the consensus auditory-perceptual evaluation of voice (CAPE-V). *Am J Speech Lang Pathol.* 2011;20(1):14. http://dx.doi.org/10.1044/1058-0360(2010/09-0105).

101. Eadie T, Sroka A, Wright DR, Merati A. Does knowledge of medical diagnosis bias auditory-perceptual judgments of dysphonia? *J Voice.* 2011;25(4):420–429. http://dx.doi.org/10.1016/j.jvoice.2009.12.009.

102. Helou LB, Solomon NP, Henry LR, Coppit GL, Howard RS, Stojadinovic A. The role of listener experience on consensus auditory-perceptual evaluation of voice (CAPE-V) ratings of postthyroidectomy voice. *Am J Speech Lang Pathol.* 2010;19(3):248. http://dx.doi.org/10.1044/1058-0360(2010/09-0012).

103. Kreiman J, Gerratt BR, Precoda K. Listener experience and perception of voice quality. *J Speech Lang Hear Res.* 1990;33(1):103. http://dx.doi.org/10.1044/jshr.3301.103.

104. Maryn Y, Roy N, De Bodt M, Van Cauwenberge P, Corthals P. Acoustic measurement of overall voice quality: a meta-analysis. *J Acoust Soc Am.* 2009;126(5):2619–2634. http://dx.doi.org/10.1121/1.3224706.

105. Behrman A. Evidence-based treatment of paralytic dysphonia: making sense of outcomes and efficacy data. *Otolaryngol Clin North Am.* 2004;37(1):75–104. http://dx.doi.org/10.1016/S0030-6665(03)00169-5.

106. Little MA, Costello DAE, Harries ML. Objective dysphonia quantification in vocal fold paralysis: comparing nonlinear with classical measures. *J Voice.* 2011;25(1):21–31. http://dx.doi.org/10.1016/j.jvoice.2009.04.004.

107. Thomas L, Stemple J. Voice therapy: does science support the art? *Commun Dis Rev.* 2007;1(1):49–77.

108. Van Houtte E, Van Lierde K, Claeys S. Pathophysiology and treatment of muscle tension dysphonia: a review of the current knowledge. *J Voice.* 2011;25:202–207. http://dx.doi.org/10.1016/j.jvoice.2009.10.009.

109. Johns MM. Update on the etiology, diagnosis, and treatment of vocal fold nodules, polyps, and cysts. *Curr Opin Otolaryngol Head Neck Surg.* 2003;11(6):456–461. http://dx.doi.org/10.1097/00020840-200312000-00009.

110. Tang SS, Thibeault SL. Timing of voice therapy: a primary investigation of voice outcomes for surgical benign vocal fold lesion patients. *J Voice.* 2017;31(1). http://dx.doi.org/10.1016/j.jvoice.2015.12.005. 129.e1–129.e7.

111. Kotby M, Baraka M, El Sady S, Ghanem M, Shoeib R. Psychogenic stress as a possible etiological factor in non-organic dysphonia. *Int Congr Ser.* 2003;1240:1251–1256. http://dx.doi.org/10.1016/S0531-5131(03)00858-6.

112. Willinger U, Völkl-Kernstock S, Aschauer HN. Marked depression and anxiety in patients with functional dysphonia. *Psychiatry Res.* 2005;134(1):85–91. http://dx.doi.org/10.1016/j.psychres.2003.07.007.

113. Andrea M, Dias Ó, Andrea M, Luísa Figueira M. Functional voice disorders: the importance of the psychologist in clinical voice assessment. *J Voice.* 2017;31(4):507.e13–507.e22. http://dx.doi.org/10.1016/j.jvoice.2016.10.013.

114. Kosokovic F, Lenarcic-Cepelja I. Surgical therapy of dysphonia plica ventricularis. *Ann Otol Rhinol Laryngol.* 1973;82(3):386–388. http://dx.doi.org/10.1177/000348947308200321.

115. Feinstein I, Hilger P, Szachowicz E, Stimson B. Laser therapy of dysphonia plica ventricularis. *Ann Otol Rhinol Laryngol.* 1987;96(1):56–57. http://dx.doi.org/10.1177/000348948709600113.

116. Kendall KA, Leonard RJ. Treatment of ventricular dysphonia with botulinum toxin. *Laryngoscope.* 1997;107(7):948–953. http://www.ncbi.nlm.nih.gov/pubmed/9217137.

117. Rosen CA, Murry T. Botox for hyperadduction of the false vocal folds: a case report. *J Voice.* 1999;13(2):234–239. http://www.ncbi.nlm.nih.gov/pubmed/10442753.

118. Maryn Y, De Bodt MS, Van Cauwenberge P. Ventricular dysphonia: clinical aspects and therapeutic options. *Laryngoscope.* 2003;113(5):859–866. http://dx.doi.org/10.1097/00005537-200305000-00016.

119. Crawley BK, Murry T, Sulica L. Injection augmentation for chronic cough. *J Voice.* 2015;29(6):763–767. http://dx.doi.org/10.1016/j.jvoice.2015.01.001.

120. Reveiz L, Cardona AF. Antibiotics for acute laryngitis in adults. In: Reveiz L, ed. *Cochrane Database of Systematic Reviews.* Chichester, UK: John Wiley & Sons, Ltd; 2015. http://dx.doi.org/10.1002/14651858.CD004783.pub5.

121. Dworkin JP. Laryngitis: types, causes, and treatments. *Otolaryngol Clin North Am.* 2008;41(2):419–436. http://dx.doi.org/10.1016/j.otc.2007.11.011.

122. Ebenfelt A, Finizia C. Absence of bacterial infection in the mucosal secretion in chronic laryngitis. *Laryngoscope.* 2000;110(11):1954–1956.http://dx.doi.org/10.1097/00005537-200011000-00035.

123. Kinnari TJ. The role of biofilm in chronic laryngitis and in head and neck cancer. *Curr Opin Otolaryngol Head Neck Surg.* 2015;23(6):448–453. http://dx.doi.org/10.1097/MOO.0000000000000200.

124. Kinnari TJ, Lampikoski H, Hyyrynen T, Aarnisalo AA. Bacterial biofilm associated with chronic laryngitis. *Arch Otolaryngol Neck Surg.* 2012;138(5):467. http://dx.doi.org/10.1001/archoto.2012.637.

125. Wo JM, Grist WJ, Gussack G, Delgaudio JM, Waring JP. Empiric trial of high-dose omeprazole in patients with posterior laryngitis: a prospective study. *Am J Gastroenterol.* 1997;92(12):2160–2165. http://www.ncbi.nlm.nih.gov/pubmed/9399745.

126. Yiu E, Xu JJ, Murry T, et al. A randomized treatment-placebo study of the effectiveness of acupuncture for benign vocal pathologies. *J Voice.* 2006;20(1):144–156. http://dx.doi.org/10.1016/j.jvoice.2004.11.007.

127. Yiu EML, Chan KMK, Kwong E, et al. Is acupuncture efficacious for treating phonotraumatic vocal pathologies? A randomized control trial. *J Voice.* 2016;30(5):611–620. http://dx.doi.org/10.1016/j.jvoice.2015.07.004.

128. Koufman JA. The otolaryngologic manifestations of gastroesophageal reflux disease (GERD): a clinical investigation of 225 patients using ambulatory 24-hour pH monitoring and an experimental investigation of the role of acid and pepsin in the development of laryngeal injury. *Laryngoscope.* 1991;101(4 Pt 2 suppl 53):1–78. http://www.ncbi.nlm.nih.gov/pubmed/1895864.

129. Guo H, Ma H, Wang J. Proton pump inhibitor therapy for the treatment of laryngopharyngeal reflux. *J Clin Gastroenterol.* 2016;50(4):295–300. http://dx.doi.org/10.1097/MCG.0000000000000324.

130. Wei C. A meta-analysis for the role of proton pump inhibitor therapy in patients with laryngopharyngeal reflux. *Eur Arch Otorhinolaryngol.* 2016;273(11):3795–3801. http://dx.doi.org/10.1007/s00405-016-4142-y.

131. Megwalu UC. A systematic review of proton-pump inhibitor therapy for laryngopharyngeal reflux. *Ear Nose Throat J.* 2013;92(8):364–371. http://www.ncbi.nlm.nih.gov/pubmed/23975490.

132. Hopkins C, Yousaf U, Pedersen M. Acid reflux treatment for hoarseness. In: Hopkins C, ed. *Cochrane Database of Systematic Reviews.* Chichester, UK: John Wiley & Sons, Ltd; 2015. http://dx.doi.org/10.1002/14651858.CD005054.pub3.

133. El-Serag HB, Lee P, Buchner A, Inadomi JM, Gavin M, McCarthy DM. Lansoprazole treatment of patients with chronic idiopathic laryngitis: a placebo-controlled trial.

Am J Gastroenterol. 2001;96(4):979–983. http://dx.doi.org/10.1111/j.1572-0241.2001.03681.x.

134. Noordzij JP, Khidr A, Evans BA, et al. Evaluation of omeprazole in the treatment of reflux laryngitis: a prospective, placebo-controlled, randomized, double-blind study. *Laryngoscope.* 2001;111(12):2147–2151. http://dx.doi.org/10.1097/00005537-200112000-00013.

135. Steward DL, Wilson KM, Kelly DH, et al. Proton pump inhibitor therapy for chronic laryngo-pharyngitis: a randomized placebo-control trial. *Otolaryngol Head Neck Surg.* 2004;131(4):342–350. http://dx.doi.org/10.1016/j.otohns.2004.03.037.

136. Fass R, Noelck N, Willis MR, et al. The effect of esomeprazole 20 mg twice daily on acoustic and perception parameters of the voice in laryngopharyngeal reflux. *Neurogastroenterol Motil.* 2010;22(2):134–e45. http://dx.doi.org/10.1111/j.1365-2982.2009.01392.x.

137. Lam PKY, Ng ML, Cheung TK, et al. Rabeprazole is effective in treating laryngopharyngeal reflux in a randomized placebo-controlled trial. *Clin Gastroenterol Hepatol.* 2010;8(9):770–776. http://dx.doi.org/10.1016/j.cgh.2010.03.009.

138. Masaany M, Marina MB, Sharifa Ezat WP, Sani A. Empirical treatment with pantoprazole as a diagnostic tool for symptomatic adult laryngopharyngeal reflux. *J Laryngol Otol.* 2011;125(5):502–508. http://dx.doi.org/10.1017/S0022215111000120.

139. Eherer AJ, Habermann W, Hammer HF, Kiesler K, Friedrich G, Krejs GJ. Effect of pantoprazole on the course of reflux-associated laryngitis: a placebo-controlled double-blind crossover study. *Scand J Gastroenterol.* 2003;38(5):462–467. http://www.ncbi.nlm.nih.gov/pubmed/12795454.

140. Reichel O, Dressel H, Wiederänders K, Issing WJ. Double-blind, placebo-controlled trial with esomeprazole for symptoms and signs associated with laryngopharyngeal reflux. *Otolaryngol Head Neck Surg.* 2008;139(3):414–420. http://dx.doi.org/10.1016/j.otohns.2008.06.003.

141. Wo JM, Koopman J, Harrell SP, Parker K, Winstead W, Lentsch E. Double-blind, placebo-controlled trial with single-dose pantoprazole for laryngopharyngeal reflux CME. *Am J Gastroenterol.* 2006;101(9):1972–1978. http://dx.doi.org/10.1111/j.1572-0241.2006.00693.x.

142. Lee YC, Na SY, Kim HJ, et al. Effect of postoperative proton pump inhibitor therapy on voice outcomes following phonomicrosurgery for vocal fold polyp: a randomized controlled study. *Clin Otolaryngol.* 2016;41(6):730–736. http://dx.doi.org/10.1111/coa.12611.

143. Weber B, Portnoy JE, Castellanos A, et al. Efficacy of anti-reflux surgery on refractory laryngopharyngeal reflux disease in professional voice users: a pilot study. *J Voice.* 2014;28(4):492–500. http://dx.doi.org/10.1016/j.jvoice.2013.12.009.

144. Carroll TL, Nahikian K, Asban A, Wiener D. Nissen fundoplication for laryngopharyngeal reflux after patient selection using dual pH, full column impedance testing: a pilot study. *Ann Otol Rhinol Laryngol.* 2016;125(9):722–728. http://dx.doi.org/10.1177/0003489416649974.

145. Scarpignato C, Gatta L, Zullo A, et al. Effective and safe proton pump inhibitor therapy in acid-related diseases – a position paper addressing benefits and potential harms of acid suppression. *BMC Med.* 2016;14(1):179. http://dx.doi.org/10.1186/s12916-016-0718-z.

146. Thomas JP, Zubiaur FM. Over-diagnosis of laryngopharyngeal reflux as the cause of hoarseness. *Eur Arch Otorhinolaryngol.* 2013;270(3):995–999. http://dx.doi.org/10.1007/s00405-012-2244-8.

147. Rafii B, Taliercio S, Achlatis S, Ruiz R, Amin MR, Branski RC. Incidence of underlying laryngeal pathology in patients initially diagnosed with laryngopharyngeal reflux. *Laryngoscope.* 2014;124(6):1420–1424. http://dx.doi.org/10.1002/lary.24483.

148. Sulica L. Hoarseness misattributed to reflux. *Ann Otol Rhinol Laryngol.* 2014;123(6):442–445. http://dx.doi.org/10.1177/0003489414527225.

149. Verdolini Abbott K, Li NYK, Branski RC, et al. Vocal exercise may attenuate acute vocal fold inflammation. *J Voice.* 2012;26(6):814.e1–814.e13. http://dx.doi.org/10.1016/j.jvoice.2012.03.008.

150. Ingle JW, Helou LB, Li NYK, Hebda PA, Rosen CA, Abbott KV. Role of steroids in acute phonotrauma: a basic science investigation. *Laryngoscope.* 2014;124(4):921–927. http://dx.doi.org/10.1002/lary.23691.

151. Russell KF, Liang Y, O'Gorman K, Johnson DW, Klassen TP. Glucocorticoids for croup. In: Klassen TP, ed. *Cochrane Database of Systematic Reviews.* Chichester, UK: John Wiley & Sons, Ltd; 2011:CD001955. http://dx.doi.org/10.1002/14651858.CD001955.pub3.

152. Eng J, Sabanathan S. Airway complications in relapsing polychondritis. *Ann Thorac Surg.* 1991;51(4):686–692. http://www.ncbi.nlm.nih.gov/pubmed/2012438.

153. Teitel AD, MacKenzie CR, Stern R, Paget SA. Laryngeal involvement in systemic lupus erythematosus. *Semin Arthritis Rheum.* 1992;22(3):203–214. http://www.ncbi.nlm.nih.gov/pubmed/1295093.

154. Dean CM, Sataloff RT, Hawkshaw MJ, Pribikin E. Laryngeal sarcoidosis. *J Voice.* 2002;16(2):283–288. http://www.ncbi.nlm.nih.gov/pubmed/12150382.

155. Ozcan KM, Bahar S, Ozcan I, et al. Laryngeal involvement in systemic lupus erythematosus: report of two cases. *J Clin Rheumatol.* 2007;13(5):278–279. http://dx.doi.org/10.1097/RHU.0b013e318157f25e.

156. Vasiliou A, Nikolopoulos TP, Manolopoulos L, Yiotakis J. Laryngeal pemphigus without skin manifestations and review of the literature. *Eur Arch Otorhinolaryngol.* 2007;264(5):509–512. http://dx.doi.org/10.1007/s00405-006-0208-6.

157. Mayerhoff RM, Pitman MJ. Atypical and disparate presentations of laryngeal sarcoidosis. *Ann Otol Rhinol Laryngol.* 2010;119(10):667–671. http://www.ncbi.nlm.nih.gov/pubmed/21049851.

158. Rennie CE, Dwivedi RC, Khan AS, Agrawal N, Ziyada W. Lichen planus of the larynx. *J Laryngol Otol.* 2011;125(4): 432–435. http://dx.doi.org/10.1017/S002221511000280X.

159. Garrett CG, Cohen SM. Otolaryngological perspective on patients with throat symptoms and laryngeal irritation. *Curr Gastroenterol Rep.* 2008;10(3):195–199. http://www.ncbi.nlm.nih.gov/pubmed/18625126.

160. Brook CD, Platt MP, Reese S, Noordzij JP. Utility of allergy testing in patients with chronic laryngopharyngeal symptoms: is it allergic laryngitis? *Otolaryngol Head Neck Surg.* 2016;154(1):41–45. http://dx.doi.org/10.1177/0194599815607850.

161. Millqvist E, Bende M, Brynnel M, Johansson I, Kappel S, Ohlsson A-C. Voice change in seasonal allergic rhinitis. *J Voice.* 2008;22(4):512–515. http://dx.doi.org/10.1016/j.jvoice.2006.12.003.

162. Simberg S, Sala E, Tuomainen J, Rönnemaa A-M. Vocal symptoms and allergy–a pilot study. *J Voice.* 2009;23(1): 136–139. http://dx.doi.org/10.1016/j.jvoice.2007.03.010.

163. Koç EAÖ, Koç B, Erbek S. Comparison of acoustic and stroboscopic findings and voice handicap index between allergic rhinitis patients and controls. *Balkan Med J.* 2014;31(4):340–344. http://dx.doi.org/10.5152/balkanmedj.2014.14511.

164. Develioglu ON, Paltura C, Koleli H, Kulekci M. The effect of medical treatment on voice quality in allergic rhinitis. *Indian J Otolaryngol Head Neck Surg.* 2013; 65(S2):426–430. http://dx.doi.org/10.1007/s12070-013-0639-5.

165. Rosen CA, Gartner-Schmidt J, Hathaway B, et al. A nomenclature paradigm for benign midmembranous vocal fold lesions. *Laryngoscope.* 2012;122(6):1335–1341. http://dx.doi.org/10.1002/lary.22421.

166. Akbulut S, Gartner-Schmidt JL, Gillespie AI, Young VN, Smith LJ, Rosen CA. Voice outcomes following treatment of benign midmembranous vocal fold lesions using a nomenclature paradigm. *Laryngoscope.* 2016;126(2):415–420. http://dx.doi.org/10.1002/lary.25488.

167. do Amaral Catani GS, Hamerschmidt R, Moreira AT, et al. Subjective and objective analyses of voice improvement after phonosurgery in professional voice users. *Med Probl Perform Art.* 2016;31(1):18–24. http://dx.doi.org/10.21091/mppa.2016.1004.

168. Leonard R. Voice therapy and vocal nodules in adults. *Curr Opin Otolaryngol Head Neck Surg.* 2009;17(6):453–457. http://dx.doi.org/10.1097/MOO.0b013e3283317fd2.

169. Murry T, Woodson GE. A comparison of three methods for the management of vocal fold nodules. *J Voice.* 1992;6(3):271–276. http://dx.doi.org/10.1016/S0892-1997(05)80153-5.

170. Hogikyan ND, Appel S, Guinn LW, Haxer MJ. Vocal fold nodules in adult singers: regional opinions about etiologic factors, career impact, and treatment. A survey of otolaryngologists, speech pathologists, and teachers of singing. *J Voice.* 1999;13(1):128–142. http://www.ncbi.nlm.nih.gov/pubmed/10223681.

171. Sulica L, Behrman A. Management of benign vocal fold lesions: a survey of current opinion and practice. *Ann Otol Rhinol Laryngol.* 2003;112(10):827–833. http://dx.doi.org/10.1177/000348940311201001.

172. Verdolini-Marston K, Burke MK, Lessac A, Glaze L, Caldwell E. Preliminary study of two methods of treatment for laryngeal nodules. *J Voice.* 1995;9(1):74–85. http://www.ncbi.nlm.nih.gov/pubmed/7757153.

173. Holmberg EB, Doyle P, Perkell JS, Hammarberg B, Hillman RE. Aerodynamic and acoustic voice measurements of patients with vocal nodules: variation in baseline and changes across voice therapy. *J Voice.* 2003;17(3):269–282. http://www.ncbi.nlm.nih.gov/pubmed/14513951.

174. McCrory E. Voice therapy outcomes in vocal fold nodules: a retrospective audit. *Int J Lang Commun Disord.* 2001;(36 suppl):19–24. http://www.ncbi.nlm.nih.gov/pubmed/11340780.

175. Pedersen M, McGlashan J. Surgical versus non-surgical interventions for vocal cord nodules. In: Pedersen M, ed. *Cochrane Database of Systematic Reviews.* Chichester, UK: John Wiley & Sons, Ltd; 2012. http://dx.doi.org/10.1002/14651858.CD001934.pub2.

176. de Vasconcelos D, de Oliveira Camargo Gomes A, Marina Tavares de Araújo C. Treatment for vocal polyps: lips and tongue trill. *J Voice.* 2017;31(2):252.e27–252.e36. http://dx.doi.org/10.1016/j.jvoice.2016.07.003.

177. Yun Y-S, Kim M-B, Son Y-I. The effect of vocal hygiene education for patients with vocal polyp. *Otolaryngol Neck Surg.* 2007;137(4):569–575. http://dx.doi.org/10.1016/j.otohns.2007.03.043.

178. Klein AM, Lehmann M, Hapner ER, Johns MM. Spontaneous resolution of hemorrhagic polyps of the true vocal fold. *J Voice.* 2009;23(1):132–135. http://dx.doi.org/10.1016/j.jvoice.2007.07.001.

179. Zhuge P, You H, Wang H, Zhang Y, Du H. An analysis of the effects of voice therapy on patients with early vocal fold polyps. *J Voice.* 2016;30(6):698–704. http://dx.doi.org/10.1016/j.jvoice.2015.08.013.

180. Lee YS, Lee DH, Jeong G-E, et al. Treatment efficacy of voice therapy for vocal fold polyps and factors predictive of its efficacy. *J Voice.* 2017;31(1):120.e9–120.e13. http://dx.doi.org/10.1016/j.jvoice.2016.02.014.

181. Cohen SM, Gaelyn Garrett C. Utility of voice therapy in the management of vocal fold polyps and cysts. *Otolaryngol Head Neck Surg.* 2007;136(5):742–746. http://dx.doi.org/10.1016/j.otohns.2006.12.009.

182. Jae Cho K, Chul Nam I, Shin Hwang Y, et al. Analysis of factors influencing voice quality and therapeutic approaches in vocal polyp patients. *Eur Arch Otorhinolaryngol.* 2011;268:1321–1327. http://dx.doi.org/10.1007/s00405-011-1618-7.

183. Barillari MR, Volpe U, Mirra G, Giugliano F, Barillari U. Surgery or rehabilitation: a randomized clinical trial comparing the treatment of vocal fold polyps via phonosurgery and traditional voice therapy with "voice therapy

expulsion" training. *J Voice.* 2016. https://www-clinicalkey-com.ezproxy.lib.ucalgary.ca/service/content/pdf/watermarked/1-s2.0-S0892199716300868.pdf?locale=en_US.

184. Wang C-T, Liao L-J, Cheng P-W, Lo W-C, Lai M-S. Intralesional steroid injection for benign vocal fold disorders: a systematic review and meta-analysis. *Laryngoscope.* 2013; 123(1):197–203. http://dx.doi.org/10.1002/lary.23551.

185. Lee SW, Park KN. Long-term efficacy of percutaneous steroid injection for treating benign vocal fold lesions: a prospective study. *Laryngoscope.* 2016;126(10):2315–2319. http://dx.doi.org/10.1002/lary.25916.

186. Lan M-C, Hsu Y-B, Chang S-Y, et al. Office-based treatment of vocal fold polyp with flexible laryngosvideostroboscopic surgery. *J Otolaryngol Head Neck Surg.* 2010;39(1):90–95. http://www.ncbi.nlm.nih.gov/pubmed/20122350.

187. Wang C-T, Lai M-S, Liao L-J, Lo W-C, Cheng P-W. Transnasal endoscopic steroid injection: a practical and effective alternative treatment for benign vocal fold disorders. *Laryngoscope.* 2013;123(6):1464–1468. http://dx.doi.org/10.1002/lary.23715.

188. Cho J-H, Kim S-Y, Joo Y-H, Park Y-H, Hwang W-S, Sun D-I. Efficacy and safety of adjunctive steroid injection after microsurgical removal of benign vocal fold lesions. *J Voice.* 2017. http://dx.doi.org/10.1016/j.jvoice.2017.01.003.

189. Wang C-T, Liao L-J, Lai M-S, Cheng P-W. Comparison of benign lesion regression following vocal fold steroid injection and vocal hygiene education. *Laryngoscope.* 2014;124(2): 510–515. http://dx.doi.org/10.1002/lary.24328.

190. Hochman II , Zeitels SM. Phonomicrosurgical management of vocal fold polyps: the subepithelial microflap resection technique. *J Voice.* 2000;14(1):112–118. http://www.ncbi.nlm.nih.gov/pubmed/10764123.

191. Noordzij JP, Woo P. Glottal area waveform analysis of benign vocal fold lesions before and after surgery. *Ann Otol Rhinol Laryngol.* 2000;109(5):441–446. http://dx.doi.org/10.1177/000348940010900501.

192. Rosen CA, Murry T, Zinn A, Zullo T, Sonbolian M. Voice handicap index change following treatment of voice disorders. *J Voice.* 2000;14(4):619–623. http://www.ncbi.nlm.nih.gov/pubmed/11130118.

193. Dursun G, Ozgursoy OB, Kemal O, Coruh I. One-year follow-up results of combined use of CO_2 laser and cold instrumentation for Reinke's edema surgery in professional voice users. *Eur Arch Otorhinolaryngol.* 2007;264(9):1027–1032. http://dx.doi.org/10.1007/s00405-007-0309-x.

194. Benninger MS. Microdissection or microspot CO_2 laser for limited vocal fold benign lesions: a prospective randomized trial. *Laryngoscope.* 2000;110(2 Pt 2 suppl 92):1–17. http://dx.doi.org/10.1097/00005537-200002001-00001.

195. Xie X, Young J, Kost K, McGregor M. KTP 532 nm laser for laryngeal lesions. a systematic review. *J Voice.* 2013;27(2): 245–249. http://dx.doi.org/10.1016/j.jvoice.2012.11.006.

196. Mouadeb DA, Belafsky PC. In-office laryngeal surgery with the 585nm pulsed dye laser (PDL). *Otolaryngol Neck Surg.* 2007;137(3):477–481. http://dx.doi.org/10.1016/j.otohns.2007.02.003.

197. Kim H-T, Auo H-J. Office-based 585 nm pulsed dye laser treatment for vocal polyps. *Acta Otolaryngol.* 2008; 128(9):1043–1047. http://dx.doi.org/10.1080/00016480701787828.

198. Mallur PS, Tajudeen BA, Aaronson N, Branski RC, Amin MR. Quantification of benign lesion regression as a function of 532-nm pulsed potassium titanyl phosphate laser parameter selection. *Laryngoscope.* 2011;121(3):590–595. http://dx.doi.org/10.1002/lary.21354.

199. Sridharan S, Achlatis S, Ruiz R, et al. Patient-based outcomes of in-office KTP ablation of vocal fold polyps. *Laryngoscope.* 2014;124(5):1176–1179. http://dx.doi.org/10.1002/lary.24442.

200. Wang C-T. Office-based potassium titanyl phosphate laser–assisted endoscopic vocal polypectomy. KTP laser–assisted endoscopic vocal polypectomy *JAMA Otolaryngol Neck Surg.* 2013;139(6):610. http://dx.doi.org/10.1001/jamaoto.2013.3052.

201. Byeon HK, Han JH, Choi BI, Hwang HJ, Kim J-H, Choi H-S. Clinical study treatment of hemorrhagic vocal polyps by pulsed dye laser-assisted laryngomicrosurgery. *BioMed Res Int.* 2015;2015. http://dx.doi.org/10.1155/2015/820654.

202. Koszewski IJ, Hoffman MR, Young WG, Lai Y-T, Dailey SH. Office-based photoangiolytic laser treatment of Reinke's edema: safety and voice outcomes. *Otolaryngol Head Neck Surg.* 2015;152(6):1075–1081. http://dx.doi.org/10.1177/0194599815577104.

203. Sheu M, Sridharan S, Kuhn M, et al. Multi-institutional experience with the in-office potassium titanyl phosphate laser for laryngeal lesions. *J Voice.* 2012;26. http://dx.doi.org/10.1016/j.jvoice.2012.04.003.

204. Pitman MJ, Lebowitz-Cooper A, Iacob C, Tan M. Effect of the 532nm pulsed KTP laser in the treatment of Reinke's edema. *Laryngoscope.* 2012;122(12):2786–2792. http://dx.doi.org/10.1002/lary.23576.

205. Mizuta M, Hiwatashi N, Kobayashi T, Kaneko M, Tateya I, Hirano S. Comparison of vocal outcomes after angiolytic laser surgery and microflap surgery for vocal polyps. *Auris Nasus Larynx.* 2015;42(6):453–457. http://dx.doi.org/10.1016/j.anl.2015.03.011.

206. Karasu MF, Gundogdu R, Cagli S, et al. Comparison of effects on voice of diode laser and cold knife microlaryngology techniques for vocal fold polyps. *J Voice.* 2014;28(3): 387–392. http://dx.doi.org/10.1016/j.jvoice.2013.10.017.

207. Rubin AD, Sataloff RT. Vocal fold paresis and paralysis. *Otolaryngol Clin North Am.* 2007;40(5):1109–1131. http://dx.doi.org/10.1016/j.otc.2007.05.012.

208. Schindler A, Bottero A, Capaccio P, Ginocchio D, Adorni F, Ottaviani F. Vocal improvement after voice therapy in unilateral vocal fold paralysis. *J Voice.* 2008;22(1):113–118. http://dx.doi.org/10.1016/j.jvoice.2006.08.004.

209. D'alatri L, Galla S, Rigante M, Antonelli O, Buldrini S, Marchese MR. Role of early voice therapy in patients affected by unilateral vocal fold paralysis. *J Laryngol Otol.* 2008;122(9):936–941. http://dx.doi.org/10.1017/S0022215107000679.

210. Mattioli F, Bergamini G, Alicandri-Ciufelli M, et al. The role of early voice therapy in the incidence of motility recovery in unilateral vocal fold paralysis. *Logop Phoniatr Vocol.* 2011;36(1):40–47. http://dx.doi.org/10.3109/14015439.2011.554433.

211. Heuer RJ, Thayer Sataloff R, Emerich K, et al. Unilateral recurrent laryngeal nerve paralysis: the importance of "preoperative" voice therapy. *J Voice.* 1997;11(1):88–94. http://dx.doi.org/10.1016/S0892-1997(97)80028-8.

212. Mattioli F, Menichetti M, Bergamini G, et al. Results of early versus intermediate or delayed voice therapy in patients with unilateral vocal fold paralysis: our experience in 171 patients. *J Voice.* 2015;29(4):455–458. http://dx.doi.org/10.1016/j.jvoice.2014.09.027.

213. Monaco GN, Brown TJ, Burgette RC, et al. Electrical stimulation and testosterone enhance recovery from recurrent laryngeal nerve crush. *Restor Neurol Neurosci.* 2015;33(4):571–578. http://dx.doi.org/10.3233/RNN-130334.

214. Busto-Crespo O, Uzcanga-Lacabe M, Abad-Marco A, et al. Longitudinal voice outcomes after voice therapy in unilateral vocal fold paralysis. *J Voice.* 2016;30(6):767.e9–767.e15. http://dx.doi.org/10.1016/j.jvoice.2015.10.018.

215. Walton C, Conway E, Blackshaw H, Carding P. Unilateral vocal fold paralysis: a systematic review of speech-language pathology management. *J Voice.* 2016. http://dx.doi.org/10.1016/j.jvoice.2016.11.002.

216. Kao Y-C, Chen S-H, Wang Y-T, Chu P-Y, Tan C-T, Diana Chang W-Z. Efficacy of voice therapy for patients with early unilateral adductor vocal fold paralysis. *J Voice.* 2017. http://dx.doi.org/10.1016/j.jvoice.2017.01.007.

217. Ford C. Voice restoration in presbyphonia. *Arch Otolaryngol Head Neck Surg.* 2004;130(9):1117. http://dx.doi.org/10.1001/archotol.130.9.1117.

218. Gartner-Schmidt J, Rosen C. Treatment success for age-related vocal fold atrophy. *Laryngoscope.* 2011;121(3):585–589. http://dx.doi.org/10.1002/lary.21122.

219. Berg EE, Hapner E, Klein A, Johns MM, Atlanta I. Voice therapy improves quality of life in age-related dysphonia: a case-control study. *J Voice.* 2008;22(1):70–74. http://dx.doi.org/10.1016/j.jvoice.2006.09.002.

220. Sauder C, Roy N, Tanner K, Houtz DR, Smith ME. Vocal function exercises for presbylaryngis: a multidimensional assessment of treatment outcomes. *Ann Otol Rhinol Laryngol.* 2010;119(7):460–467. http://journals.sagepub.com.ezproxy.lib.ucalgary.ca/doi/pdf/10.1177/000348941011900706.

221. Gorman S, Weinrich B, Lee L, Stemple JC. Aerodynamic changes as a result of vocal function exercises in elderly men. *Laryngoscope.* 2008;118(10):1900–1903. http://dx.doi.org/10.1097/MLG.0b013e31817f9822.

222. Mau T, Jacobson BH, Garrett CG. Factors associated with voice therapy outcomes in the treatment of presbyphonia. *Laryngoscope.* 2010. http://dx.doi.org/10.1002/lary.20890.

223. Rosen CA, Smith L, Young V, Krishna P, Muldoon MF, Munin MC. Prospective investigation of nimodipine for acute vocal fold paralysis. *Muscle Nerve.* 2014;50(1):114–118. http://dx.doi.org/10.1002/mus.24111.

224. Sridharan SS, Rosen CA, Smith LJ, Young VN, Munin MC. Timing of nimodipine therapy for the treatment of vocal fold paralysis. *Laryngoscope.* 2015;125(1):186–190. http://dx.doi.org/10.1002/lary.24903.

225. Sulica L, Rosen CA, Postma GN, et al. Current practice in injection augmentation of the vocal folds: indications, treatment principles, techniques, and complications. *Laryngoscope.* 2010;120(2):319–325. http://dx.doi.org/10.1002/lary.20737.

226. Mathison CC, Villari CR, Klein AM, Johns MM. Comparison of outcomes and complications between awake and asleep injection laryngoplasty: a case-control study. *Laryngoscope.* 2009;119(7):1417–1423. http://dx.doi.org/10.1002/lary.20485.

227. Siu J, Tam S, Fung K. A comparison of outcomes in interventions for unilateral vocal fold paralysis: a systematic review. *Laryngoscope.* 2016;126(7):1616–1624. http://dx.doi.org/10.1002/lary.25739.

228. Tam S, Sun H, Sarma S, Siu J, Fung K, Sowerby L. Medialization thyroplasty versus injection laryngoplasty: a cost minimization analysis. *J Otolaryngol Head Neck Surg.* 2017;46(1):14. http://dx.doi.org/10.1186/s40463-017-0191-5.

229. Yung KC, Likhterov I, Courey MS. Effect of temporary vocal fold injection medialization on the rate of permanent medialization laryngoplasty in unilateral vocal fold paralysis patients. *Laryngoscope.* 2011;121(10):2191–2194. http://dx.doi.org/10.1002/lary.21965.

230. Arviso LC, Johns MM, Mathison CC, Klein AM. Long-term outcomes of injection laryngoplasty in patients with potentially recoverable vocal fold paralysis. *Laryngoscope.* 2010;120(11):2237–2240. http://dx.doi.org/10.1002/lary.21143.

231. Mortensen M, Carroll L, Woo P. Arytenoid adduction with medialization laryngoplasty versus injection or medialization laryngoplasty: the role of the arytenoidopexy. *Laryngoscope.* 2009;119(4):827–831. http://dx.doi.org/10.1002/lary.20171.

232. Li AJ, Johns MM, Jackson-Menaldi C, et al. Glottic closure patterns: type I thyroplasty versus type I thyroplasty with arytenoid adduction. *J Voice.* 2011;25(3):259–264. http://dx.doi.org/10.1016/j.jvoice.2009.11.001.

233. Murata T, Yasuoka Y, Shimada T, et al. A new and less invasive procedure for arytenoid adduction surgery: endoscopic-assisted arytenoid adduction surgery. *Laryngoscope.* 2011;121(6):1274–1280. http://dx.doi.org/10.1002/lary.21762.

234. Aynehchi BB, McCoul ED, Sundaram K. Systematic review of laryngeal reinnervation techniques. *Otolaryngol Head Neck Surg.* 2010;143(6):749–759. http://dx.doi.org/10.1016/j.otohns.2010.09.031.

235. Lynch J, Parameswaran R. Management of unilateral recurrent laryngeal nerve injury after thyroid surgery: a review. *Head Neck.* 2017. http://dx.doi.org/10.1002/hed.24772.

236. Paniello RC, Edgar JD, Kallogjeri D, Piccirillo JF. Medialization vs. reinnervation for unilateral vocal fold paralysis: a multicenter randomized clinical trial. *Laryngoscope.* 2011;121(10):2172–2179. http://dx.doi.org/10.1002/lary.21754.

237. Isshiki N, Shoji K, Kojima H, Hirano S. Vocal fold atrophy and its surgical treatment. *Ann Otol Rhinol Laryngol.* 1996;105(3):182–188. http://dx.doi.org/10.1177/000348949610500303.

238. Lu FL, Casiano RR, Lundy DS, Xue JW. Vocal evaluation of thyroplasty type I in the treatment of nonparalytic glottic incompetence. *Ann Otol Rhinol Laryngol.* 1998;107(2):113–119. http://dx.doi.org/10.1177/000348949810700206.

239. Davids T, Klein AM, Johns MM. Current dysphonia trends in patients over the age of 65: is vocal atrophy becoming more prevalent? *Laryngoscope.* 2012;122(2):332–335. http://dx.doi.org/10.1002/lary.22397.

240. Kwon T-K, An S-Y, Ahn J-C, Kim KH, Sung M-W. Calcium hydroxylapatite injection laryngoplasty for the treatment of presbylaryngis: long-term results. *Laryngoscope.* 2010;120(2):326–329. http://dx.doi.org/10.1002/lary.20749.

241. Overton L, Adams K, Shah RN, Buckmire RA. Longitudinal voice outcomes after type I gore-tex thyroplasty for nonparalytic glottic incompetence. *Ann Otol Rhinol Laryngol.* 2017;126(1):14–19. http://dx.doi.org/10.1177/0003489416672475.

242. Mallur PS, Morrison MP, Postma GN, Amin MR, Rosen CA. Safety and efficacy of carboxymethylcellulose in the treatment of glottic insufficiency. *Laryngoscope.* 2012;122(2):322–326. http://dx.doi.org/10.1002/lary.21930.

243. Carroll TL, Rosen CA. Trial vocal fold injection. *J Voice.* 2010;24(4):494–498. http://dx.doi.org/10.1016/j.jvoice.2008.11.001.

244. Dumberger LD, Overton L, Buckmire RA, Shah RN. Trial vocal fold injection predicts thyroplasty outcomes in nonparalytic glottic incompetence. *Ann Otol Rhinol Laryngol.* 2017;126(4):279–283. http://dx.doi.org/10.1177/0003489416688479.

245. Young VN, Gartner-Schmidt J, Rosen CA. Comparison of voice outcomes after trial and long-term vocal fold augmentation in vocal fold atrophy. *Laryngoscope.* 2015;125(4):934–940. http://dx.doi.org/10.1002/lary.25043.

246. Johns MM, Gaelyn Garrett E, Ossoff RH, Nashville M, Hwang J, Courey MS. Quality-of-life outcomes following laryngeal endoscopic surgery for non-neoplastic vocal fold lesions. *Ann Otol Rhinol Laryngol.* 2004;113(8):597–601. http://journals.sagepub.com.ezproxy.lib.ucalgary.ca/doi/pdf/10.1177/000348940411300801.

247. Kishimoto Y, Hirano S, Kojima T, Kanemaru S-I, Ito J. Implantation of an atelocollagen sheet for the treatment of vocal fold scarring and sulcus vocalis. *Ann Otol Rhinol Laryngol.* 2009;118(9):613–620. http://dx.doi.org/10.1177/000348940911800902.

248. Mortensen M. Laryngeal steroid injection for vocal fold scar. *Curr Opin Otolaryngol Head Neck Surg.* 2010;18(6):487–491. http://dx.doi.org/10.1097/MOO.0b013e32833fe112.

249. Pontes P, Behlau M. Sulcus mucosal slicing technique. *Curr Opin Otolaryngol Head Neck Surg.* 2010;18(6):512–520. http://dx.doi.org/10.1097/MOO.0b013e3283402a3b.

250. Prufer N, Woo P, Altman KW. Pulse dye and other laser treatments for vocal scar. *Curr Opin Otolaryngol Head Neck Surg.* 2010;18(6):492–497. http://dx.doi.org/10.1097/MOO.0b013e32833f890d.

251. Sataloff RT. Autologous fat implantation for vocal fold scar. *Curr Opin Otolaryngol Head Neck Surg.* 2010;18(6):503–506. http://dx.doi.org/10.1097/MOO.0b013e32833f8c21.

252. Welham NV, Choi SH, Dailey SH, Ford CN, Jiang JJ, Bless DM. Prospective multi-arm evaluation of surgical treatments for vocal fold scar and pathologic sulcus vocalis. *Laryngoscope.* 2011;121(6):1252–1260. http://dx.doi.org/10.1002/lary.21780.

253. Mallur PS, Gartner-Schmidt J, Rosen CA. Voice outcomes following the gray minithyrotomy. *Ann Otol Rhinol Laryngol.* 2012;121(7):490–496. http://dx.doi.org/10.1177/000348941212100711.

254. Pitman MJ, Rubino SM, Cooper AL. Temporalis fascia transplant for vocal fold scar and sulcus vocalis. *Laryngoscope.* 2014;124(7):1653–1658. http://dx.doi.org/10.1002/lary.24536.

255. Ohno S, Hirano S, Yasumoto A, Ikeda H, Takebayashi S, Miura M. Outcome of regenerative therapy for age-related vocal fold atrophy with basic fibroblast growth factor. *Laryngoscope.* 2016;126(8):1844–1848. http://dx.doi.org/10.1002/lary.25578.

256. Hirano S, Tateya I, Kishimoto Y, Kanemaru S, Ito J. Clinical trial of regeneration of aged vocal folds with growth factor therapy. *Laryngoscope.* 2012;122(2):327–331. http://dx.doi.org/10.1002/lary.22393.

257. Hirano S, Kishimoto Y, Suehiro A, Kanemaru S, Ito J. Regeneration of aged vocal fold: first human case treated with fibroblast growth factor. *Laryngoscope.* 2008;118(12):2254–2259. http://dx.doi.org/10.1097/MLG.0b013e3181845720.

CHAPTER 12

Evidence-Based Practice: Endoscopic Skull Base Resection for Malignancy

CRISTINE N. KLATT-CROMWELL, MD • THEODORE A. SCHUMAN, MD •
BRIAN D. THORP, MD • CHARLES S. EBERT, MD, MPH •
DEANNA M. SASAKI-ADAMS, MD • MATTHEW G. EWEND, MD •
ADAM M. ZANATION, MD

OVERVIEW OF SINONASAL AND SKULL BASE MALIGNANCY

Endoscopic skull base surgery is a progressive and evolving area of otolaryngology that has become extensively broad and diversified in recent years. With the expansion of endonasal techniques, approaches can now incorporate not only the traditional paramedian skull base, but also the upper cervical spine and orbits. Permitted by improving technology and a more thorough understanding of anatomic relationships in this area, endoscopic endonasal surgery has revolutionized how sinonasal and skull base malignancies are approached and managed. From the patient perspective, endoscopic approaches provide consistently safe outcomes that have decreased morbidity and easier recovery. With these techniques, interdisciplinary care incorporating otolaryngologists, neurosurgeons, medical and radiation oncologists, and nutritionists has become the standard of care. As surgeons became more comfortable with these techniques, endoscopic resection came to the forefront of cancer treatment.[1]

Traditionally, sinonasal and skull base malignancies were treated with transfacial approaches with an emphasis on negative margins. From the perspective of oncologic surgery, endoscopic surgery has not deterred from that fundamental principle.[2] Advancing endoscopy techniques have provided the opportunity to protect vital structures and normal anatomy while providing complete and oncologic resections with significantly less cosmetic morbidity to the patient.[3] In addition, patient-reported quality of life outcomes show improved outcomes with endoscopic approaches compared with open transfacial approaches and are represented in the literature.[4,5] These benefits do not come without a unique set of challenges, including mastery of endoscopic dissection techniques and the need for complex yet reliable reconstructive options.

Criticisms toward endoscopic surgery for malignancy include the inability to obtain oncologic en bloc resections, with the concern that removal in pieces leaves a risk for residual tumor.[6]

Sinonasal and skull base malignancies incorporate a wide variety of pathologies and make up approximately 3%–5% of all head and neck cancer, with an incidence of 5–10 million/year.[7] Pathologies in this group are diverse, with a multitude of different etiologies, histologic attributes, and management characteristics. Diagnosis for these patients can be especially challenging given the nonspecific set of signs and symptoms noted on initial presentation. Patients can complain of vague nasal congestion, rhinorrhea, and pain that is undistinguishable from chronic sinusitis. Progression of symptoms to include facial numbness, diplopia, Eustachian tube obstruction, and extraocular muscle limitations causes increased alarm and typically indicates more advanced disease. In addition, evidence of lymph node enlargement may expedite further imaging and also tends to portend further disease. With the diversity of pathology incorporated into sinonasal and skull base malignancies, we have emphasized the most common diagnoses in this review.

ESTHESIONEUROBLASTOMA

Incidence and Epidemiology

Esthesioneuroblastoma, a neuroendocrine malignancy otherwise known as olfactory neuroblastoma, arises from the specialized sensory cells in the olfactory epithelium. It originates in the upper portion of the nasal septum, superior turbinate, roof of the nose, and cribriform plate and represents 3%–5% of malignancies of the nasal cavity.[8,9] Esthesioneuroblastomas typically present with bimodal distribution, with peaks in the second and sixth decades of life.

Clinical Assessment

Esthesioneuroblastoma staging was initially proposed in 1976 by Kadish based on the presence of metastasis.[10] These data were then modified further by Morita and colleagues to describe four different subtypes based on the different areas of tumor involvement.[11] Since that time, several other systems have been described in the literature. Biller and colleagues described a system that required craniotomy for staging,[12] whereas Dulguerov and Calceterra described a system based on imaging.[13] Hyams went on to describe a staging system based on histopathologic characteristics. Although there is still significant controversy regarding the role of these staging systems in prognostication, recent studies have shown stronger recommendations.[14] In a study by Bell and colleagues, the prognostic utility of the Kadish and Hyams grading systems was compared in their prediction of outcomes for patients with esthesioneuroblastoma.[15] In this prospective study, the authors validated the two separate systems as tools to prognosticate and guide treatment decisions. The study assessed 124 cases and found an overall survival rate of 75% at 5 years. Within that, the overall survival of patients with metastatic esthesioneuroblastoma was much worse. In addition, the disease-free survival was worse for high grade versus low grade based on the Hyams staging system. Based on the Kadish system, it was found that recurrence, distant metastasis, and 5-year survival rates were not significantly different between patients with stage A, B, or C disease. Overall, the study notes that high-grade esthesioneuroblastoma associated with the Hyams grading was more predictive of poor outcome, whereas advanced stage-based was not. Grading based on the Hyams system should thus be considered in the prognostication and treatment of patients with esthesioneuroblastoma.[15] In a separate study by Van Gompel and colleagues, the role of pathologic grading was assessed in regards to patient outcomes.[16] Overall, the study assessed 109 patients and concluded that the extent of disease at presentation (Kadish stage and lymph node metastasis) and higher Hyams pathologic grade were associated with poorer outcomes.[16]

Evaluation of patients with any nasal symptoms begins with a comprehensive head and neck evaluation as well as nasal endoscopy. Further imaging incorporates the use of fine-cut computed tomography (CT) and magnetic resonance imaging (MRI) modalities to further evaluate the initial stage of all tumors. The use of positron emission tomography (PET) in the assessment of esthesioneuroblastoma has always been an area of question. Previously the use of PET was described only in case reports[17,18]; a study by Broski and colleagues found that PET imaging was useful in initial staging for detecting small nodal and distant metastatic disease.[19] The study assessed 28 patients and ultimately upstaged 11 of those based on PET results. All imaging modalities contribute to the evaluation of the neck, as nodal positivity plays a role in patient survival. Overall, esthesioneuroblastomas tend to metastasize first to cervical lymph nodes, typically in approximately 20%–25% of all tumors.[20,21] A meta-analysis completed by Zanation and colleagues noted that, with radiologic or clinical evidence of disease, the neck should be treated with neck dissection followed by radiotherapy.[22] In the recent literature, further support of management of the neck has become more widely accepted. In a study by Jiang and colleagues, 71 patients were evaluated with a diagnosis of esthesioneuroblastoma. The role of the elective neck dissection in a node-negative neck was evaluated in regards to nodal relapse. The study found that elective neck dissection at the time of primary surgery reduced the risk of cervical nodal recurrence. However, this did not translate into long-term survival benefit.[23] Similarly, in a study in *Larynogoscope* by Banuchi and colleagues, a retrospective review of 57 patients showed that the overall survival was negatively affected by intracranial tumor extension, neck metastasis, and positive resection margins. Overall, 17% of patients developed nodal recurrence, more than half of which had distant metastasis up to 40 months after the initial surgery. They also noted that nodal recurrence was not associated with Kadish stage. Overall, patients with esthesioneuroblastoma were at risk for regional and distant metastasis in a delayed fashion, thus the group recommended elective nodal irradiation of the N0 neck for improved locoregional control.[24]

Surgical Management of Esthesioneuroblastoma

Consistent with the goals of oncologic surgery, surgical management of esthesioneuroblastoma includes resection of the entire cribriform plate and crest galli and subfrontal dura with the goal of negative margins and complete resection.[25] This procedure is traditionally done through open approaches, and there are multiple studies that compare this resection with new endoscopic techniques. A meta-analysis conducted by Devaiah and Andreoli in 2009 assessed a total of 1170 cases of esthesioneuroblastoma from 49 different journals from 1992 to 2008. The study overall showed that endoscopic techniques were traditionally used more often with Kadish A and B tumors, whereas traditional approaches were used with Kadish C or D staged tumors.[26] More recently, a new meta-analysis assessed

609 cases of esthesioneuroblastoma in 36 different studies from 2000 to 2014.[27] This study compared outcomes for traditional open approaches with those for endoscopic approaches for all patients, Kadish C/D only, and Hyams III/IV only. The study found no significant difference in the locoregional control or metastasis-free survival between the two techniques. In addition, endoscopic approaches were associated with improved overall disease-specific survival for all patients. With these more recent reviews, endoscopic approaches are validated from an oncologic perspective in the management of these patients. Multimodality therapy has also become the standard of practice for the management of esthesioneuroblastoma. In an effort to improve disease control and overall survival, several studies evaluate the role of radiation therapy in the postoperative period. In a retrospective study by Ow and colleagues, 70 patients with T3 or T4 tumors were evaluated.[28] Over 90% of these patients had surgery as the first-line treatment. Of those, 66% received postoperative radiation or chemoradiation. Overall, the cohort was followed up for 7.6 years. The study found that patients treated with surgery alone had a median disease-specific survival of 87.9 months, whereas those with postoperative radiation had a disease-specific survival of 218.5 months. This emphasizes the significant impact that surgery followed by radiation can have on overall survival and is therefore recommended in treatment algorithms. In a separate Chinese study, Xiong and colleagues again confirmed that combined modality therapy including surgery with postoperative radiation or chemoradiation improved the overall survival and disease-free survival in patients at all stages.[29] Recommendations for multimodality therapy are also made for patients with known oncologic risk factors, including positive margins, intracranial or orbital involvement, or known residual tumor.[30]

Surgical management of esthesioneuroblastoma has been extensively discussed with a beneficial role for postoperative radiation to the tumor bed; however, the role of elective neck irradiation when clinically negative is an ongoing area of controversy. As previously discussed, Jiang and colleagues assessed 71 patients with N0 neck disease who were treated with elective neck irradiation. Outcomes were assessed by recurrence rate and overall survival. They found that selective neck irradiation significantly reduced cervical nodal recurrence but did not affect overall survival.[23] The study went on to describe the greatest benefit for elective neck irradiation in young patients who presented with more advanced disease. Further studies into the role of elective radiation continue to be performed.

In patients with esthesioneuroblastoma, previous studies have emphasized long-term monitoring for recurrent or metastatic disease.[31] In a more recent study, Rimmer and colleagues developed a long-term follow-up protocol for patients with esthesioneuroblastoma.[30] The group assessed 95 patients and found the disease recurrence typically occurred in the first 4 years following the initial management. However, they did see very late recurrence as well, 19.4 years after the initial diagnosis. Because of this, lifelong follow-up is recommended for patients with this diagnosis. Other groups have emphasized the need for ongoing endoscopic surveillance for at least 10 years to assess the clinical efficacy of all treatment.[32–34] Because of the late risk of metastasis, the role of salvage therapy was also assessed. As discussed previously, the study by Banuchi and colleagues evaluated the risk factors for metastatic disease with esthesioneuroblastoma and effectiveness of salvage therapy. Overall, patient survival was 85% at 5 years and 75% at 10 years. Significant factors affecting overall survival were found to include intracranial extension, neck metastasis, and positive margins. The study did see a significant number of patients with late neck metastasis, which was addressed separately. Patients noted to have nodal recurrence were significantly more likely to develop distant metastasis. Overall, distant metastases were found in 39% of patients up to 40 months after diagnosis.[24] The study concluded that patients presenting with more advanced disease had a higher risk of distant failure, and patients with nodal metastasis were more likely to develop distant metastasis, which can present in a delayed fashion. Because of these findings, the authors recommend the use of elective neck irradiation in patients with an N0 neck to help improve outcomes. Further analysis of these outcomes is ongoing at multiple institutions.

SINONASAL MELANOMA
Incidence and Epidemiology
Sinonasal mucosal melanoma is a rare entity that accounts for only 1.3% of all new melanoma diagnoses.[35] This tumor arises from melanocytes originating from the neural crest, traditionally thought to be of cutaneous origin. However, it can develop in pigment cells of the mucosal surfaces of the upper respiratory tract as well. More recently, the World Health Organization found that sinonasal melanoma was the most common site of mucosal melanoma in the head and neck (66%), whereas the oral cavity accounted for only 25%. The incidence of mucosal melanoma is about 2/2 new diagnosis per million, compared with

153.5 per million for cutaneous sites. Overall, mucosal melanoma is more commonly found in women, and the incidence increases with age.[36] The incidence of this tumor varies greatly between different geographic locations, and the tumor is known to be more common in Japan. In addition, there is varying incidence depending upon race.[37] The peak incidence for patients is between 60 and 80 years, with a mean of 64.3 years.[38]

Histologic features of mucosal melanomas of the head and neck can vary greatly and can include spindled, epithelioid, plasmacytoid, and undifferentiated, among others. In addition, a large portion of these lesions are amelanotic (50%), making diagnosis and differentiation from other sinonasal tumors more difficult.[34] Even with all the histologic variability, the overall prognosis of patients with sinonasal melanoma is poor. The 5-year survival rates range from 14% to 25%, and up to one-third of patients will develop regional or distant metastasis.[39–41] Most patients with distant metastasis succumb to the disease in a mean of 3 months.[42] Overall, the disease is most common in the nasal cavity; however, it does present in the maxillary and ethmoid sinuses as well.[41]

Clinical Assessment

As previously described with esthesioneuroblastoma, there is no single staging system that is accepted as the gold standard for staging mucosal melanomas.[43] However, the seventh edition of The American Committee on Cancer (AJCC) Staging Manual developed a formal tumor-node-metastasis (TNM) staging system for mucosal melanoma of the head and neck[44] (see Table 12.1). It should be noted that this most recent system does not use factors such as tumor thickness and ulceration into consideration for prognosis.[34] Mucosal melanoma has also been noted to have multiple distinct molecular alterations compared with traditional cutaneous melanoma, including the presence of CD117 (C-kit) mutations. A common mutation, BRAF V600E, traditionally associated with >50% of cutaneous malignancies, is rare in mucosal melanoma (<6%).[34]

Patients in this group present in a manner similar to patients with esthesioneuroblastoma, with unilateral nasal obstruction, mass lesion in the nasal cavity, or recurrent nosebleeds.[45] Eye symptoms and cranial neuropathies are typically associated with more advanced disease. A portion of these tumors are associated with a pigmented lesion; however, up to 50% can be amelanotic, instead of presenting more like other nasal masses.[45] Patients are assessed using multiple imaging modalities, including sinus CT and MRI imaging. PET has also been used in this patient population.

Goerres and colleagues previously assessed the role of whole-body PET in mucosal melanoma for the evaluation of distant metastasis.[46] The use of PET to evaluate posttreatment response has been studied by Samstein and colleagues, and they demonstrated that patients showing PET response had a greater overall survival.[47] Studies have shown fludeoxyglucose-PET to be the gold-standard imaging modality for the evaluation of patients with cutaneous melanoma. Although this method is commonly used, further studies are required before making this reservation specifically for mucosal melanoma.

Surgical Management of Sinonasal Mucosal Melanoma

The management of malignant mucosal melanoma has traditionally encompassed primary surgery. Although these methods typically required open resections, the recent literature has emphasized the role of endoscopic surgery for the management of these tumors. In a study by Miglani and colleagues, patients were retrospectively reviewed comparing open and endoscopic outcomes in regards to local control and overall survival following surgery.[48] The group found that, in some patients with sinonasal melanoma, endoscopic surgery offers comparable survival and local control without the morbidity of open procedures. In addition, a small case series by Lund and colleagues showed ongoing support for endoscopic management of sinonasal melanomas.[49]

Owing to the aggressive nature of mucosal melanomas and their propensity to recur and metastasize, the role of radiation therapy in these patients has also been extensively evaluated. A meta-analysis conducted by Li and colleagues assessed 12 different cohort studies including 1593 patients. This study recommended primary surgical management in patients who could be considered stable surgical candidates. They also recommended that surgery be combined with postoperative radiotherapy for dramatic improvement in control of local disease at the primary site; however, this did not significantly affect the overall death risk because of its inability to control distant metastasis. The study also recommended that, in efforts to improve control of distant metastasis and lower the overall death risk, immunologic therapy should be considered after primary treatment.[50]

Overall, treatment of sinonasal melanoma remains difficult with poor outcomes. Patients typically have advanced disease at the time of diagnosis and tend to have a high rate of recurrence and distant metastasis after treatment. Although previous studies supported the use of surgery for mucosal melanoma as a palliative

TABLE 12.1 AJCC Classification for Mucosal Melanoma			
PRIMARY TUMOR			
T3	Mucosal disease		
T4a	Moderately advanced disease. Tumor involving deep soft tissue, cartilage, bone, or overlying skin		
T4b	Very advanced disease. Tumor involving brain, dura, skull base, lower cranial nerves (IX, X, XI, XII), masticator space, carotid artery, prevertebral space, or mediastinal structures		
REGIONAL LYMPH NODES			
NX	Regional lymph nodes cannot be assessed		
N0	No regional lymph node metastases		
N1	Regional lymph node metastases present		
DISTANT METASTASIS			
M0	No distant metastasis		
M1	Distant metastasis present		
CLINICAL STAGE			
Stage III	T3	N0	M0
Stage IVA	T4a	N0	M0
	T3-T4a	N1	M0
Stage IVB	T4b	Any N	M0
Stage IVC	Any T	Any N	M1

AJCC, American Joint Committee on Cancer.
From Edge SB, Byrd DR, Compton CC, eds. *AJCC Cancer Staging Manual.* 7th ed. New York, NY: Springer; 2009.

option, the newer literature supports improved locoregional control with surgery and improved outcomes when combined with long-term immunotherapy.

NASOPHARYNGEAL CARCINOMA

Incidence and Epidemiology

Nasopharyngeal carcinoma is the most common cancer of the nasopharynx, traditionally originating in the fossa of Rosenmuller. It arises from the epithelial lining of the nasopharynx and is largely categorized based on histology (see Table 12.2). This tumor is influenced by a variety of factors, including viral exposure, environmental exposure, as well as geography and ethnicity.[51] Nasopharyngeal carcinoma has been noted to be highly endemic to the Cantonese in the Guangdong Province in China, supporting the geographic and ethnic correlation.[52] The disease is rare in the United States, with an incidence of 1 per 100,000 person-years.[51] This malignancy has a bimodal age distribution, associated with a first peak in late childhood, whereas the second peak

does not affect individuals typically until the fifth and sixth decades.[53] Both groups demonstrate a male-to-female ration of 2:1. Unique to this disease process is its close association with Epstein-Barr virus (EBV) infection. Although this virus is one of the most common worldwide, genetic predisposition precludes transformation into malignancy in only certain patients. External environmental factors such as the consumption of salted fish and exposure to carcinogenic chemicals such as in smoking contribute to this conversion. Risk factors associated with nasopharyngeal carcinoma included high EBV antibody titers, family history, exposure to formaldehyde and wood dust, consumption of salted fish, and cigarettes.

Clinical Assessment

Staging for nasopharyngeal carcinoma is done via the tumor node metastasis system developed by the AJCC[54] (see Table 12.3). Much like other nasal tumors, patients present with nonspecific nasal symptoms, including nasal obstruction, bleeding, or drainage. In addition,

TABLE 12.2
World Health Organization Classification of NPC

Stage	Histopathology
I	Keratinizing squamous cell carcinoma
II	Nonkeratinizing squamous cell carcinoma
III	Basaloid/undifferentiated squamous cell carcinoma

NPC, nasopharyngeal carcinoma.

patients with nasopharyngeal carcinoma can present with unilateral ear complaints or a neck mass. Patients are evaluated using both CT and MRI to assess tumor infiltration into surrounding soft tissues, orbit, or intracranially. Imaging is also vital in completely staging the tumor before treatment considerations.[55] Biopsy is vital to the diagnosis and may typically be done in clinic endoscopically or may involve a fine-needle aspiration of a suspicious neck node. In addition, the use of PET/CT can help diagnose the presence of additional metastasis as a component of the initial evaluation. A meta-analysis by Xu and colleagues pooled data on 1276 patients and found that 174 (13.7%) had evidence of metastatic disease at the time of diagnosis, supporting the use of PET in this role.[56] Upon completion of initial imaging, patients with a diagnosis of nasopharyngeal carcinoma should have EBV antibody titers drawn, as this has been shown to correlate with risk stratification.[57,58]

Surgical Management of Nasopharyngeal Carcinoma

The gold standard of primary treatment for nasopharyngeal carcinoma is chemoradiation, because of the locations, affected structures, and morbidity associated with surgical resection. However, because of recurrence, the role for salvage surgery in the management of patients with recurrent or persistent disease has come to the forefront. In a meta-analysis conducted by Na'ara, a review of outcomes for patients requiring salvage surgery for the management of nasopharyngeal carcinoma was conducted with a review of 17 studies. In this review, prognostic factors that improved outcomes for patients needing salvage surgery were identified. In this study, 779 patients were reviewed. Of these, 83% were T1-T2, 16.6% were T3-4, and 88 patients had evidence of nodal disease. In this study, more than half the patients with recurrent disease could be successfully treated with surgery. Margin status, nodal status, and overall tumor bulk significantly contributed to outcomes. The study went further to recommend endoscopic surgery

because this offered better outcomes than open procedures for more advanced disease.[59] If patients were eligible for reirradiation, outcomes improved even further. In a separate study by You and colleagues, salvage endoscopic nasopharyngectomy was compared with intensity-modulated radiation therapy (IMRT) for local recurrence. The study found the 5-year overall survival was 77.1% for surgery and 55.5% for IMRT and recommended that surgical management of recurrence was associated with quality of life, lower complication rate, and lower overall cost.[60] Previously, similar findings were found by Chen and colleagues, who studied 37 patients who underwent salvage nasopharyngectomy in 2009. Although this study had a selection bias for lower stage tumors, it still showed excellent local control and disease-free survival for patients undergoing surgical management for recurrent disease.[61] The role of surgery has yet to be thoroughly studied for recurrence in patients with very advanced disease.

SINONASAL ADENOCARCINOMA
Incidence and Epidemiology

Sinonasal adenocarcinoma (SNAC) refers to a variety of different tumors and comprises 11.4% of all sinonasal tumors.[62] SNAC can be divided into nonintestinal-type adenocarcinoma (non-ITAC) and intestinal-type adenocarcinoma (ITAC). Of these, further categorization can occur into low- and high-grade types.[63,64] Sinonasal ITAC has previously been classified by Barnes and comprises a mix of different tumors[65] (see Table 12.4). Although the individual epidemiology and clinical behavior of each subtype is different, the overall prognosis of SNAC is poor, with 5-year survival between 20% and 50%.[66]

There is evidence that ITAC is associated with occupational exposures, including wood and leather dust exposure. Patients can present up to 40 years after exposure.[67] Individuals typically working in the furniture-making industry have more than 500 times the risk of getting ITAC as the general population.[68] Because of the work-related exposure that occurs with this disease, ITAC affects males up to three times more than women and presents during their mid-sixties.[69] Owing to the method of exposure, typically the middle and inferior turbinates are the most affected.[70]

Sinonasal non-ITAC can be divided into low- and high-grade tumors with unique tumor characteristics. Like most high-grade tumors, there is associated high mitotic activity, tissue necrosis, and cytologic atypic associated with these tumors.[53] With high-grade tumors, the disease course is much faster, and 3-year survival is

TABLE 12.3
AJCC TNM Staging for Nasopharyngeal Carcinoma

PRIMARY TUMOR (T)

TX	Primary tumor cannot be assessed
T0	No evidence of primary tumor
Tis	Carcinoma in situ
T1	Tumor confined to the nasopharynx or tumor extends to the oropharynx and/or nasal cavity without parapharyngeal extension
T2	Tumor with parapharygeal extension
T3	Tumor involves bony structures of skull base and/or paranasal sinuses
T4	Tumor with intracranial extension and/or involvement of cranial nerves, hypopharynx, orbit, or with extension to the infratemporal fossa/masticator space

REGIONAL LYMPH NODES (N)

This site is different from other head and neck sites

NX	Regional lymph nodes cannot be assessed
N0	No regional lymph node metastasis
N1	Unilateral metastasis in cervical lymph node(s), 6 cm or less in greatest dimension, above the supraclavicular fossa, and/or unilateral or bilateral retropharyngeal lymph nodes, 6 cm or less in greatest dimension[a]
N2	Bilateral metastasis in cervical lymph node(s), 6 cm or less in greatest dimension, above the supraclavicular fossa[a]
N3	Metastasis in lymph node[a] >6 cm and/or to supraclavicular fossa[a]
N3a	Greater than 6 cm in dimension
N3b	Extension to the supraclavicular fossa

STAGE GROUPING

This stage grouping is unique to regional lymph nodes

Stage 0	Tis	N0	M0
Stage I	T1	N0	M0
Stage II	T2	N1	M0
	T2	N0	M0
	T2	N1	M0
Stage III	T1	N2	M0
	T2	N2	M0
	T3	N0	M0
	T3	N1	M0
	T3	N2	M0
Stage IVA	T4	N0	M0
	T4	N1	M0
	T4	N2	M0
Stage IVB	Any T	N3	M0
Stage IVC	Any T	Any N	M1

AJCC, American Joint Committee on Cancer.
From Edge SB, Byrd DR, Compton CC, eds. *AJCC Cancer Staging Manual*. 7th ed. New York, NY: Springer; 2009.
[a]Midline nodes are considered ipsilateral nodes.

TABLE 12.4
Classification and Survival for Intestinal-Type SNACs

Barnes	Klesinasser and Schroede	3-year Cumulative Survival (%)
Papillary	Papillary tubular cylinder cell—I	82
Colonic	Papillary tubular cylinder cell—II	54
Solid	Papillary tubular cylinder cell—III	35
Mucinous	Alveolar goblet	48
	Signet ring	0
Mixed	Transitional	71

Data from Barnes L. Intestinal-type adenocarcinoma of the nasal cavity and paranasal sinuses. *Am J Surg Pathol*. 1986;10(3):192–202 and Kleinsasser O, Schroeder HG. Adenocarcinomas of the inner nose after exposure to wood dust. Morphological findings and relationships between histo-pathology and clinical behavior in 79 cases. *Arch Otorhinolaryngol*. 1988;245:1–15.

around 20%.[71] Conversely, low-grade tumors typically have excellent prognosis associated with a 5-year survival of 85%.[72] Low- and high-grade tumors are also differentiated by the location of the tumor. High-grade tumors are typically in the maxillary sinus,[72] whereas low-grade tumors are primarily in the nasal cavity, followed by the ethmoid and maxillary sinus.[64]

Clinical Assessment

The key to diagnosis of SNAC is biopsy to differentiate the different types of salivary, intestinal, and nonintestinal SNAC. It is vital for all tumors to be imaged properly, including CT and MRI, to identify the extent of disease.[73] Because of the risk factors described earlier, the ITACs typically present with clinically advanced disease, usually T3 or T4 at the time of diagnosis. Because of the variety of different tumors, a unified staging system for these pathologies is not in common practice.

Surgical Management of Sinonasal Adenocarcinoma

An overall consensus for the surgical management of SNAC is difficult to obtain because most studies do not separate results based on histology. With the completely diverse set of tumors and clinical behavior within this tumor group, a unified management strategy is challenging. The surgical approaches to SNAC management, including endoscopic, combined open and endoscopic, and traditional craniofacial resection, remain controversial throughout the literature. In a study by Mortuaire and colleagues, endoscopic approaches were compared with external approaches in the management of SNAC. Patients in this study were limited to those with ITAC of the ethmoid sinus. The study sites the previous gold-standard approach,

which included a lateral rhinotomy approach to tumor resection. In this study, two groups that underwent disease management with either the endoscopic or open approach were compared. Overall, endoscopic approaches did not have significantly different local control and disease-free survival when compared with traditional open approaches. The endoscopic group was noted to have a shorter hospital stay.[74] A meta-analysis by Meccariello and colleagues reviewed 1826 patients and compared outcomes of endoscopic with traditional open surgical technique. In this study, the authors found that the endoscopic group overall had lower complication rates and a lower incidence of local failures. The article concludes that endoscopic management is both safe and beneficial in the management of patients with SNAC.[75]

The role of multimodality therapy in the management of SNAC must also be assessed. In a separate study by Turri-Zanoni and colleagues multiple treatment strategies for SNAC were evaluated. Here, 61 patients were followed up for over 60 months and were treated with surgery alone or surgery plus postoperative radiotherapy. Overall, the study showed that endoscopic endonasal surgery could be used as a single-modality treatment for low-grade early-stage tumors with negative resection margins.[76] For high-grade lesions, surgery with postoperative radiation therapy offered the best hope for disease-free survival.

Long-term survival for patients with SNAC varies greatly depending on specific histology. However, Camp and colleagues assessed the long-term outcomes for patients with intestinal-type SNAC when treated with endoscopic resection and postoperative radiation therapy. In this study, 123 patients were followed up for a mean of 66 months. From this review, 5-year overall survival was found to be 68%, disease-specific survival was 82%, and recurrence-free survival was 62%.[77] When reviewed at 10 years, these numbers shift to 51%, 74%, and 45%, respectively. This study concluded that outcomes were most strongly influenced by local recurrence, T classification, histologic classification, and development of distant metastasis.[77] In a separate study by D'Aguillo, review of the SEER database identified 1270 cases of SNAC. In this group, disease-specific survival at 5, 10, 15, and 20 years was 65.2%, 50.9%, 40.9% and 36.5%, respectively. Overall, the data showed that females had higher survival than males and the condition was more common in whites than in other ethnicities. The data from the SEER database may be more reflective, as it includes the more aggressive subtypes of SNAC into the analysis.[78] Overall, SNAC is a rare tumor that can be associated with occupational risk factors, that has been noted to be well treated with endoscopic surgical techniques and possible postoperative radiation therapy.

SINONASAL UNDIFFERENTIATED CARCINOMA

Incidence and Epidemiology

Sinonasal undifferentiated carcinoma (SNUC) is a recently described tumor type that is aggressive and difficult to treat. It was first described in 1986, and the survival time was once reported as 4 months after diagnosis.[79] More recent studies have extended the number to about 1 year from the time of diagnosis but do not show significant improvement.[80] The average age of diagnosis for most patients is between 50 and 60 years, although the disease can present from age 20 to 80 years.[81] The cause of SNUC is completely unknown and noted to have no association with EBV.[82] As with most aggressive tumors, worse prognosis is typically associated with orbital involvement, dural invasion, or neck metastasis.[83]

Clinical Assessment

There is no standard staging system used independently for SNUC. However, previously described systems, including the Kadish staging system and the AJCC staging system for nasal cavity and ethmoid sinus tumors, are used interchangeably.[11,12] As with all other sinonasal pathologies, biopsy and staining is key to diagnosis. Standard imaging must be performed, including a CT and MRI, although most patients undergo a PET/CT at diagnosis to improve the detection of distant disease before any intervention.[83] It is important to note that the neck must also be included in this evaluation. Traditionally, a CT chest was used

for staging; however, this has largely shifted to PET/CT when it is available.[84,85]

Surgical Management of Sinonasal Undifferentiated Carcinoma

SNUC is a very aggressive malignancy with known poor outcomes. Because of this, multimodality therapy, including surgical resection, chemotherapy, and radiation therapy, is considered required for management. Khan and colleagues published a study that assessed the different treatment modalities for the management of SNUC. For this study, the authors reviewed the National Cancer Data Base and found 460 patients to include in the study. Results showed that 60.2% of the patients were diagnosed (based on AJCC) with stage 3 or 4 disease and the overall 5-year survival was 42.2%. The study concluded that surgery followed by adjuvant chemoradiotherapy was better than chemoradiotherapy alone. Overall, the margin status played the most critical role in survival, as they saw no patients with positive margins survive to 5 years. Therefore, the study recommended aggressive management, with surgical resection first with negative margins followed by chemoradiation therapy, especially in advanced disease.[86] Another study by Kuo and colleagues further assessed survival outcomes for combined modality therapy. This multiinstitutional study assessed 435 patients who had been treated with either single-modality or multimodality therapy for SNUC. The study found that the surgery followed by chemoradiotherapy group had significant improved 5-year survival when compared with the surgery followed by radiation therapy alone or radiation alone group.[87]

With the known aggressiveness of SNUC, we have already discussed the role of multimodality therapy. However, Kuan and colleagues assessed the role of T staging for SNUC and overall outcomes. Using the SEER database, the group identified 328 patients with SNUC. Mean overall survival at 2, 5, and 10 years was 43%, 30%, and 25%, respectively. Several factors were assessed in relation to overall survival, and the group found that tumor stage as determined by the Kadish system was associated with worse survival.[88] In addition, a study by Ahn and colleagues assessed the role of nodal metastasis in SNUC and again assessed overall survival. Again using the SEER database, the study revealed that of 141 patients, 31 (22%) had gross nodal involvement at presentation, typically in levels 2–3.[89] Because of this point, elective treatment of the neck should be considered.

Endoscopic management of SNUC has not been widely described in the literature. Revenaugh and colleagues published the only study assessing the role of endoscopic technique in the management of SNUC. This small study assessed patients treated with endoscopic resection and concurrent chemoradiation and found the overall survival rate at 2 years was 85.7%.[90] Although this number is higher than that cited elsewhere, no obvious selection bias was noted, as the majority of patients had T4 disease at the time of diagnosis.

SUMMARY AND CONCLUSIONS

Overall, the literature regarding the use of endoscopic techniques in the management of sinonasal malignancies is largely supportive. No single prospective study has compared endoscopic techniques with traditional gold-standard open techniques in a head-to-head fashion. Because of this, the surgeon must be facile with both endoscopic and open approaches in an effort to keep the best interest of the patients at the center of the decision tree. In a meta-analysis by Rawal and Zanation, the role of endoscopic resection of sinonasal malignancies was further reviewed. A total of 35 studies with 952 patients were included in the study.[91] Overall 2- and 5-year survival for patients was 87.5% and 72.3%, respectively. Follow-up was on average of 34 months. The study found that, of the 759 patients ultimately included in the analysis, 90% had purely endoscopic surgical management of their disease. The study found that there was a statistically significant difference in outcomes between low- and high-grade tumors. The most common pathologies managed with endoscopic surgery included SNAC, sinonasal melanoma, and squamous cell carcinoma. In the pooled analysis, most of the patients (63%) had low-stage cancer, including esthesioneuroblastoma, SNAC, and squamous cell carcinoma with or without inverted papilloma. Carcinomas comprised the majority of high-stage malignancies. No significant difference in overall survival was found between the low-stage and the high-stage cancers, which illustrates the low level of application of the current staging systems to our endoscopic outcomes. This meta-analysis was one of those that included primary squamous cell carcinoma.[91] Although squamous cell carcinoma is the most common sinus cancer, its presence in the sinuses is complicated by oral cavity extension and the differences between primary maxillary and ethmoidal carcinomas. These differences make combining squamous carcinoma outcomes difficult, and most tumors cannot be resected endoscopically. Because primary ethmoidal squamous cell carcinoma, which would be the most amenable to purely endoscopic techniques, is rare, there are little data regarding its outcomes.

From this meta-analysis, there is strong evidence supporting the use of endoscopic techniques for sinonasal malignancies. These techniques provide oncologic resection, while improving cosmetic deformity, an overall decrease in complication rate, and shorter hospital stays. Comparison of endoscopic data to the gold-standard open approach is difficult because of confounders, including clinical stage, histologic diagnosis, and time frame of diagnosis. A specific group of patients, those with squamous cell carcinoma, were included in this meta-analysis but were not previously described in this chapter. Squamous cell carcinoma encompasses a wide array of heterogenous tumors. These tumors have a variety of presentations originating from multiple etiologies, making careful comparison difficult. However, this meta-analysis includes this pathology into a group of high-grade tumors, thus illustrating that it should be treated similarly to other aggressive malignancies. In addition, it can be concluded from other high-grade malignancies that endoscopic resection (if the tumor was ideal) was preferred over traditional open resection and postoperative radiation was frequently implemented as well.

Sinonasal and skull base malignancies encompass a vast array of different tumors with variable clinical and histopathologic behaviors. The surgeon must review this literature and incorporate the use of endoscopic techniques, as there is a clear support for this across histologies throughout the literature. However, the surgeon must be prepared to convert to traditional open techniques should conditions warrant. The overall goal should be oncologic resection with the same principles established in traditional surgery.

REFERENCES

1. Luong A, Citardi MJ, Batra PS. Management of sinonasal malignant neoplasms: defining the role of endoscopy. *Am J Rhinol Allergy.* 2010;24(2):150–155.
2. Lund VJ, Stammberger H, Nicolai P, et al. European position paper on endoscopic management of tumours of the nose, paranasal sinuses and skull base. *Rhinol Suppl.* 2010;22:1–143.
3. Chen MK. Minimally invasive endoscopic resection of sinonasal malignancies and skull base surgery. *Acta Otolaryngol.* 2006;126(9):981–986.
4. de Almeida JR, Witterick IJ, Vescan AD. Functional outcomes for endoscopic and open skull base surgery: an evidence-based review. *Otolaryngol Clin North Am.* 2011;44(5):1185–1200.

5. Tay HN, Leong JL, Sethi DS. Long-term results of endoscopic resection of naso-pharyngeal tumours. *Med J Malays.* 2009;64(2):159–162.

6. Roh HJ, Batra PS, Citardi MJ, et al. Endoscopic resection of sinonasal malignancies: a preliminary report. *Am J Rhinol.* 2004;18(4):239–246.

7. Thompson L. WHO 2005 World Health Organization classification of tumours: pathology and genetics of head and neck tumours. *Ear Nose Throat J.* 2006;85:74.

8. Komotar RJ, Starke RM, Raper DM, Anand VK, Schwartz TH. Endoscopic endonasal compared with anterior craniofacial and combined cranianasal resection of esthesioneuroblastomas. *World Neurosurg.* 2013;80:148–159.

9. McCormack LJ, Harris HE. Neurogenic tumors of the nasal fossa. *JAMA.* 1955;157:318–321.

10. Kadish S, Goodman M, Wang CC. Olfactory neuroblastoma. A clinical analysis of 17 cases. *Cancer.* 1976;37(3):1571–1576.

11. Morita A, Ebersold MJ, Olsen KD, et al. Esthesioneuroblastoma: prognosis and management. *Neurosurgery.* 1993;32(5):706–714. [Discussion: 714–5].

12. Biller HF, Lawson W, Sachdev VP, et al. Esthesioneuroblastoma: surgical treatment without radiation. *Laryngoscope.* 1990;100:1199–1201.

13. Dulguerov P, Calcaterra T. Esthesioneuroblastoma: the UCLA experience 1970–1990. *Laryngoscope.* 1992;102(8):843–849.

14. Hyams VJ. Tumors of the upper respiratory tract and ear. In: Hyams VJ, Batsakis JG, Michaels L, eds. *Atlas of Tumor Pathology.* Second Series, Fascicle 25; Washington, DC: Armed Forces Institute of Pathology; 1988:240–248.

15. Bell D, Saade R, Roberts D, et al. Prognostic utility of Hyams histological grading and Kadish-Morita staging systems for esthesioneuroblastoma outcomes. *Head Neck Pathol.* 2015;9(1):51–59.

16. Van Gompel JJ, Giannini C, Olsen KD, et al. Long-term outcome of esthesioneuroblastoma: hyams grade predicts patient survival. *J Neurol Surg B Skull Base.* 2012;73(5):331–336.

17. Nguyen BD, Roarke MC, Nelson KD, et al. F-18 FDG PET/CT staging and post-therapeutic assessment of esthesioneuroblastoma. *Clin Nucl Med.* 2006;31(3):172–174.

18. Yu J, Koch CA, Patsalides A, et al. Ectopic Cushing's syndrome caused by an esthesioneuroblastoma. *Endocr Pract.* 2004;10:119–124.

19. Broski SM, Hunt CH, Johnson GB, Subramaniam RM, Peller PJ. The added value of 18F-FDG PET/CT for evaluation of patients with esthesioneuroblastoma. *J Nucl Med.* 2012;53(8):1200–1206.

20. Gore MR, Zanation AM. Salvage treatment of late neck metastasis in esthesioneuroblastoma: a meta-analysis. *Arch Otolaryngol Head Neck Surg.* 2009;135:1030–1034.

21. Davis RE, Weissler MC. Esthesioneuroblastoma and neck metastasis. *Head Neck.* 1992;14:477–482.

22. Zanation AM, Ferlito A, Rinaldo A, et al. When, how and why to treat the neck in patients with esthesioneuroblastoma: a review. *Eur Arch Otorhinolaryngol.* 2010;267(11):1667–1671.

23. Jiang W, Mohamed AS, Fuller CD, et al. The role of elective nodal irradiation for esthesioneuroblastoma patients with clinically negative neck. *Pract Radiat Oncol.* 2016;6(4):241–247.

24. Banuchi VE, Dooley L, Lee NY, et al. Patterns of regional and distant metastasis in esthesioneuroblastoma. *Laryngoscope.* 2016;126(7):1556–1561.

25. Harvey RJ, Winder M, Parmar P, et al. Endoscopic skull base surgery for sinonasal malignancy. *Otolaryngol Clin North Am.* 2011;44(5):1081–1140.

26. Devaiah AK, Andreoli MT. Treatment of esthesioneuroblastoma: a 16-year meta-analysis of 361 patients. *Laryngoscope.* 2009;119(7):1412–1416.

27. Fu TS, Monteiro E, Muhanna N, Goldstein DP, de Almeida JR. Comparison of outcomes for open versus endoscopic approaches for olfactory neuroblastoma: a systematic review and individual participant data meta-analysis. *Head Neck.* 2016;38(suppl 1):E2306–E2316.

28. Ow TJ, Hanna EY, Roberts DB, et al. Optimization of long-term outcomes for patients with esthesioneuroblastoma. *Head Neck.* 2014;36(4):524–530.

29. Xiong L, Zeng XL, Guo CK, Liu AW, Huang L. Optimal treatment and prognostic factors for esthesioneuroblastoma: retrospective analysis of 187 Chinese patients. *BMC Cancer.* 2017;17(1):254.

30. Rimmer J, Lund VJ, Beale T, Wei WI, Howard D. Olfactory neuroblastoma: a 35-year experience and suggested follow-up protocol. *Laryngoscope.* 2014;124(7):1542–1549.

31. Bachar G, Goldstein DP, Shah M, et al. Esthesioneuroblastoma: the princess Margaret hospital experience. *Head Neck.* 2008;30(12):1607–1614.

32. de Gabory L, Abdulkhaleq HM, Darrouzet V, et al. Long-term results of 28 esthesioneuroblastomas managed over 35 years. *Head Neck.* 2011;33(1):82–86.

33. Chang AE, Karnell LH, Menck HR. The national cancer data base report on cutaneous and noncutaneous melanoma: a summary of 84,836 cases from the past decade. The American College of Surgeons Commission on Cancer and the American Cancer Society. *Cancer.* 1998;83(8):1664–1678.

34. Williams MD. Update from the 4th edition of the world health organization classification of head and neck tumours: mucosal melanomas. *Head Neck Pathol.* 2017;11(1):110–117.

35. Simard EP, Ward EM, Siegel R, Jemal A. Cancers with increasing incidence trends in the United States: 1999 through 2008. *CA Cancer J Clin.* 2012;62(2):118–128.

36. McLaughlin CC, Wu XC, Jemal A, Martin HJ, Roche LM, Chen VW. Incidence of noncutaneous melanomas in the U.S. *Cancer.* 2005;103(5):1000–1007.

37. Papaspyrou G, Garbe C, Schadendorf D, et al. Mucosal melanomas of the head and neck: new aspects of the clinical outcome, molecular pathology, and treatment with c-kit inhibitors. *Melanoma Res.* 2011;21(6):475–482.

38. Clifton N, Harrison L, Bradley PJ, et al. Malignant melanoma of nasal cavity and paranasal sinuses: report of 24 patients and literature review. *J Laryngol Otol.* 2011;125(5):479–485.

39. Yii NW, Eisen T, Nicolson M, et al. Mucosal malignant melanoma of the head and neck: the Marsden experience over half a century. *Clin Oncol (R Coll Radiol)*. 2003;15(4):199–204.
40. Manolidis S, Donald PJ. Malignant mucosal melanoma of the head and neck: review of the literature and report of 14 patients. *Cancer*. 1997;80(8):1373–1386.
41. Gal TJ, Silver N, Huang B. Demographics and treatment trends in sinonasal mucosal melanoma. *Laryngoscope*. 2011;121(9):2026–2033.
42. Dauer EH, Lewis JE, Rohlinger AL, et al. Sinonasal melanoma: a clinicopathologic review of 61 cases. *Otolaryngol Head Neck Surg*. 2008;138(3):347–352.
43. Mihajlovic M, Vlajkovic S, Jovanovic P, Stefanovic V. Primary mucosal melanomas: a comprehensive review. *Int J Clin Exp Pathol*. 2012;5(8):739–753.
44. Edge SB, Compton CC. The American Joint Committee on Cancer: the 7th edition of the AJCC cancer staging manual and the future of TNM. *Ann Surg Oncol*. 2010;17(6):1471–1474.
45. Thompson LD, Wieneke JA, Miettinen M. Sinonasal tract and nasopharyngeal melanomas: a clinicopathologic study of 115 cases with a proposed staging system. *Am J Surg Pathol*. 2003;27(5):594–611.
46. Goerres GW, Stoeckli SJ, von Schulthess GK, et al. FDG PET for mucosal malignant melanoma of the head and neck. *Laryngoscope*. 2002;112(2):381–385.
47. Samstein RM, Carvajal RD, Postow MA, et al. Localized sinonasal mucosal melanoma: outcomes and associations with stage, radiotherapy, and positron emission tomography response. *Head Neck*. 2016;38(9):1310–1317.
48. Miglani A, Patel SH, Kosiorek HE, Hinni ML, Hayden RE, Lal D. Endoscopic resection of sinonasal mucosal melanoma has comparable outcomes to open approaches. *Am J Rhinol Allergy*. 2017;31(3):200–204.
49. Lund V, Howard DJ, Wei WI. Endoscopic resection of malignant tumors of the nose and sinuses. *Am J Rhinol*. 2007;21(1):89–94.
50. Li W, Yu Y, Wang H, Yan A, Jiang X. Evaluation of the prognostic impact of postoperative adjuvant radiotherapy on head and neck mucosal melanoma: a meta-analysis. *BMC Cancer*. 2015;15:758.
51. Chang ET, Adami HO. The enigmatic epidemiology of nasopharyngeal carcinoma. *Cancer Epidemiol Biomarkers Prev*. 2006;15(10):1765–1777.
52. Yu MC, Yuan JM. Epidemiology of nasopharyngeal carcinoma. *Semin Cancer Biol*. 2002;12(6):421–429.
53. Barnes L, Eveson JW, Reichart P, et al. *Pathology and Genetics of Head and Neck Tumors*. Lyon, France: IARC Press; 2005.
54. Edge SE, Byrd DR, Compton CC, et al. *AJCC Cancer Staging Manual*. New York: Springer; 2009.
55. Liao XB, Mao YP, Liu LZ, et al. How does magnetic resonance imaging influence staging according to AJCC staging system for nasopharyngeal carcinoma compared with computed tomography? *Int J Radiat Oncol Biol Phys*. 2008;72(5):1368.
56. Xu GZ, Guan DJ, He ZY. (18)FDG-PET/CT for detecting distant metastases and second primary cancers in patients with head and neck cancer. A meta-analysis. *Oral Oncol*. 2011;47(7):560–565. [Epub 2011 May 28].
57. Lin JC, Wang WY, Chen KY, et al. Quantification of plasma Epstein-Barr virus DNA in patients with advanced nasopharyngeal carcinoma. *N Engl J Med*. 2004;350(24):2461–2470.
58. Leung SF, Zee B, Ma BB, et al. Plasma Epstein-Barr viral deoxyribonucleic acid quantitation complements tumor-node-metastasis staging prognostication in nasopharyngeal carcinoma. *J Clin Oncol*. 2006;24(34):5414–5418.
59. Na'ara M, Amit M, Billan S, Cohen JT, Gil Z. Outcome of patients undergoing salvage surgery for recurrent nasopharyngeal carcinoma: a meta-analysis. *Ann Surg Oncol*. 2014;21(9):3056–3062.
60. You R, Zou X, Hua YJ, et al. Salvage endoscopic nasopharyngectomy is superior to intensity-modulated radiation therapy for local recurrence of selected T1-T3 nasopharyngeal carcinoma—a case-matched comparison. *Radiother Oncol*. 2015;115(3):399–406.
61. Chen MY, Wen WP, Guo X, et al. Endoscopic nasopharyngectomy for locally recurrent nasopharyngeal carcinoma. *Laryngoscope*. 2009;119(3):516–522.
62. Dulgerov P, Jacobsen MS, Allal AS, et al. Nasal and paranasal sinus carcinoma: are we making progress? A series of 220 patients and a systematic review. *Cancer*. 2002;92:3012–3029.
63. Bhaijee F, Carron J, Bell D. Low-grade nonintestinal sinonasal adenocarcinoma: a diagnosis of exclusion. *Ann Diagn Pathol*. 2011;15(3):181–184.
64. Franchi A, Santucci M, Wenig B. Adenocarcinoma. In: Barnes L, Eveson JW, Reichart P, Sidransky D, eds. *World Health Organization Classification of Tumors. Pathology and Genetics of Head and Neck Tumors*. Lyon, France: IARC; 2005:20–23.
65. Barnes L. Intestinal-type adenocarcinoma of the nasal cavity and paranasal sinuses. *Am J Surg Pathol*. 1986;10(3):192–202.
66. Klintenberg C, Olofsson J, Hellquist H, et al. Adenocarcinoma of the ethmoid sinuses. A review of 28 cases with special reference to wood dust exposure. *Cancer*. 1984;54(3):482–488.
67. Macbeth R. Malignant disease of the paranasal sinuses. *J Laryngol Otol*. 1965;79:592–612.
68. Acheson ED. Nasal cancer in the furniture and boot and shoe manufacturing industries. *Prev Med*. 1976;5(2):295–315.
69. Abecasis J, Viana G, Pissarra C, et al. Adenocarcinomas of the nasal cavity and paranasal sinuses: a clinicopathological and immunohistochemical study of 14 cases. *Histopathology*. 2004;45(3):254–259.
70. Thompson LD. Intestinal-type sinonasal adenocarcinoma. *Ear Nose Throat J*. 2010;89(1):16–18.
71. Heffner DK, Hyams VJ, Hauck KW, et al. Low-grade adenocarcinoma of the nasal cavity and paranasal sinuses. *Cancer*. 1982;50(2):312–322.

72. Knegt PP, Ah-See KW, vd Velden LA, et al. Adenocarcinoma of the ethmoidal sinus complex: surgical debulking and topical fluorouracil may be the optimal treatment. *Arch Otolaryngol Head Neck Surg.* 2001;127(2):141–146.

73. Raghavan P, Phillips CD. Magnetic resonance imaging of sinonasal malignancies. *Top Magn Reson Imaging.* 2007;18(4):259–267.

74. Mortuaire G, Leroy X, Vandenhende-Szymanski C, Chevalier D, Thisse AS. Comparison of endoscopic and external resections for sinonasal intestinal-type adenocarcinoma. *Eur Arch Otorhinolaryngol.* 2016;273(12):4343–4350. [Epub 2016 June 30].

75. Meccariello G, Deganello A, Choussy O, et al. Endoscopic nasal versus open approach for the management of sinonasal adenocarcinoma: a pooled-analysis of 1826 patients. *Head Neck.* 2016;38(suppl 1).

76. Turri-Zanoni M, Battaglia P, Lambertoni A, et al. Treatment strategies for primary early-stage sinonasal adenocarcinoma: a retrospective bi-institutional case-control study. *Head Neck.* 2016;38(suppl 1):E2267–E2274.

77. Camp S, Van Gerven L, Poorten VV, et al. Long-term follow-up of 123 patients with adenocarcinoma of the sinonasal tract treated with endoscopic resection and postoperative radiation therapy. *Head Neck.* 2016;38(2):294–300.

78. D'Aguillo CM, Kanumuri VV, Khan MN, et al. Demographics and survival trends of sinonasal adenocarcinoma from 1973 to 2009. *Int Forum Allergy Rhinol.* 2014;4(9):771–776.

79. Frierson HF, Mills S, Fechner R, et al. Sinonasal undifferentiated carcinoma: an aggressive neoplasm derived from schneiderian epithelium and distinct from olfactory neuroblastoma. *Am J Surg Pathol.* 1986;10:771–779.

80. Gorelick J, Ross D, Marentette L, et al. Sinonasal undifferentiated carcinoma: case series and review of the literature. *Neurosurgery.* 2000;47(3):750–754. [Discussion: 754–5].

81. Rischin D, Coleman A. Sinonasal malignancies of neuroendocrine origin. *Hematol Oncol Clin North Am.* 2008;22(6):1297–1316, xi.

82. Cerilli LA, Holst VA, Brandwein MS, et al. Sinonasal undifferentiated carcinoma: immunohistochemical profile and lack of EBV association. *Am J Surg Pathol.* 2001;25(2):156–163.

83. O'Reilly AG, Wismayer DJ, Moore EJ. Prognostic factors for patients with sinonasal undifferentiated carcinoma. *Laryngoscope.* 2010;120(suppl 4):S173.

84. Enepekides DJ. Sinonasal undifferentiated carcinoma: an update. *Curr Opin Otolaryngol Head Neck Surg.* 2005; 13(4):222–225.

85. Smullen JL, Amedee RG. Sinonasal undifferentiated carcinoma: a review of the literature. *J La State Med Soc.* 2001;153(10):487–490.

86. Khan MN, Konuthula N, Parasher A, et al. Treatment modalities in sinonasal undifferentiated carcinoma: an analysis from the national cancer database. *Int Forum Allergy Rhinol.* 2017;7(2):205–210.

87. Kuo P, Manes RP, Schwam ZG, Judson BL. Survival outcomes for combined modality therapy for sinonasal undifferentiated carcinoma. *Otolaryngol Head Neck Surg.* 2017;156(1):132–136.

88. Kuan EC, Arshi A, Mallen-St Clair J, Tajudeen BA, Abemayor E, St John MA. Significance of tumor stage in sinonasal undifferentiated carcinoma survival: a population-based analysis. *Otolaryngol Head Neck Surg.* 2016;154(4).

89. Ahn PH, Mitra N, Alonso-Basanta M, et al. Nodal metastasis and elective nodal level treatment in sinonasal small-cell and sinonasal undifferentiated carcinoma: a surveillance, epidemiology and end results analysis. *Otolaryngol Head Neck Surg.* 2016;154(4):667–673.

90. Revenaugh PC, Seth R, Pavlovich JB, et al. Minimally invasive endoscopic resection of sinonasal undifferentiated carcinoma. *Am J Otolaryngol.* 2011;32(6):464–469.

91. Rawal RB, Farzal Z, Federspiel JJ, Sreenath SB, Thorp BD, Zanation AM. Endoscopic resection of sinonasal malignancy: a systematic review and meta-analysis. *Otolaryngol Head Neck Surg.* 2016;155(3):376–386.

FURTHER READING

1. Rinne D, Baum RP, Hör G, et al. Primary staging and follow-up of high risk melanoma patients with whole-body 18F-fluorodeoxyglucose positron emission tomography. *Cancer.* 1998;82:1664–1671.

2. Berry MP, Smith CR, Brown TC, et al. Nasopharyngeal carcinoma in the young. *Int J Radiat Oncol Biol Phys.* 1980;6(4):415–421.

CHAPTER 13

Evidence-Based Practice: Management of Glottic Cancer

DANA M. HARTL, MD, PHD • INGRID BREUSKIN, MD, PHD • DANIEL F. BRASNU, MD

KEY POINTS

The following points provide the highest level of evidence for curative treatment based on the Oxford Center for Evidence-Based Medicine.[1] Each issue is expanded in the text and summarized at the end of this chapter.

Tis: Transoral surgery or radiation therapy (level 3 evidence). Surgery may be preferable for younger patients to "save" radiation therapy for local failure or second primary lesions (level 5 evidence).

T1a and T1b: Surgery (transoral) or radiation therapy (level 3 evidence). Laryngeal preservation and overall survival may be higher in patients treated initially with surgery (metaanalyses of retrospective studies) (level 3 evidence).

T2 with normal vocal fold mobility: Surgery or radiation therapy (level 3 evidence).

T2 with impaired vocal fold mobility: Surgery provides higher rates of local control than radiation therapy alone (level 3 evidence). There are no data regarding the outcomes of these lesions treated with chemoradiation, however.

T3T4: Surgery or radiation therapy. When a nonsurgical organ preservation strategy is chosen, concurrent cisplatin with radiation therapy optimizes local control and survival as compared with radiation therapy alone or induction chemoradiation (even with taxanes) (level 1 evidence).

Advanced T4 tumors with cartilage invasion and/or tongue base involvement: Surgery may provide higher survival rates as compared with chemoradiation (level 3 evidence).

DISEASE OVERVIEW: MAIN QUESTIONS IN GLOTTIC CARCINOMA

Evidence-based medicine is the "conscientious, explicit, and judicious use of current best evidence in making decisions about the care of individual patients," and "integrating experience with the best available data in decision-making."[2] The goal in oncology is to optimize disease-free survival while maintaining the best quality of life as possible and, in the case of glottic carcinoma, preserving voice and swallowing. For early stage tumors, only one treatment modality—surgery or radiation therapy (RT)—is generally required to attain this goal. For advanced tumors, combining cisplatin with RT provides high rates of organ preservation and survival. Disease-specific survival for these tumors is not only related to locoregional control but also to metastatic disease that may appear years later and that may be affected by the choice of initial therapy. Finally, and contrary to other cancers, in head and neck cancer patients, overall survival is not always related to the cancer being treated, because of associated comorbidities that determine a large part of overall survival.

EVIDENCE-BASED INITIAL WORKUP

Evaluation of glottic cancer requires a complex evaluation in three dimensions: laryngeal cancer spreads outwardly, like other cancers, but takes specific paths along muscles and perichondrium, with sometimes unexpected paraglottic, subglottic, and supraglottic extensions. Evaluation of the depth of tumor invasion and cartilage involvement is required to optimize the treatment choice.

Clinical Examination

Today, the clinical examination is most often performed using fiberoptic laryngoscopy or a rigid endoscope, but no study has ever prospectively compared mirror laryngoscopy (by experienced physicians) with these technologies. Fiberoptic laryngoscopy is less operator-dependent, provides a magnified view, and allows for archiving of images and videos for multidisciplinary tumor board evaluation.[3]

Evaluation under general anesthesia is performed systematically by most teams, but then again, there are no randomized trials to "prove" that this is better than not doing it. The anterior commissure (AC) and subglottis are generally seen with more precision under general anesthesia. Studies of newer imaging techniques, such as narrow band imaging, near-infrared imaging, and confocal imaging, have found, in some cases, higher sensitivities for the diagnosis of early stage cancer (level 4 evidence), but for now there is no high-level evidence showing an improvement in oncologic outcomes with their use.[4,5]

General health and comorbidities should also be thoroughly evaluated, particularly respiratory comorbidities that may be affected by aspiration that can be a temporary or permanent side effect to treating glottic carcinoma and renal and cardiovascular comorbidities that may preclude some chemotherapeutic agents.

Laryngeal mobility is a main clinical sign of tumor depth and extensions. Dr. Kirchner's seminal study of whole-organ sections has shown that decreased vocal fold motion may be caused not only by a bulky tumor, but also by a tumor invading the paraglottic space.[6] In retrospective studies, laryngeal mobility was the only predictor of minor thyroid cartilage invasion by T1-T3 tumors treated with conservation laryngeal surgery and for early stage to midstage tumors involving the AC (level 3 evidence).[7,8]

Imaging Studies

Contrast-enhanced computed tomography (CT) scan, magnetic resonance imaging (MRI), and 18-fluorodeoxyglucose positron emission tomography combined with CT scan (PET-CT) are the three main imaging modalities for glottic carcinoma. Adding CT and/or MRI to the clinical and endoscopic workup improves diagnostic accuracy (level 2 evidence).[9,10] Using CT, diagnostic accuracy improved from 58% to 80%, and using MRI, accuracy improved from 58% to 88%. The difference between adding CT versus MRI was not significant. Using pathology as the gold standard, reported sensitivities of CT scan for predicting cartilage invasion by laryngeal carcinoma range from 46% to 67% and can be as low as 10% for early stage to midstage tumors (level 3 evidence).[7] Reported specificities range from 87% to 94% (level 4 evidence).[11] A recent systematic review of studies comparing CT with pathology found that CT had a 44%–80% positive predictive value and an 85%–100% negative predictive value for thyroid cartilage invasion (level 4 evidence).[12] MRI has been shown to be not only significantly more sensitive than CT (89% vs. 66%) but also significantly less specific than CT (84% vs. 94%) (level 3 evidence).[13] Thus, there is no evidence favoring CT over MRI for the initial staging of laryngeal

cancer; CT may have a tendency to underestimate, whereas MRI may tend to overestimate.

For the diagnosis of laryngeal primary tumors, clinical examination and CT were found to be superior to PET-CT.[14] In the evaluation of the neck, CT, MRI, ultrasound, and PET-CT are clearly more sensitive and specific than neck palpation alone for the diagnosis of metastatic lymphadenopathy (level 3 evidence).[15–17] However, for the diagnosis of metastatic neck nodes for head and neck cancers in general, two recent metaanalyses have shown PET-CT to be more sensitive and specific than conventional imaging, with a pooled sensitivity of 89% versus 71% and a pooled specificity of 89% versus 79%.[18,19] Diagnostic performance decreases in the clinically N0 neck, but PET-CT remains superior to CT (level 3 evidence).[20]

MANAGEMENT OF EARLY STAGE GLOTTIC CANCER (TIST1)

For glottic Tis initial local control ranges from 56% to 92% with surgery (transoral) and from 79% to 98% with RT. The final local control after salvage ranges from 90% to 100% for both modalities, with ultimate laryngeal preservation ranging from 85% to 100% for surgery and 88%–98% for RT (level 4 evidence).[21–29] Retrospective comparative studies have shown that ultimate local control and ultimate laryngeal preservation were not significantly different between these two modalities (level 3 evidence).[21,30] However, level 3 evidence (retrospective studies and a metaanalysis of retrospective studies) has shown that involvement of the AC by the tumor is a significant factor for local control, using any treatment modality.[21,31]

For T1 lesions, two systematic reviews and metaanalyses of retrospective studies (level 3 evidence) found no difference in terms of local control between transoral laser surgery and RT, but both found a higher rate of ultimate laryngeal preservation in patients treated with transoral laser surgery.[32,33] The most recent metaanalysis of 11 retrospective studies also found a significantly better overall survival rate for patients treated with transoral laser surgery (odds ratio 1.35, 95% confidence interval 1.02, 1.79, $P = .04$).[33] The biases inherent in retrospective studies must be considered, however. Patients selected for RT in these retrospective studies were perhaps in worse general health with more comorbidities, which may contribute to the difference observed. Involvement of the AC may also have been a confounding factor in these studies, with patients chosen for RT because of the technical difficulties and voice problems involved with transoral laser surgery of the AC.

AC involvement by early stage tumors has been shown in retrospective cohort studies to be a factor for decreased local control as compared with tumors without AC invasion, whether treated surgically or with RT (level 3 evidence).[29,34–39] The few retrospective studies (level 3 evidence) directly comparing these two treatment modalities for AC tumors found that open or transoral surgery provided higher rates of local control than RT.[40–42] A systematic review of retrospective studies (level 3 evidence) compared local control with RT for T1b tumors versus transoral laser surgery. Local control ranged from 72% to 96% for RT versus 43%–100% for transoral laser surgery.[43] No statistical analysis was performed, however, because of the study heterogeneity. This study did not particularly evaluate AC involvement; it only took into consideration the initial local control rates, not final local control rates with treatment for failures, and laryngeal preservation was not evaluated. There is thus very little strong evidence favoring a particular treatment specifically for T1 lesions involving the AC. The data from the two aforementioned metaanalyses would favor transoral laser resection for any T1 glottic carcinoma.

In a recent systematic review and metaanalysis of eight retrospective studies (level 3 evidence), voice outcomes, using the Voice Handicap Index, for T1 glottic carcinoma (including T1b), were found to be equivalent between transoral laser surgery and RT, after a mean follow-up of 47 months.[44] There is currently no evidence that robot assistance for transoral surgery for glottic carcinoma confers an oncologic or functional advantage over traditional transoral laser surgery.

Finally, the long-term effects of treatment and the possibility of metachronous second primary head and neck cancer in these patients should be considered. In the study by Holland et al., after a median follow-up of 68 months, 21% of the patients with early laryngeal cancer treated by RT developed a second primary head and neck cancer (level 4 evidence).[45] The American Broncho-Esophagological Association recommended favoring surgery when possible for younger patients, to "save" RT as a future treatment option (level 5 evidence).[46]

MANAGEMENT OF T2 GLOTTIC CANCER

If AC involvement is an important prognostic factor for T1 lesions, laryngeal mobility is the main prognostic factor for T2 lesions. For T2 tumors with normal vocal fold mobility treated with open conservation surgery, transoral laser resection, or RT, initial local control rates range from 84% to 95% (level 4 evidence).[47–53] Five retrospective comparative studies and one systematic

review (level 3 evidence) comparing RT with open or transoral surgery found no significant difference in terms of local control or survival.[54–59] For T2 tumors with impaired vocal fold mobility, local control rates are lower than for T2 tumors with normal mobility, whether the treatment be RT, transoral laser resection, or open surgery, with local control rates falling as low as 50%.[29,42,48,52,55,60–68]

Tumors with impaired vocal fold mobility are at higher risk of minor cartilage invasion (28% histopathologic invasion, in one retrospective study), which is often missed on pretherapeutic CT evaluation (level 4 evidence).[8] Paraglottic space invasion and subglottic extension are also factors for decreased local control for T2 lesions (level 3 evidence).[57,69] For tumors with impaired vocal fold mobility, level 3 evidence shows high rates of local control and preservation of a functional larynx with open surgery, in experienced hands for selected patients, albeit with the voice and swallowing outcomes inherent to this type of surgery.[57,59,69–71]

Thus, for T2 tumors with decreased vocal fold mobility, organ preservation surgery is more effective than RT alone for local control (level 3 evidence), but there is currently no data comparing surgery with combined modality therapy (concurrent chemoradiation with cisplatin), for these tumors. Concurrent chemoradiation remains an organ preservation option for these tumors, but with currently unreported oncologic and functional outcomes in this particular setting (level 5 UK guidelines).

MANAGEMENT OF THE NECK IN T1T2CN0 GLOTTIC CANCER

Without elective treatment of the neck, nodal recurrence rates for early stage (T1T2) glottic carcinoma are in the range of 4%.[72,73] There is no evidence that elective treatment of the neck improves regional control or disease-free survival. One retrospective cancer registry study analyzed the outcomes of 73 patients with pT2cN0 glottic cancer.[74] About half of the patients had undergone elective neck dissection, with occult metastatic nodes found in 10%. Multivariate analysis did not find neck dissection or adjuvant treatment to be significantly related to recurrence-free or overall survival, however (level 3 evidence). Metastatic Delphian nodes were found in 7.5% of patients with T1b or T2 cancers with AC involvement treated with supracricoid partial laryngectomy in the study by Wierzbicka et al.[75] Delphian node involvement was a significant prognostic factor for locoregional failure, lower larynx preservation, and lower overall survival (level 3 evidence). This evidence, however, does not confirm the necessity for neck dissection in all patients, but only encourages particular vigilance when treating this specific subtype of cancer and may be an argument (low-level evidence) in favor of open surgery in these cases. Clinical studies using sentinel node biopsy for staging in the neck for T1T2 laryngeal cancers are currently under way, but there are currently insufficient data to support this approach. There is currently no high-level evidence to guide treatment of the neck for T1T2 glottic tumors, but the low rate of occult disease and regional recurrence would favor the current practice of not treating the neck electively, as suggested in several current guidelines (level 5 evidence).[76–78]

MANAGEMENT OF ADVANCED LESIONS T3T4

Ever since the seminal study by the veterans' association, using induction chemotherapy and RT for larynx preservation in responders, as opposed to an up-front total laryngectomy, with no adverse effect on survival, nonsurgical organ preservation has become a major goal in the treatment of advanced laryngeal tumors.[79] One must keep in mind, however, that organ preservation surgery may still be an option for selected tumors staged T3 and T4a. There are no studies directly comparing organ preservation surgery with nonsurgical organ preservation protocols for advanced stage laryngeal tumors, in a prospective manner with comparable patient groups. Retrospective noncomparative studies (level 4 evidence) show high rates of local control and organ preservation for selected patients treated with open surgery (supracricoid partial laryngectomy)[80,81] or with transoral laser resection.[82,83] As for T1 and T2 tumors, not all T3 or T4 lesions are the same. Vilaseca et al. reported a 5-year larynx preservation of 59% for T3 tumors treated with transoral laser resection, citing vocal fold fixation and laryngeal cartilage invasion as significant prognostic factors for lower local control.[82] Thus, organ preservation surgery remains an option for selected patients in specialized centers.[71,78,84]

The highest level evidence that currently exists for laryngeal cancer is in favor of better locoregional control, organ preservation, and overall survival if concomitant chemoradiation with cisplatin is used as a nonsurgical means of organ preservation, as compared with RT alone or induction chemotherapy protocols.[85,86] The 3-arm prospective randomized trial conducted by Forastiere et al. comparing RT, induction chemotherapy (cisplatin and 5-fluorouracil) and radiation, and concurrent chemoradiation with cisplatin for advanced laryngeal cancer (level 2 evidence) showed a higher 2-year locoregional control rate for the group treated with concurrent chemoradiation (78% vs. 61% for the group treated with induction chemotherapy and 56% for the group treated with RT alone).[85] The 2-year laryngeal preservation rate was 88% for the chemoradiation arm, versus 75% for the induction chemotherapy group and 70% for the RT group. This study excluded large-volume lesions, and T4 laryngeal carcinoma represented only 10% of the cohort.

In the metaanalysis of randomized controlled trials (level 1 evidence) by Blanchard et al., overall survival improved from 42.5% to 47% in the group of 3216 patients with laryngeal cancer treated with concomitant chemoradiation.[86] The benefit was not significant, however, for adjuvant or neoadjuvant chemotherapy. This study included only randomized controlled trials and compared locoregional treatment alone (RT +/- surgery) with locoregional treatment and chemotherapy. This evidence also implies that accelerated RT regimens alone do not provide the survival advantage of concurrent chemoradiation for laryngeal cancer. Current evidence, then, is in favor of concurrent chemoradiation when a nonsurgical organ preservation strategy is chosen. It is important to note that in this metaanalysis, only 28% of the tumors were T4. When the administration of cisplatin is not possible, level 1 evidence (randomized trial) is in favor of concomitant cetuximab with RT, which significantly improved survival as compared with RT alone.[87]

Adding taxanes (T) to neoadjuvant chemotherapy with cisplatin (P) and 5-fluorouracil (F) significantly improves response rates and organ preservation rates for laryngeal cancer, as compared with induction PF alone, and induction TPF results in a higher rate of functional larynx preservation after a median follow-up of almost 9 years as compared with induction PF (level 2 evidence)[88–90]. However, a recent metaanalysis of five randomized trials comparing induction chemotherapy with TPF followed by concurrent chemoradiation with concurrent chemoradiation alone—all tumor sites, with 18.7% laryngeal tumors—failed to show superiority of the induction regimen (level 1 evidence).[91]

The evidence does not show, however, that concurrent chemoradiation is superior to initial total laryngectomy followed by RT: no studies directly comparing these modalities have been performed. The functional results of chemoradiation must also be considered, with high rates of tracheostomy and dysphagia.[92] In the update of the EORTC 24954 phase III trial, only half of the survivors were deemed to have a functional larynx after a median follow-up of 10 years.[93] Another question is exactly what does one mean by "advanced" laryngeal cancer. T-stage takes into account the tumor volume and extensions, cartilage invasion, and resectability. Global staging (stages I-IVc) takes into account nodal disease and distant metastases, in addition to T-stage. As pointed out earlier, prospective randomized trials tend to exclude particularly advanced tumors with extensive invasion of the thyroid cartilage or tongue base, for example.[85]

The results of these randomized trials can thus only be applied to these selected patient and tumor subgroups.[94] For extensive stage IV tumors, in fact, current evidence shows an overall survival advantage with a total laryngectomy as compared with definitive chemoradiation. In the database study by Chen et al., 7019 patients with advanced laryngeal cancer (stage III or IV) were evaluated. Those with stage IV cancer treated with total laryngectomy had a significantly better overall survival than those treated with chemoradiation, who had a hazard ratio for death of 1.43 (level 3 evidence).[95] Another large retrospective study by Gourin et al. included 451 patients of which 195 had stage IV laryngeal cancer.[54] Survival was better for patients treated surgically as compared with those treated using chemoradiation (hazard ratio 3.5) (level 3 evidence). A Canadian database study of 258 patients found similar results.[94] A recent large US National Cancer Database Analysis (level 2 evidence) of 1559 patients treated for T4 laryngeal carcinoma, confirming an earlier National Cancer Database study,[96] found that overall survival was higher in patients treated with laryngectomy followed by RT as compared with concurrent chemoradiation (hazard ratio 1.55), an advantage that persisted even when limiting the analysis to T4a lesions.[97] This study also found that the induction chemotherapy regimen provided a higher rate of overall survival than concurrent chemoradiation (hazard ratio 1.25). Large database studies are, however, limited in scope by possible biases in coding and reporting and by an inherent lack of detail concerning specific chemotherapeutic agents, their doses, and duration of administration, all which may affect the results of the analysis. Finally, a recent metaanalysis including 16 retrospective studies and 8308 patients also concluded that total laryngectomy provided an overall and disease-specific survival advantage for T4 tumors (level 3 evidence).[98] Indeed, low-level evidence has shown that tumor volume is a prognostic factor for local control in patients treated with chemoradiation, whereas tumor volume was not a prognostic factor for patients treated with total laryngectomy (level 4 evidence).[99] These results are compelling and represent the highest level of evidence

currently available regarding the outcomes for patients with advanced T4 lesions, comparing surgery and nonsurgical organ preservation strategies. Currently, only T-stage has been used for prognostication in these studies; other biomarkers or radiologic characteristics are needed for patient selection for nonsurgical organ preservation protocols.

In conclusion, for advanced stage tumors (T3, and some T4), selected tumors may be amenable to conservation surgery (open or endoscopic) or concurrent chemoradiation with cisplatin. For more advanced tumors, a total laryngectomy should still be considered as an important treatment option. The results of protocols with taxanes and cetuximab are encouraging, and eligible patients should be enrolled in clinical trials when possible.[84]

EVIDENCE BASE FOR EXCLUSIVE CHEMOTHERAPY FOR GLOTTIC CARCINOMA

Since the introduction of platinum-based chemotherapy, and more recently with taxane-based treatments, it has become clear that glottic cancer is chemosensitive, with one-fourth to one-third of patients being complete responders and one-half to two-thirds of patients being partial responders.[79,88,100-102] In light of the advantages of chemotherapy and the high response rates, seven published studies have investigated using chemotherapy exclusively for treating early stage, midstage, and advanced stage glottic cancer.[103-109] Five of these studies were retrospective studies of complete responders after three cycles of induction chemotherapy (cisplatin and 5-fluorouracil), who were then allowed to decide if they preferred locoregional treatment or to pursue chemotherapy (level 4 evidence).[103-107] Four studies were from the same hospital.[103-106] Four of the studies included only tumors initially considered amenable to conservation laryngeal surgery.[103,105,106,108] In these studies, between 29 and 65 patients were treated with exclusive chemotherapy, for a rate of local control with chemotherapy alone ranging from 54% to 72% and an ultimate larynx preservation rate ranging from 90% to 100%. Toxicity was acceptable, and no chemotherapy deaths were recorded, but chemotherapy was prematurely stopped in 1% of patients because of toxicity.

To date, only two published studies have prospectively treated all complete responders with exclusive chemotherapy (level 3 evidence).[108,109] The study by Holsinger et al. included 30 patients with stage II-IVa glottic (n = 14) or supraglottic (n = 16) carcinoma considered amenable to conservation laryngeal surgery.[108]

Eleven patients, four glottic tumors and seven supra-glottic tumors, were complete responders after three to four cycles of chemotherapy (37%) and received three more cycles. Of the 11 patients, 10 had no locoregional recurrence after a median follow-up of 5 years, for a local control rate with chemotherapy alone of 91% among the complete responders.

Divi et al. prospectively studied 32 patients with stage III-IVb laryngeal and hypopharyngeal tumors.[109] Four patients were complete responders after one cycle (two hypopharyngeal cancers and two supraglottic cancers) and received additional chemotherapy. All of the patients recurred during the additional cycles, three in the neck and one locally and regionally. For advanced stage tumors, exclusive chemotherapy does not provide long-term locoregional control.

Thus, low-level evidence shows that highly selected patients with early stage glottic cancer may undergo complete remission after exclusive chemotherapy. However, the initial local control rates for these highly selected patients, initially amenable to conservation laryngeal surgery, are not better than other conservation protocols using open surgery, transoral laser resection, or RT (see above). In addition, we currently have no means of preselecting tumors that are more biologically susceptible to respond to chemotherapy, so that many patients need to be treated (between 3 and 17[110]) to select the few complete responders (corresponding to 5.8%–33% of patients). Higher-level evidence is needed before exclusive chemotherapy can become a standard of care.

EVIDENCE BASE FOR THE ROLE OF HUMAN PAPILLOMAVIRUS IN LARYNGEAL SQUAMOUS CELL CARCINOMA

The human papillomavirus (HPV) has been shown to be a major etiologic factor in head and neck squamous cell carcinoma, and particularly for sites in the oropharynx. The implication of HPV in laryngeal cancer seems to be less prevalent than in oropharyngeal tumors, but the rate of detection of HPV in laryngeal cancers varies from 1% to 30% in the literature (level 4 evidence).[111-114] This heterogeneity in the reported prevalence of HPV-related cancer in the larynx is at least in part related to the geographic region of the population studied (level 4 evidence).[115,116] A large study with a homogeneous tissue processing technique (3680 patients) found a prevalence of HPV involvement in only 1.5%–3.5% of the laryngeal cancers studied.[117] Another similar study of 1420 samples of head and neck cancers found a prevalence of 0%

of HPV-related laryngeal cancer in Brazilian samples, as compared with a prevalence of 2.8% for samples from the United States and 5.2% of samples from Europe.[115] A recent metaanalysis of 179 studies comprising 7347 samples of only laryngeal squamous cell carcinoma found a 25% prevalence of HPV positivity, related only to geographic origin, with no statistical evidence in favor of differences related to detection method (level 4 evidence).[116] A metaanalysis of all tumor sites, including 148 studies with 12,163 cases of head and neck squamous cell carcinoma from 44 countries, found a prevalence of HPV detection in 22.1% of laryngeal + hypopharyngeal tumors (level 4 evidence).[112] Finding signs of HPV in sample from laryngeal carcinoma, however, is not the same as showing its involvement in the oncogenesis of these tumors.

WHAT DOES THE EVIDENCE REALLY SAY?

We place the highest value on evidence obtained from randomized controlled trials, which provide the best objective, a statistically sound evidence to guide decisions for treatment of individual patients. Much has been written, however, about the defects inherent in this approach. Patients enrolled in randomized controlled trials are highly selected not only in terms of their tumor, but also in terms of comorbidities. Enrolled patients tend to be more often white, educated, insured, health conscious, and younger than the general population of cancer patients.[118] Moreover, the self-selection of patients for clinical trials may in and of itself constitute a bias toward globally better results than one could expect in the general population.[119]

For glottic carcinoma, we have seen that in the randomized controlled trials comparing different nonsurgical organ preservation strategies, widely invasive tumors with extensive tongue base involvement and/or cartilage invasion were excluded. Thus, we must always be careful when applying the results of these trials to our general patient population and regularly reevaluate our outcomes in "real-life."

Treatment choices for early stage glottic cancer are still currently based on low-level evidence. Conservation surgery (open or transoral laser resection) and RT are all still valid options for treating Tis, T1, and selected T2 glottic lesions. A higher overall laryngeal preservation rate and possibly a higher survival rate have been associated with surgery for these tumors, but this is based only on metaanalyses of retrospective studies. Subjective selection criteria are still the basis for treatment choice for these lesions. For advanced lesions not amenable to conservation surgery, high-level evidence favors concurrent chemoradiation with cisplatin for nonsurgical organ preservation. With the increasing use of taxanes and cetuximab, and the advent of immune checkpoint blockers, however, the optimal combination of chemotherapy, targeted therapy, and RT is currently unknown. Finally, for large tumors with extensive cartilage and/or tongue base invasion, total laryngectomy followed by RT is still the treatment of choice for optimization of oncologic outcomes.

In the treatment of glottic carcinoma, the evidence in favor of one type of treatment as opposed to another is globally low level. For now, bias and opinion may still mar our decision-making, even in the context of multidisciplinary tumor boards. The opportunities for conservation laryngeal surgery depend on the experience and expertise of the local surgical oncology organ specialists. Guidelines based on expert opinion may be useful but generally do not provide details on appropriate criteria for patient selection for various treatment modalities (particularly conservation laryngeal surgery). Conservation surgery, and particularly transoral surgery, is often an "à la carte" procedure, and patient heterogeneity can impede coherent evaluation of patient groups. Prospective surgical registries may improve our options for outcomes analysis according to tumor subtypes and "atypical" surgeries.[120]

To optimize patient outcome, current evidence must be combined with experience of the multidisciplinary team managing these patients,[121] along with maintenance of a high regard for the patient-physician relationship, with an honest, open discussion regarding all of the aspects of different treatment options.

- Initial workup should include CT and/or MRI of the larynx (level 2 evidence).
- Curative treatment for Tis: Transoral surgery or RT. Possibly prefer surgery for younger patients. Save radiotherapy for failure of a surgical approach.
- Curative treatment for T1: Surgery (transoral laser surgery if technically feasible) may provide a higher rate of laryngeal preservation and survival as compared with RT (level 3 evidence). Voice outcomes seem to be comparable between these treatment options (level 3 evidence).
- Curative treatment for T2: T2 with normal vocal fold mobility may be treated by surgery or RT (level 3 evidence); surgery provides better outcomes for tumors with impaired vocal fold mobility as compared with RT alone (level 3 evidence). There are no specific data on outcomes of chemoradiation for T2 tumors with impaired laryngeal mobility.
- Curative treatment for T3T4: Conservation laryngeal surgery remains an option for selected tumors (level 4 evidence). When a nonsurgical organ preservation strategy is chosen, concurrent chemoradiation with cisplatin still provides better outcomes than RT alone or induction chemotherapy with cisplatin, 5-fluorouracil, and taxanes (level 1 evidence). Eligible patients should be referred for inclusion in clinical trials.
- For locally advanced tumors (T4), survival seems to be better with initial total laryngectomy followed by RT (level 3 evidence).
- HPV does not seem to be present in the majority of laryngeal squamous cell carcinomas but with regional differences in prevalence. The prevalence of its oncogenic role in laryngeal squamous cell carcinoma has yet to be elucidated.

REFERENCES

1. OCEBM Levels of Evidence Working Group, Howick J, Chalmers I, et al. *The Oxford 2011 Levels of Evidence.* Oxford Centre for Evidence-Based Medicine; 2011. http://wwwcebmnet/indexaspx?o=5653.
2. Elstein AS. On the origins and development of evidence-based medicine and medical decision making. *Inflamm Res.* 2004;53(suppl 2):S184–S189.
3. Paul BC, Rafii B, Achlatis S, Amin MR, Branski RC. Morbidity and patient perception of flexible laryngoscopy. *Ann Otol Rhinol Laryngol.* 2012;121(11):708–713.
4. Shoffel-Havakuk H, Lahav Y, Meidan B, et al. Does narrow band imaging improve preoperative detection of glottic malignancy? A matched comparison study. *Laryngoscope.* 2017;127(4):894–899.
5. Mannelli G, Cecconi L, Gallo O. Laryngeal preneoplastic lesions and cancer: challenging diagnosis. Qualitative literature review and meta-analysis. *Crit Rev Oncol Hematol.* 2016;106:64–90.
6. Kirchner JA. Fifteenth Daniel C. Baker, Jr, memorial lecture. What have whole organ sections contributed to the treatment of laryngeal cancer? *Ann Otol Rhinol Laryngol.* 1989;98(9):661–667.
7. Hartl DM, Landry G, Hans S, Marandas P, Brasnu DF. Organ preservation surgery for laryngeal squamous cell carcinoma: low incidence of thyroid cartilage invasion. *Laryngoscope.* 2010;120(6):1173–1176.
8. Hartl DM, Landry G, Hans S, et al. Thyroid cartilage invasion in early-stage squamous cell carcinoma involving the anterior commissure. *Head Neck.* 2011;34.
9. Zbaren P, Becker M, Lang H. Pretherapeutic staging of laryngeal carcinoma. Clinical findings, computed tomography, and magnetic resonance imaging compared with histopathology. *Cancer.* 1996;77(7):1263–1273.
10. Zbaren P, Becker M, Lang H. Staging of laryngeal cancer: endoscopy, computed tomography and magnetic resonance versus histopathology. *Eur Arch Otorhinolaryngol.* 1997;254(suppl 1):S117–S122.

11. Becker M, Burkhardt K, Dulguerov P, Allal A. Imaging of the larynx and hypopharynx. *Eur J Radiol.* 2008;66(3):460–479.

12. Adolphs AP, Boersma NA, Diemel BD, et al. A systematic review of computed tomography detection of cartilage invasion in laryngeal carcinoma. *Laryngoscope.* 2015;125(7):1650–1655.

13. Becker M, Zbaren P, Laeng H, Stoupis C, Porcellini B, Vock P. Neoplastic invasion of the laryngeal cartilage: comparison of MR imaging and CT with histopathologic correlation. *Radiology.* 1995;194(3):661–669.

14. Jeong HS, Chung MK, Baek CH, et al. Combined 18F-FDG PET/CT imaging for the initial evaluation of glottic cancer. *Clin Exp Otorhinolaryngol.* 2008;1(1):35–40.

15. Hao SP, Ng SH. Magnetic resonance imaging versus clinical palpation in evaluating cervical metastasis from head and neck cancer. *Otolaryngol Head Neck Surg.* 2000;123(3):324–327.

16. King AD, Tse GM, Ahuja AT, et al. Necrosis in metastatic neck nodes: diagnostic accuracy of CT, MR imaging, and US. *Radiology.* 2004;230(3):720–726.

17. Wax MK, Myers LL, Gona JM, Husain SS, Nabi HA. The role of positron emission tomography in the evaluation of the N-positive neck. *Otolaryngol Head Neck Surg.* 2003;129(3):163–167.

18. Sun R, Tang X, Yang Y, Zhang C. (18)FDG-PET/CT for the detection of regional nodal metastasis in patients with head and neck cancer: a meta-analysis. *Oral Oncol.* 2015;51(4):314–320.

19. Rohde M, Dyrvig AK, Johansen J, et al. 18F-fluoro-deoxy-glucose-positron emission tomography/computed tomography in diagnosis of head and neck squamous cell carcinoma: a systematic review and meta-analysis. *Eur J Cancer.* 2014;50(13):2271–2279.

20. Roh JL, Park JP, Kim JS, et al. 18F fluorodeoxyglucose PET/CT in head and neck squamous cell carcinoma with negative neck palpation findings: a prospective study. *Radiology.* 2014;271(1):153–161.

21. Le QT, Takamiya R, Shu HK, et al. Treatment results of carcinoma in situ of the glottis: an analysis of 82 cases. *Arch Otolaryngol Head Neck Surg.* 2000;126(11):1305–1312.

22. Garcia-Serra A, Hinerman RW, Amdur RJ, Morris CG, Mendenhall WM. Radiotherapy for carcinoma in situ of the true vocal cords. *Head Neck.* 2002;24(4):390–394.

23. Spayne JA, Warde P, O'Sullivan B, et al. Carcinoma-in-situ of the glottic larynx: results of treatment with radiation therapy. *Int J Radiat Oncol Biol Phys.* 2001;49(5):1235–1238.

24. Damm M, Sittel C, Streppel M, Eckel HE. Transoral CO_2 laser for surgical management of glottic carcinoma in situ. *Laryngoscope.* 2000;110(7):1215–1221.

25. Sengupta N, Morris CG, Kirwan J, Amdur RJ, Mendenhall WM. Definitive radiotherapy for carcinoma in situ of the true vocal cords. *Am J Clin Oncol.* 2010;33(1):94–95.

26. Fein DA, Mendenhall WM, Parsons JT, Stringer SP, Cassisi NJ, Million RR. Carcinoma in situ of the glottic larynx: the role of radiotherapy. *Int J Radiat Oncol Biol Phys.* 1993;27(2):379–384.

27. Hartl DM, de Mones E, Hans S, Janot F, Brasnu D. Treatment of early-stage glottic cancer by transoral laser resection. *Ann Otol Rhinol Laryngol.* 2007;116(11):832–836.

28. Peretti G, Nicolai P, Piazza C, Redaelli de Zinis LO, Valentini S, Antonelli AR. Oncological results of endoscopic resections of Tis and T1 glottic carcinomas by carbon dioxide laser. *Ann Otol Rhinol Laryngol.* 2001;110(9):820–826.

29. Smee RI, Meagher NS, Williams JR, Broadley K, Bridger GP. Role of radiotherapy in early glottic carcinoma. *Head Neck.* 2010;32(7):850–859.

30. Nguyen C, Naghibzadeh B, Black MJ, Rochon L, Shenouda G. Carcinoma in situ of the glottic larynx: excision or irradiation? *Head Neck.* 1996;18(3):225–228.

31. Eskiizmir G, Baskin Y, Yalcin F, Ellidokuz H, Ferris RL. Risk factors for radiation failure in early-stage glottic carcinoma: a systematic review and meta-analysis. *Oral Oncol.* 2016;62:90–100.

32. Abdurehim Y, Hua Z, Yasin Y, Xukurhan A, Imam I, Yuqin F. Transoral laser surgery versus radiotherapy: systematic review and meta-analysis for treatment options of T1a glottic cancer. *Head Neck.* 2012;34(1):23–33.

33. Mo HL, Li J, Yang X, et al. Transoral laser microsurgery versus radiotherapy for T1 glottic carcinoma: a systematic review and meta-analysis. *Lasers Med Sci.* 2017;32(2):461–467.

34. Sachse F, Stoll W, Rudack C. Evaluation of treatment results with regard to initial anterior commissure involvement in early glottic carcinoma treated by external partial surgery or transoral laser microresection. *Head Neck.* 2009;31(4):531–537.

35. Chone CT, Yonehara E, Martins JE, Altemani A, Crespo AN. Importance of anterior commissure in recurrence of early glottic cancer after laser endoscopic resection. *Arch Otolaryngol Head Neck Surg.* 2007;133(9):882–887.

36. Bradley PJ, Rinaldo A, Suarez C, et al. Primary treatment of the anterior vocal commissure squamous carcinoma. *Eur Arch Otorhinolaryngol.* 2006;263(10):879–888.

37. Nozaki M, Furuta M, Murakami Y, et al. Radiation therapy for T1 glottic cancer: involvement of the anterior commissure. *Anticancer Res.* 2000;20(2B):1121–1124.

38. Maheshwar AA, Gaffney CC. Radiotherapy for T1 glottic carcinoma: impact of anterior commissure involvement. *J Laryngol Otol.* 2001;115(4):298–301.

39. Rodel RM, Steiner W, Muller RM, Kron M, Matthias C. Endoscopic laser surgery of early glottic cancer: involvement of the anterior commissure. *Head Neck.* 2009;31(5):583–592.

40. Rucci L, Gallo O, Fini-Storchi O. Glottic cancer involving anterior commissure: surgery vs radiotherapy. *Head Neck.* 1991;13(5):403–410.

41. Zohar Y, Rahima M, Shvili Y, Talmi YP, Lurie H. The controversial treatment of anterior commissure carcinoma of the larynx. *Laryngoscope.* 1992;102(1):69–72.

42. Bron LP, Soldati D, Zouhair A, et al. Treatment of early stage squamous-cell carcinoma of the glottic larynx: endoscopic surgery or cricohyoidoepiglottopexy versus radiotherapy. *Head Neck*. 2001;23(10):823–829.

43. O'Hara J, Markey A, Homer JJ. Transoral laser surgery versus radiotherapy for tumour stage 1a or 1b glottic squamous cell carcinoma: systematic review of local control outcomes. *J Laryngol Otol*. 2013;127(8):732–738.

44. Greulich MT, Parker NP, Lee P, Merati AL, Misono S. Voice outcomes following radiation versus laser microsurgery for T1 glottic carcinoma: systematic review and meta-analysis. *Otolaryngol Head Neck Surg*. 2015;152(5):811–819.

45. Holland JM, Arsanjani A, Liem BJ, Hoffelt SC, Cohen JI, Stevens Jr KR. Second malignancies in early stage laryngeal carcinoma patients treated with radiotherapy. *J Laryngol Otol*. 2002;116(3):190–193.

46. Burns JA, Har-El G, Shapshay S, Maune S, Zeitels SM. Endoscopic laser resection of laryngeal cancer: is it oncologically safe? Position statement from the American Broncho-Esophagological Association. *Ann Otol Rhinol Laryngol*. 2009;118(6):399–404.

47. Ambrosch P. The role of laser microsurgery in the treatment of laryngeal cancer. *Curr Opin Otolaryngol Head Neck Surg*. 2007;15(2):82–88.

48. Peretti G, Piazza C, Cocco D, et al. Transoral CO_2 laser treatment for T(is)-T(3) glottic cancer: the University of Brescia experience on 595 patients. *Head Neck*. 2010;32(8):977–983.

49. Laccourreye O, Laccourreye L, Garcia D, Gutierrez-Fonseca R, Brasnu D, Weinstein G. Vertical partial laryngectomy versus supracricoid partial laryngectomy for selected carcinomas of the true vocal cord classified as T2N0. *Ann Otol Rhinol Laryngol*. 2000;109(10 Pt 1):965–971.

50. Peretti G, Piazza C, Mensi MC, Magnoni L, Bolzoni A. Endoscopic treatment of cT2 glottic carcinoma: prognostic impact of different pT subcategories. *Ann Otol Rhinol Laryngol*. 2005;114(8):579–586.

51. Peretti G, Piazza C, Bolzoni A, et al. Analysis of recurrences in 322 Tis, T1, or T2 glottic carcinomas treated by carbon dioxide laser. *Ann Otol Rhinol Laryngol*. 2004;113(11):853–858.

52. Mendenhall WM, Amdur RJ, Morris CG, Hinerman RW. T1-T2N0 squamous cell carcinoma of the glottic larynx treated with radiation therapy. *J Clin Oncol*. 2001;19(20):4029–4036.

53. Smee RI, Meagher NS, Williams JR, Broadley K, Bridger GP. Role of radiotherapy in early glottic carcinoma. *Head Neck*. 2010 Jul;32(7):850–9.

54. Gourin CG, Conger BT, Sheils WC, Bilodeau PA, Coleman TA, Porubsky ES. The effect of treatment on survival in patients with advanced laryngeal carcinoma. *Laryngoscope*. 2009;119(7):1312–1317.

55. Jones DA, Mendenhall CM, Kirwan J, et al. Radiation therapy for management of t1-t2 glottic cancer at a private practice. *Am J Clin Oncol*. 2010;33(6):587–590.

56. Stoeckli SJ, Schnieper I, Huguenin P, Schmid S. Early glottic carcinoma: treatment according patient's preference? *Head Neck*. 2003;25(12):1051–1056.

57. Marandas P, Hartl DM, Charffedine I, Le RA, Schwaab G, Luboinski B. T2 laryngeal carcinoma with impaired mobility: subtypes with therapeutic implications. *Eur Arch Otorhinolaryngol*. 2002;259(2):87–90.

58. Warner L, Lee K, Homer JJ. Transoral laser microsurgery versus radiotherapy for T2 glottic squamous cell carcinoma: a systematic review of local control outcomes. *Clin Otolaryngol*. 2017;42(3):629–636.

59. Gorphe P, Blanchard P, Breuskin I, Temam S, Tao Y, Janot F. Vocal fold mobility as the main prognostic factor of treatment outcomes and survival in stage II squamous cell carcinomas of the glottic larynx. *J Laryngol Otol*. 2015;129(9):903–909.

60. Motta G, Esposito E, Motta S, Tartaro G, Testa D. CO(2) laser surgery in the treatment of glottic cancer. *Head Neck*. 2005;27(7):566–573. Discussion 73–74.

61. Gallo A, de Vincentiis M, Manciocco V, Simonelli M, Fiorella ML, Shah JP. CO2 laser cordectomy for early-stage glottic carcinoma: a long-term follow-up of 156 cases. *Laryngoscope*. 2002;112(2):370–374.

62. Tucker HM, Benninger MS, Roberts JK, Wood BG, Levine HL. Near-total laryngectomy with epiglottic reconstruction. Long-term results. *Arch Otolaryngol Head Neck Surg*. 1989;115(11):1341–1344.

63. Brasnu DF. Supracricoid partial laryngectomy with cricohyoidopexy in the management of laryngeal carcinoma. *World J Surg*. 2003;27(7):817–823.

64. Dinshaw KA, Sharma V, Agarwal JP, Ghosh S, Havaldar R. Radiation therapy in T1-T2 glottic carcinoma: influence of various treatment parameters on local control/complications. *Int J Radiat Oncol Biol Phys*. 2000;48(3):723–735.

65. Howell-Burke D, Peters LJ, Goepfert H, Oswald MJ. T2 glottic cancer. Recurrence, salvage, and survival after definitive radiotherapy. *Arch Otolaryngol Head Neck Surg*. 1990;116(7):830–835.

66. Karim AB, Kralendonk JH, Yap LY, et al. Heterogeneity of stage II glottic carcinoma and its therapeutic implications. *Int J Radiat Oncol Biol Phys*. 1987;13(3):313–317.

67. Harwood AR, DeBoer G. Prognostic factors in T2 glottic cancer. *Cancer*. 1980;45(5):991–995.

68. Ansarin M, Cattaneo A, De Benedetto L, et al. Retrospective analysis of factors influencing oncologic outcome in 590 patients with early-intermediate glottic cancer treated by transoral laser microsurgery. *Head Neck*. 2017;39(1):71–81.

69. Chevalier D, Laccourreye O, Brasnu D, Laccourreye H, Piquet JJ. Cricohyoidoepiglottopexy for glottic carcinoma with fixation or impaired motion of the true vocal cord: 5-year oncologic results with 112 patients. *Ann Otol Rhinol Laryngol*. 1997;106(5):364–369.

70. Laccourreye O, Diaz Jr EM, Bassot V, Muscatello L, Garcia D, Brasnu D. A multimodal strategy for the treatment of patients with T2 invasive squamous cell carcinoma of the glottis. *Cancer*. 1999;85(1):40–46.

71. Thomas L, Drinnan M, Natesh B, Mehanna H, Jones T, Paleri V. Open conservation partial laryngectomy for laryngeal cancer: a systematic review of English language literature. *Cancer Treat Rev.* 2012;38(3):203–211.

72. Smee R, Bridger GP, Williams J, Fisher R. Early glottic carcinoma: results of treatment by radiotherapy. *Australas Radiol.* 2000;44(1):53–59.

73. Chera BS, Amdur RJ, Morris CG, Kirwan JM, Mendenhall WM. T1N0 to T2N0 squamous cell carcinoma of the glottic larynx treated with definitive radiotherapy. *Int J Radiat Oncol Biol Phys.* 2010;78(2):461–466.

74. Pantel M, Wittekindt C, Altendorf-Hofmann A, et al. Diversity of treatment of T2N0 glottic cancer of the larynx: lessons to learn from epidemiological cancer registry data. *Acta Otolaryngol.* 2011;131(11):1205–1213.

75. Wierzbicka M, Leszczynska M, Mlodkowska A, Szyfter W, Bartochowska A. The impact of prelaryngeal node metastases on early glottic cancer treatment results. *Eur Arch Otorhinolaryngol.* 2012 Jan;269(1):193–9.

76. Pfister DG, Spencer S, Brizel DM, et al. Head and neck cancers, version 2.2014. Clinical practice guidelines in oncology. *J Natl Compr Cancer Netw.* 2014;12(10):1454–1487.

77. Korean Society of T-H, Neck Surgery Guideline Task Force, Ahn SH, Hong HJ, et al. Guidelines for the surgical management of laryngeal cancer: Korean Society of Thyroid-Head and Neck Surgery. *Clin Exp Otorhinolaryngol.* 2017;10(1):1–43.

78. Jones TM, De M, Foran B, Harrington K, Mortimore S. Laryngeal cancer: United Kingdom national multidisciplinary guidelines. *J Laryngol Otol.* 2016;130(S2):S75–S82.

79. Wolf GT, Hong WK, Fischer SG, et al. Induction chemotherapy plus radiation compared with surgery plus radiation in patients with advanced laryngeal cancer. *N Engl J Med.* 1991;324(24):1685–1690.

80. Dufour X, Hans S, De Mones E, Brasnu D, Menard M, Laccourreye O. Local control after supracricoid partial laryngectomy for "advanced" endolaryngeal squamous cell carcinoma classified as T3. *Arch Otolaryngol Head Neck Surg.* 2004;130(9):1092–1099.

81. Laccourreye O, Salzer SJ, Brasnu D, Shen W, Laccourreye H, Weinstein GS. Glottic carcinoma with a fixed true vocal cord: outcomes after neoadjuvant chemotherapy and supracricoid partial laryngectomy with cricohyoidoepiglottopexy. *Otolaryngol Head Neck Surg.* 1996;114(3):400–406.

82. Vilaseca I, Bernal-Sprekelsen M, Luis Blanch J. Transoral laser microsurgery for T3 laryngeal tumors: prognostic factors. *Head Neck.* 2010;32(7):929–938.

83. Hinni ML, Salassa JR, Grant DG, et al. Transoral laser microsurgery for advanced laryngeal cancer. *Arch Otolaryngol Head Neck Surg.* 2007;133(12):1198–1204.

84. Forastiere AA, Weber RS, Trotti A. Organ preservation for advanced larynx cancer: issues and outcomes. *J Clin Oncol.* 2015;33(29):3262–3268.

85. Forastiere AA, Goepfert H, Maor M, et al. Concurrent chemotherapy and radiotherapy for organ preservation in advanced laryngeal cancer. *N Engl J Med.* 2003;349(22):2091–2098.

86. Blanchard P, Baujat B, Holostenco V, et al. Meta-analysis of chemotherapy in head and neck cancer (MACH-NC): a comprehensive analysis by tumour site. *Radiother Oncol.* 2011;100(1):33–40.

87. Bonner JA, Harari PM, Giralt J, et al. Radiotherapy plus cetuximab for locoregionally advanced head and neck cancer: 5-year survival data from a phase 3 randomised trial, and relation between cetuximab-induced rash and survival. *Lancet Oncol.* 2010;11(1):21–28.

88. Pointreau Y, Garaud P, Chapet S, et al. Randomized trial of induction chemotherapy with cisplatin and 5-fluorouracil with or without docetaxel for larynx preservation. *J Natl Cancer Inst.* 2009;101(7):498–506.

89. Posner MR, Norris CM, Wirth LJ, et al. Sequential therapy for the locally advanced larynx and hypopharynx cancer subgroup in TAX 324: survival, surgery, and organ preservation. *Ann Oncol.* 2009;20(5):921–927.

90. Janoray G, Pointreau Y, Garaud P, et al. Long-term results of a multicenter randomized phase III trial of induction chemotherapy with cisplatin, 5-fluorouracil, +/– docetaxel for larynx preservation. *J Natl Cancer Inst.* 2016;108(4).

91. Budach W, Bolke E, Kammers K, et al. Induction chemotherapy followed by concurrent radio-chemotherapy versus concurrent radio-chemotherapy alone as treatment of locally advanced squamous cell carcinoma of the head and neck (HNSCC): a meta-analysis of randomized trials. *Radiother Oncol.* 2016;118(2):238–243.

92. Rosenthal DI, Mohamed AS, Weber RS, et al. Long-term outcomes after surgical or nonsurgical initial therapy for patients with T4 squamous cell carcinoma of the larynx: a 3-decade survey. *Cancer.* 2015;121(10):1608–1619.

93. Henriques De Figueiredo B, Fortpied C, Menis J, et al. Long-term update of the 24954 EORTC phase III trial on larynx preservation. *Eur J Cancer.* 2016;65:109–112.

94. Sanabria A, Chaves AL, Kowalski LP, et al. Organ preservation with chemoradiation in advanced laryngeal cancer: the problem of generalizing results from randomized controlled trials. *Auris Nasus Larynx.* 2017;44(1):18–25.

95. Chen AY, Halpern M. Factors predictive of survival in advanced laryngeal cancer. *Arch Otolaryngol Head Neck Surg.* 2007;133(12):1270–1276.

96. Grover S, Swisher-McClure S, Mitra N, et al. Total laryngectomy versus larynx preservation for T4a larynx cancer: patterns of care and survival outcomes. *Int J Radiat Oncol Biol Phys.* 2015;92(3):594–601.

97. Stokes WA, Jones BL, Bhatia S, et al. A comparison of overall survival for patients with T4 larynx cancer treated with surgical versus organ-preservation approaches: a National Cancer Data Base analysis. *Cancer.* 2017;123(4):600–608.

98. Fu X, Zhou Q, Zhang X. Efficacy comparison between total laryngectomy and nonsurgical organ-preservation modalities in treatment of advanced stage laryngeal cancer: a meta-analysis. *Medicine*. 2016;95(14):e3142.

99. Timmermans AJ, Lange CA, de Bois JA, et al. Tumor volume as a prognostic factor for local control and overall survival in advanced larynx cancer. *Laryngoscope*. 2016;126(2):E60–E67.

100. Urba S, Wolf G, Eisbruch A, et al. Single-cycle induction chemotherapy selects patients with advanced laryngeal cancer for combined chemoradiation: a new treatment paradigm. *J Clin Oncol*. 2006;24(4):593–598.

101. Rapidis AD, Trichas M, Stavrinidis E, et al. Induction chemotherapy followed by concurrent chemoradiation in advanced squamous cell carcinoma of the head and neck: final results from a phase II study with docetaxel, cisplatin and 5-fluorouracil with a four-year follow-up. *Oral Oncol*. 2006;42(7):675–684.

102. Vermorken JB. A new look at induction chemotherapy in locally advanced head and neck cancer. *Oncologist*. 2010;15(suppl 3):1–2.

103. Laccourreye O, Brasnu D, Bassot V, Menard M, Khayat D, Laccourreye H. Cisplatin-fluorouracil exclusive chemotherapy for T1-T3N0 glottic squamous cell carcinoma complete clinical responders: five-year results. *J Clin Oncol*. 1996;14(8):2331–2336.

104. Laccourreye O, Veivers D, Hans S, Menard M, Brasnu D, Laccourreye H. Chemotherapy alone with curative intent in patients with invasive squamous cell carcinoma of the pharyngolarynx classified as T1-T4N0M0 complete clinical responders. *Cancer*. 2001;92(6):1504–1511.

105. Laccourreye O, Veivers D, Bassot V, Menard M, Brasnu D, Laccourreye H. Analysis of local recurrence in patients with selected T1-3N0M0 squamous cell carcinoma of the true vocal cord managed with a platinum-based chemotherapy-alone regimen for cure. *Ann Otol Rhinol Laryngol*. 2002;111(4):315–321. Discussion 21–22.

106. Vachin F, Hans S, Atlan D, Brasnu D, Menard M, Laccourreye O. Long term results of exclusive chemotherapy for glottic squamous cell carcinoma complete clinical responders after induction chemotherapy. *Ann Otolaryngol Chir Cervicofac*. 2004;121(3):140–147.

107. Bonfils P, Trotoux J, Bassot V. Chemotherapy alone in laryngeal squamous cell carcinoma. *J Laryngol Otol*. 2007;121(2):143–148.

108. Holsinger FC, Kies MS, Diaz Jr EM, et al. Durable long-term remission with chemotherapy alone for stage II to IV laryngeal cancer. *J Clin Oncol*. 2009;27(12):1976–1982.

109. Divi V, Worden FP, Prince ME, et al. Chemotherapy alone for organ preservation in advanced laryngeal cancer. *Head Neck*. 2010;32(8):1040–1047.

110. Hartl DM, Brasnu DF. Chemotherapy alone for glottic carcinoma: a need for higher-level evidence. *Ann Otol Rhinol Laryngol*. 2009;118(8):543–545.

111. Gheit T, Anantharaman D, Holzinger D, et al. Role of mucosal high-risk human papillomavirus types in head and neck cancers in central India. *Int J Cancer*. 2017;141.

112. Ndiaye C, Mena M, Alemany L, et al. HPV DNA, E6/E7 mRNA, and p16INK4a detection in head and neck cancers: a systematic review and meta-analysis. *Lancet Oncol*. 2014;15(12):1319–1331.

113. Taberna M, Resteghini C, Swanson B, et al. Low etiologic fraction for human papillomavirus in larynx squamous cell carcinoma. *Oral Oncol*. 2016;61:55–61.

114. Betiol JC, Sichero L, Costa HO, et al. Prevalence of human papillomavirus types and variants and p16(INK4a) expression in head and neck squamous cells carcinomas in Sao Paulo, Brazil. *Infect Agents Cancer*. 2016;11:20.

115. Anantharaman D, Abedi-Ardekani B, Beachler DC, et al. Geographic heterogeneity in the prevalence of human papillomavirus in head and neck cancer. *Int J Cancer*. 2017;140(9):1968–1975.

116. Gama RR, Carvalho AL, Longatto Filho A, et al. Detection of human papillomavirus in laryngeal squamous cell carcinoma: systematic review and meta-analysis. *Laryngoscope*. 2016;126(4):885–893.

117. Castellsague X, Alemany L, Quer M, et al. HPV involvement in head and neck cancers: comprehensive assessment of biomarkers in 3680 patients. *J Natl Cancer Inst*. 2016;108(6):djv403.

118. Al Refaie W, Vickers S, Zhong W, Parsons H, Rothenberger D, Habermann E. Cancer trials versus the real world in the United States. *Ann Surg*. 2011;254(3):438–442.

119. Clark A, Lammiman M, Goode K, Cleland J. Is taking part in clinical trials good for your health? A cohort study. *Eur J Heart Fail*. 2009;11(11):1078–1083.

120. Korenkov M, Troidl H, Sauerland S. Individualized surgery in the time of evidence-based medicine. *Ann Surg*. 2014 May;259(5):e76–7.

121. Marshall J. Surgical decision-making: integrating evidence, inference, and experience. *Surg Clin North Am*. 2006;86(1):201–215.

CHAPTER 14

Evidence-Based Practice: Management of Well-Differentiated Thyroid Cancer

LOURDES QUINTANILLA-DIECK, MD • MAISIE SHINDO, MD, FACS

INTRODUCTION

Thyroid cancer occurs in 7%–15% of patients with detected thyroid nodules, and incidence estimates for thyroid cancer in the year 2015 exceed 62,000.[1,2] The incidence of this cancer continues to rise worldwide, and is thought to be mostly a result of increased use of diagnostic imaging and surveillance. In spite of this, mortality from this disease has changed minimally over the last 50 years decades.[2] The incidence varies according to age, sex, and other risk factors such as a history of radiation exposure or a family history of thyroid malignancy.[1] The incidence of papillary thyroid cancer (PTC) has been increasing yearly, and thyroid cancers are being identified at an earlier stage. This may be attributed to the rising use of ultrasonography and other imaging modalities, where thyroid nodules are found incidentally.

Differentiated thyroid cancer (DTC) constitutes the vast majority (over 90%) and originates from thyroid follicular epithelial cells. Under the classification of DTC are PTC, follicular thyroid cancer (FTC), and the histologic variants of FTC, which include Hürthle cell or oncocytic thyroid cancer, clear cell, and insular (poorly differentiated).[1-3] DTC arises from follicular epithelial cells and accounts for over 90% of thyroid cancers. PTC accounts for approximately 85% of cases as compared with the 12% of follicular origin. PTC is frequently multifocal and bilateral and can metastasize to regional neck lymph nodes more commonly than with FTC, especially in pediatric patients. FTC is typically unifocal and more prone to initial hematogenous metastasis to the lungs and bones.[3] Of note, a 2016 publication proposed a change to the terminology used when describing the noninvasive encapsulated follicular variant of PTC that has a low risk of adverse outcomes.[4] The authors of this study suggested reclassifying this group of tumors as "noninvasive follicular thyroid neoplasm with papillary-like nuclear features" or NIFTP. This study was based on a sample size of 109 patients and will likely lead to larger studies with longer follow-up.

Overall, the majority of patients with DTC have an excellent clinical outcome when they receive appropriate treatment. However, 5%–10% experience a more aggressive clinical course, characterized by recurrent disease, early metastasis, resistance to radioactive iodine (RAI), and increased mortality.[5]

The emphasis on evidence-based medicine has resulted in development of management guidelines. The first treatment guidelines for patients with thyroid nodules and DTC were published in 1996 by the American Thyroid Association (ATA).[6] The most recent revision is from 2015. This review includes evidence-based recommendations from the most recent treatment guidelines for DTC, incorporating any additional moderate- to high-quality evidence studies that have been published in recent years. It is important to keep in mind that not all recommendations in the guidelines have grade A evidence, and there are still many areas of controversy regarding management of DTC.

CLINICAL ASSESSMENT FOR THYROID CANCER
Clinical Examination Including Voice Assessment

Several societies have published guidelines or statements regarding preoperative voice assessment on patients undergoing thyroid surgery.[1,7,8] There is some variability, however, on the recommendations when it comes to preoperative laryngeal examination. The ATA strongly recommends preoperative laryngoscopy in the presence of voice abnormalities, history of neck or upper chest surgery, and known thyroid cancer with posterior extrathyroidal extension (ETE) or extensive central neck lymphadenopathy.[1] The American Head and Neck Society and the German Association of Endocrine Surgeons practice guidelines recommend preoperative laryngeal examination in all cases of surgery for thyroid cancer.[7,8] The evaluation should consist of both the patient's and the physician's assessment of voice. Preoperative diagnosis of vocal cord function is essential in surgical planning and patient counseling, as it may be the first finding implicating locally invasive disease. Approximately 10%–15% of thyroid cancer presents with ETE, with involvement of the larynx in 12% of cases.[8–11] It may guide planning the extent of surgery and perioperative airway management.[9,12,13] In addition, the surgeon should be aware that any injury to the contralateral nerve could lead to airway compromise and the need for tracheostomy.

Imaging
Ultrasonography
Ultrasound (US) is the most important imaging modality in the evaluation of thyroid nodules and thyroid cancer. Cervical lymph node metastases are found in 20%–50% of patients with DTC.[14,15] Preoperative US identified suspicious cervical adenopathy in 20%–31% of cases, leading to a change in surgical approach in up to 20% of cases.[1] These findings led to the guideline recommendation to perform preoperative neck US in all patients undergoing thyroidectomy for malignant or suspicious for malignancy cytologic findings. This preoperative imaging study is specifically for evaluating central and lateral cervical lymph nodes in search for atypical features or characteristics that are suspicious for metastasis and may require further evaluation or treatment. Furthermore, US-guided fine needle aspiration (FNA) of any suspicious lymph nodes 8 mm in diameter or larger should be done to confirm malignancy if this would change surgical management.

Sonographic lymph node characteristics that should raise suspicion for metastatic disease include loss of fatty hilum (the most sensitive criterion in multiple papers),[16,17] enlargement, rounded shape, cystic changes, hyperechogenicity, peripheral vascularity, and the presence of calcifications (the most specific characteristic in one reference).[18] The lymph nodes at highest risk for metastasis from thyroid cancer are at levels III, IV, and VI,[17,18] although PTC tumors that arise in the upper pole have a higher propensity to demonstrate metastases to levels II and III.[19]

Computed tomography, magnetic resonance imaging, and positron emission tomography
In patients with advanced disease including an invasive primary tumor (where invasion into the trachea or esophagus is suspected) or bulky lymphadenopathy, preoperative use of a cross-sectional imaging study is recommended.[1] This could consist of either computed tomography (CT) or magnetic resonance imaging (MRI) of the neck with contrast. This additional workup helps identify nodal involvement in regions that are difficult to visualize with US, such as the mediastinum, infraclavicular space, retropharynx, and parapharyngeal space. One study showed that combined preoperative mapping with US and CT was superior to US alone in detecting nodal disease, especially in the central neck where US visualization can be challenging due to the presence of the thyroid gland.[20] The sensitivities of MRI and positron emission tomography (PET) scan for detecting cervical lymph node metastases are low (30%–40%).[21] The use of intravenous (IV) contrast is important to help delineate the anatomic relationship between metastatic disease and other structures including the primary tumor. Some physicians have concern about iodine burden from IV contrast causing a delay in postsurgical whole-body scans or RAI treatment, but iodine generally clears within 4–8 weeks.[1] Routine preoperative PET scan is not recommended. However, it is important to keep in mind that hypermetabolic thyroid lesions identified incidentally on PET have an associated risk of malignancy of 33.2%.[22]

Genetic Testing
The most frequent mutation in DTC is the *BRAF* mutation that results in *BRAF^{V600E}* mutant kinase[2]; research shows that 50%–70% of PTCs harbor this mutation.[23,24] Mutations in the *RAS* family of oncogenes are also a frequent finding in thyroid cancer, especially FTC and follicular variant of PTC. Chromosomal translocations can also occur, which lead to expression of novel fusion oncogenes. One example is the *PAX8-peroxisome proliferator-activated receptor † (PPAR†)* translocation, found in approximately 30% of FTCs. Radiation-related PTCs typically present with a higher frequency of *RET* chromosomal rearrangements. Sporadic PTCs, on the other hand, have a higher prevalence of *BRAF Val600Glu* or *RAS* point mutations.[25]

Molecular markers now play a very important role in both diagnosis and treatment of DTC. Although recent reports observed large interinstitutional variation in the cost-effectiveness of genetic tests, genetic testing of FNA specimens can be used as an additional diagnostic evaluation for thyroid nodules that are indeterminate on cytology.[1,26–28] There are two approaches in use: gene mutation profiling panels and a 167 gene expression classifier.[29–31] The 167 gene expression classifier (known as Afirma) offers a strong sensitivity of 90% and negative predictive value (NPV) of 95% (a good "rule-out" test). However, a suspicious result is predictive of thyroid cancer in less than 50% of cases, given a low specificity of 52% and a low positive predictive value (PPV) in several studies.[29,31] In contrast, gene mutation profiling (also called ThyroSeq) panels offer a PPV of 77% (higher than the gene expression classifier, therefore a better "rule-in" test) when positive for a mutation. It also showed 91% sensitivity, 92% specificity, and 97.2% NPV.[32] A more recent expanded mutation panel seems to improve the poor NPV of early seven-gene mutation testing.[31,32]

Genetic testing on both FNAs and surgical specimens can also help in patient counseling and for determining prognosis. Several studies suggest propensity for higher aggressiveness of cancer in tumors bearing a *BRAF* mutation[1,33–36] and a *TERT* mutation.[37–39] One study analyzed more than 400 DTCs and found that the presence of a *TERT* mutation was an independent predictor of mortality for all differentiated cancers.[40]

TREATMENT OF DIFFERENTIATED THYROID CANCER

DTC has an overall very favorable prognosis and long-term survival rates. It is important to keep this in mind when reviewing goals of treatment, which include improving overall and disease-specific survival, reducing risk of persistent or recurrent disease, and permitting accurate disease staging and risk stratification. Given this disease's favorable prognosis in most cases, minimizing treatment-related morbidity and unnecessary therapies are also important targets of treatment planning. The latest 2015 guidelines place more emphasis than its older 2009 version on consideration for less extensive surgery (thyroid lobectomy vs. total thyroidectomy) and reduced use of RAI with a lower dose of ^{131}I for ablation of low-risk DTCs. For the first time, the guidelines discuss active surveillance as a safe and effective alternative to immediate surgical treatment in properly selected patients.[25] These developments are a result of studies suggesting a very low likelihood of progression in patients with low-risk asymptomatic PTC < 1 cm in diameter, particularly in patients over the age of 60 years.[41,42]

Treatment of DTC has several components to consider—surgical, radiation, and possible adjunct therapies. The primary goal of surgery is removal of the primary tumor, any disease that has extended beyond the thyroid capsule, and lymph nodes that are affected or significantly at risk of having disease. Several studies have shown that completeness of surgical resection is an indicator for outcomes.[1] To minimize risk of disease recurrence and metastasis, adjunct treatment, such as RAI treatment and thyroid-stimulating hormone suppression, may be necessary. Risk stratification based on accurate staging is essential to determine the appropriate patient-specific long-term surveillance plan.

Surgical Therapy
Thyroid surgery
The extent of thyroidectomy for DTC depends on the extent of disease based on clinical findings and preoperative imaging as well as the presence of risk factors that may be associated with multifocality or more aggressive behavior. Such risk factors include prior head and neck or bone marrow irradiation, strong family history of DTC, personal history of familial adenomatous polyposis, Cowden syndrome, or *BRAF*-positive melanoma. Recommendations on the extent of resection have shifted more toward conservatism in the latest 2015 guidelines for the management of DTC.[1] These changes in the guideline recommendations are based on several evidence-based studies. Two different studies analyzed the Surveillance, Epidemiology, and End Results (SEER) database: one by Barney et al. that included 23,605 DTC patients diagnosed between 1983 and 2002, and the other by Mendelsohn et al. that analyzed 22,724 PTC patients diagnosed between 1998 and 2001.[43,44] Neither study found a difference in 10-year overall survival or 10-year cause-specific survival between patients undergoing total thyroidectomy versus lobectomy. Furthermore, a study by Matsuzu et al. reported a cause-specific survival rate of 98% after a median of 17 years of follow-up in properly selected PTC patients treated with lobectomy and ipsilateral neck dissection.[45] One of the supporting arguments for total thyroidectomy in the past was the propensity for PTC to be multifocal, often involving both thyroid lobes. However, with proper patient selection, locoregional recurrence rates of less than 1%–4% and completion thyroidectomy rates of less than 10% can be achieved after a lobectomy.[46,47] Even if there is a recurrence, this can be readily detected and treated with no decrease in survival rates.[45–47]

Thus, for microcarcinomas of the thyroid (<1 cm) without evidence of ETE or metastatic lymphadenopathy in a person without risk factors, a thyroid lobectomy is the recommended surgical approach. For low-volume (>1 and <4 cm) thyroid tumors without evidence of ETE or lymph node (LN) metastases, a thyroid lobectomy alone may be sufficient.[1] However, total thyroidectomy may instead be appropriate if the patient has risk factors such as history of radiation exposure or strong family history of thyroid cancer, or based on patient preference. For patients with primary tumor above 4 cm in maximal diameter, with gross ETE, or with clinically apparent cervical lymph node metastasis, or metastases to distant sites, near-total or total thyroidectomy should constitute the initial surgical approach.[1]

Tumor involvement of the recurrent laryngeal nerve

Invasive DTC occurs in about 16% of patients.[48] One area of debate in thyroid surgery for cancer is how to manage invasion of the recurrent laryngeal nerve (RLN). Although this finding is a marker of aggressiveness of the cancer, high long-term survival rates are seen in patients with known preoperative vocal cord paralysis and complete nerve transection caused by gross involvement.[49] The RLN has been found to be involved in 33%–61% of invasive thyroid cancers, but this factor does not independently affect survival rates, in contrast to invasion of the trachea and the esophagus.[48] In 2014, the American Head and Neck Society put forth an evidence-based consensus statement on management of invasive thyroid cancer, including laryngeal nerve invasion.[50] If the tumor involvement of the RLN is minimal, the nerve should be spared. If the RLN is encased by tumor and the patient has vocal fold paralysis preoperatively, the RLN should be resected; however, if the vocal cord is functioning preoperatively, the tumor may be shaved off if gross tumor removal can be achieved. In the rare setting where the contralateral RLN is paralyzed and the tumor encases the functioning nerve, it would be reasonable to shave the tumor in an attempt to avoid bilateral vocal cord paralysis and use adjuvant therapy for local control. If the RLN is resected, laryngeal reinnervation with ansa hypoglossi to the distal RLN stump should be performed if feasible, as it has been shown to improve voice outcomes.[51]

Management of the central lymph node compartment

The most common site of nodal metastases is in the central neck, cervical level VI, given that this is the main zone of lymphatic drainage for the majority of thyroid cancers.[52] Therapeutic central compartment (Level VI) neck dissection is recommended in patients with central nodes that are clinically involved (cN1), and this should accompany a total thyroidectomy to provide clearance from the central neck.[1] There has been a change in the new guidelines based on newer studies.

The rationale for complete compartment-oriented lymph node clearance is to minimize recurrence and thus reduce the need for repeated treatments and their associated morbidity.

However, in many cases, lymph node metastases to the central neck are not apparent on preoperative imaging or by inspection at the time of surgery[53,54]; this defines a clinically N0 (cN0) group. The value of prophylactic central neck dissection (CND) is more controversial. Several studies have shown no improvement in long-term patient outcomes, while the procedure may portend increased temporary or permanent morbidity, including hypoparathyroidism and RLN injury.[1,5] Based on imperfect data, the benefits of a prophylactic CND are thought to be improvement in disease-specific survival, decrease in local recurrence, posttreatment thyroglobulin levels, and decrease in the need for repeated RAI treatments.[1] Proponents of this procedure point to the high rate of positive nodes found in clinically N0 patients; several studies quote rates between 31% and 64%.[55–59]

Lymph node metastasis has been shown in many studies to affect the rate of recurrence in DTC. Harwood and colleagues compared the records of DTC patients, half of whom were N0 at the time of diagnosis, and found that patients with nodal involvement had significantly more recurrences those without.[59] Mazzaferri and Jhiang analyzed 1355 patients above the age of 40 years up to 91 years and discovered a significant correlation between the presence of lymph node metastases and higher recurrence rates at 30 years, regardless of cancer type.[60] A study by Hay and colleagues on patients with papillary thyroid microcarcinoma found higher recurrence rates in node-positive patients, with more than 80% of all recurrences localizing to regional lymph nodes.[61]

In addition to its impact on recurrence, lymph node metastasis has an independently significant effect on survival. Harwood et al. found that when matching for age, nodal metastasis resulted in a worse survival prognosis, especially in older populations.[59] Scheumann and colleagues reported a decrease in survival for node-positive patients, after controlling for age, tumor invasion, and distant metastasis.[62] Lundgren et al. performed a large population-based study on 5123 patients showing cervical metastases to have an odds ratio of 2.5 on mortality, after adjusting for TNM stage.[63] Grant and colleagues examined 420 patients who underwent thyroidectomy with or without neck dissection based on the 2009 ATA guideline recommendations and saw only a 5% nodal recurrence rate.[64] A recent comprehensive study of the National Cancer Data Base and

SEER also showed a small but significantly increased risk of death for patients younger than 45 years with lymph node metastases compared with younger patients without involved lymph nodes; in addition, having more metastatic lymph nodes, up to six positive nodes, confers additional mortality risk in this age group.[65] Another SEER registry study found that cervical lymph node metastasis was an independent risk factor for decreased survival in patients with PTC above the age of 45 years and those with FTC.[66]

As of yet, preoperative characteristics have not been seen to accurately predict PTCs that are associated with increased risk of lymph node metastasis. Many papers have tried to address this issue, as identifying risk factors could help tailor decisions related to prophylactic CNDs. The usefulness of $BRAF^{V600E}$ and other genetic findings in the predictive presence of lymph node metastasis remains questionable. In an attempt to further elucidate this question, Han and colleagues performed a multiinstitutional prospective study at four tertiary endocrine surgery centers, looking at 237 patients who underwent total thyroidectomy and routine CND.[5] They found that patients with all PTC subtypes who were $BRAF^{V600E}$-positive had a 48% chance of harboring central lymph node metastases, whereas those who were negative had a 28% chance. This gave the $BRAF^{V600E}$ mutation a PPV of 47.6% and NPV of 71.8%. These low numbers, however, limit its validity as a stand-alone marker for aggressiveness or metastasis. Importantly, when they looked at the subset of patients with classic variant PTC only, the $BRAF^{V600E}$ mutation was not associated with central lymph node metastases, although a tumor size > 2 cm was significantly associated ($P < .05$). Elevated levels of microRNAs including miR146b-3p, mi-146b-5p, and miR-222 were seen to be independent predictors of the presence of central lymph node metastases.

Management of the lateral lymph node compartment

Lateral neck lymph nodes are also at risk for metastasis from thyroid cancer, specifically compartments II–V, VII (anterior mediastinum), and rarely level I.[53,67] Thyroid cancers involving the upper pole, pyramidal lobe, and isthmus are more likely to drain to levels II and III of the lateral neck. In addition, the lateral portion of the hemithyroid lobe may drain toward lateral neck levels III and IV.[68] For patients with clinically positive lateral nodal disease on preoperative US with FNA cytologic confirmation or thyroglobulin washout measurement, surgical resection by compartmental node dissection may reduce the risk of recurrence and

possibly mortality risk.[69,70] The 2015 ATA guidelines recommend that "therapeutic lateral neck compartmental lymph node dissection should be performed for patients with biopsy-proven metastatic lateral cervical lymphadenopathy."[1] Risk factors for involvement of the lateral compartment are younger age, gender, tumor multifocality, tumor calcifications, upper pole tumor location, larger tumor size, ETE, central node positivity, ipsilateral involvement of other lateral neck levels, and contralateral lateral involvement.[71–75]

There is still some controversy and no real consensus on whether performing lateral neck dissection requires full clearance of levels II–V, or whether selective dissection may be performed based on clinical data. Caron and colleagues found a low rate of recurrence to levels I and V (3% for both levels combined) in a population that had had previous resection rates of 3.9% for level I and 18.6% for level V.[76] However, two other studies by Kupferman et al. and Farrag et al. showed high rates of level V metastases, at 21% and 40%, respectively.[72,77] In the latter study, all metastases were found in level V. Several studies have shown that multilevel involvement is common in the lateral neck. There are also some questions about how sensitive preoperative imaging is for finding involved lymph nodes. Many investigators advocate for a thorough neck dissection for any known lateral involvement.

Although skip metastases can occur, patients with positive lateral neck metastasis have a very high risk of having central compartment involvement. Roh et al. performed a review of 22 patients who presented with lateral neck recurrences, none of whom had had a previous CND with the initial thyroid surgery. At reoperation, elective CND revealed that 86% of patients had central metastases.[78]

Indications for Postoperative Radioactive Iodine Treatment

There are three main goals of postoperative administration of RAI after surgical treatment:

1. *RAI remnant ablation*, which would facilitate detection of recurrent disease and initial staging by tests such as thyroglobulin measurements or whole-body RAI scans;

2. *RAI adjuvant therapy*, intended to improve long-term outcomes by destroying occult microscopic foci of residual neoplastic cells within a thyroid remnant or elsewhere in the body; and

3. *RAI therapy*, by treating persistent disease, such as distant metastases, in higher-risk patients.[1,2]

There is still much higher-level research to be done in the area of indications for postoperative RAI

TABLE 14.1
ATA 2009 Risk Stratification System With Proposed Modifications in the 2015 American Thyroid Association (ATA) Guideline

ATA Risk Category	Primary Tumor	Metastasis	Surveillance Findings
Low risk	Papillary thyroid cancer (PTC) with: • No local or distant metastases • Macroscopic tumor fully resected • No tumor invasion of locoregional tissues or structures • No aggressive histology (e.g., tall cell, hobnail variant, columnar cell carcinoma) • No vascular invasion Intrathyroidal, encapsulated follicular variant of PTC[a] Intrathyroidal, well-differentiated FTC with capsular invasion and no or minimal (<4 foci) vascular invasion[a] Intrathyroidal, papillary microcarcinoma, unifocal or multifocal, including BRAF[V600E] mutated[a]	Clinical N0, or ≤5 positive nodes characterized as micrometastasis based on a size of <2 mm[a]	If ^{131}I is given, there are no RAI-avid metastatic foci outside the thyroid bed on the first posttreatment whole-body RAI scan
Intermediate risk	Microscopic ETE Aggressive tumor histology (e.g., tall cell, hobnail variant, columnar cell carcinoma) PTC with vascular invasion Multifocal papillary microcarcinoma with ETE and BRAF[V600E] mutated[a]	Clinical N1 or >5 pathologic nodes with metastasis, but all LNs measuring <3 cm in greatest dimension[a]	RAI-avid metastatic foci in the neck on the first posttreatment whole-body RAI scan
High risk	Gross ETE Incomplete tumor resection FTC with extensive vascular invasion (>4 foci)[a]	Any pathologic LN≥3 cm in greatest dimension.[a] Distant metastases	Postoperative serum thyroglobulin suggestive of distant metastases

ETE, extrathyroidal extension; FTC, follicular thyroid cancer; LN, lymph node; PTC, papillary thyroid cancer; RAI, radioactive iodine.
[a]Modification from 2015 ATA guidelines.
Data from 2015 American Thyroid Association management guidelines for adult patients with thyroid nodules and differentiated thyroid cancer.

treatment for thyroid cancer. Over recent years, the indications for RAI treatment have been questioned, and the current trend is for selective use of RAI, based on individual risk, with the lowest activity needed to ensure successful treatment.[2] It is important to keep in mind the adverse effects including short-term morbidity and possible increases in the risk of second cancers, especially in children.[2,3] The following are the current recommendations in terms of RAI treatment[1]:

• *Not routinely recommended*: for ATA low-risk DTC patients; after surgical treatment for unifocal or multifocal papillary microcarcinoma in the absence of other adverse features.
• *Should be considered in*: ATA intermediate-risk level DTC patients.
• *Routinely recommended for*: ATA high-risk DTC patients.

STAGING SYSTEMS AND RISK STRATIFICATION

The American Joint Committee on Cancer/Union for International Cancer Control (AJCC/UICC) TNM staging system for thyroid cancer is broadly used and recommended in the latest ATA guidelines. Several studies have demonstrated that this system, along with the MACIS system from the Mayo clinic, provides some of the highest proportion of variance explained: a statistical measure of how well a staging system can predict an outcome of interest, when applied to a broad range of patient cohorts.[1]

In the 2015 guidelines, the ATA has incorporated lymph node metastasis information into a three-tiered clinic-pathologic risk stratification system (Table 14.1). Several studies have retrospectively validated the 2009 system and reported the estimates of patients who subsequently had no evidence of disease (NED) in each category after total thyroidectomy and RAI remnant ablation: (1) low risk, 78%–91% NED; (2) intermediate risk, 52%–64% NED; and (3) high risk, 31%–32% NED.[1] NED is defined as a stimulated thyroglobulin <1 ng/mL with no other radiologic or clinical evidence of disease. There are several modifications mentioned in the 2015 guidelines that were based on new, albeit not high-quality, data. One big change is that in the 2009 system, any positive cervical lymph node metastasis would place a patient into the intermediate-risk category. The new guidelines mention that if there are five or less positive lymph nodes and they have micrometastases, they can be placed into the low-risk category because of lower risk of recurrence.[1,79] The mere presence of a positive node is no longer deemed to confer an intermediate level of risk. Rather, other factors carry more weight: the number and size of lymph nodes, the ability to detect the lymph node clinically, and the presence of extranodal extension.[79] As described in a metaanalysis by Randolph et al., clinically evident nodes as determined by preoperative imaging or physical examination, as well as intraoperative inspection, had an average risk of recurrence of 22% (10%–42%) compared with an average risk of recurrence of 2% (0%–9%) for patients without clinically evident nodes.[53] The number of positive nodes was also an important factor: if fewer than five nodes were positive for metastasis, the average recurrence rate was 4% (range 3%–8%), compared with patients with five or more positive nodes who had an average recurrence rate of 19% (range 7%–21%). The presence of extranodal extension conferred a recurrence risk of 24% (range 15%–32%).

The decision to include lymph node features in risk profile has significant implications in the management of patients with DTC. It can influence the decision to administer RAI, the degree of thyrotropin suppression, and the schedule for surveillance testing.[79]

MANAGEMENT OF RECURRENCE

Studies have shown patients with CND to have reduced thyroglobulin levels and decreased overall recurrence rates as defined by positive radioiodine scan or rising thyroglobulin. However, there are currently few studies that show a significant difference in recurrence between patients who receive neck dissection and those who do not.

- A study by Leboulleux and colleagues showed central nodes to be a risk factor for persistent disease but did not find them to also be significant for recurrence.[80] The same group found overall survival rates in their patients to be high, 99% at 10 years, regardless of whether a neck dissection was performed or not.
- Mazzaferri and Jhiang performed a study indicating nodal disease to negatively affect survival only in patients with the follicular subtype but not with other thyroid cancers.[60]
- A Korean study by So et al. found a reduction in postoperative thyroglobulin levels with elective CND, but this difference disappeared after RAI therapy and, at a 3-year follow-up, no significant difference in locoregional control rates was found.[81]

REFERENCES

1. Haugen BRM, Alexander EK, Bible KC, et al. 2015 American Thyroid Association management guidelines for adult patients with thyroid nodules and differentiated thyroid cancer. *Thyroid*. 2016;26:1–133.
2. Cabanillas ME, McFadden DG, Durante C. Thyroid cancer. *Lancet*. 2016;388:2783–2795.
3. Francis GL, Waguespack SG, Bauer AJ, et al. Management guidelines for children with thyroid nodules and differentiated thyroid cancer. The American Thyroid Association guidelines task force on pediatric thyroid cancer. *Thyroid*. 2015;25(7):716–759.
4. Nikiforov YE, Seethala RR, Tallini G, et al. Nomenclature revision for encapsulated follicular variant of papillary thyroid carcinoma: a paradigm shift to reduce overtreatment of indolent tumors. *JAMA Oncol*. 2016;2(8):1023–1029.
5. Han PA, Kim HS, Cho S, et al. Association of *BRAF^{V600E}* mutation and microRNA expression with central lymph node metastases in papillary thyroid cancer: a prospective study from four endocrine surgery centers. *Thyroid*. 2016;26(4):532–542.
6. Cooper DS, Doherty GM, Haugen BR, et al. Revised American Thyroid Association management guidelines for patients with thyroid nodules and differentiated thyroid cancer. *Thyroid*. 2009;19:1167–1214.
7. Musholt TJ, Clerici T, Dralle H, et al. German Association of Endocrine Surgeons practice guidelines for the surgical treatment of benign thyroid disease. *Langenbecks Arch Surg*. 2011;396:639–649.
8. Shindo ML, Caruana S, Kandil E, et al. Management of invasive well-differentiated thyroid cancer an American Head and Neck Society consensus statement. *Head Neck*. 2014;36:1379–1390.
9. Randolph GW, Kamani D. The importance of preoperative laryngoscopy in patients undergoing thyroidectomy: voice, vocal cord function, and the preoperative detection of invasive thyroid malignancy. *Surgery*. 2006;139:357–362.
10. Terris DJ, Snyder S, Carneiro-Pla D, et al. American Thyroid Association statement on outpatient thyroidectomy. *Thyroid*. 2013;23:1193–1202.

11. Dralle H, Sekulla C, Haerting J, et al. Risk factors of paralysis and functional outcome after recurrent laryngeal nerve monitoring in thyroid surgery. *Surgery*. 2004;136:1310–1322.

12. Farrag TY, Samlan RA, Lin FR, Tufano RP. The utility of evaluating true vocal fold motion before thyroid surgery. *Laryngoscope*. 2006;116:235–238.

13. Roh JL, Yoon YH, Park CI. Recurrent laryngeal nerve paralysis in patients with papillary thyroid carcinomas: evaluation and management of resulting vocal dysfunction. *Am J Surg*. 2009;197:459–465.

14. Chow SM, Law SC, Chan JK, Au SK, Yau S, Lau WH. Papillary microcarcinoma of the thyroid-prognostic significance of lymph node metastasis and multifocality. *Cancer*. 2003;98:31–40.

15. Ito Y, Uruno T, Nakano K, et al. An observation trial without surgical treatment in patients with papillary microcarcinoma of the thyroid. *Thyroid*. 2003;13:381–387.

16. Frasoldati A, Valcavi R. Challenges in neck ultrasonography: lymphadenopathy and parathyroid glands. *Endocr Pract*. 2004;10:261–268.

17. Kuna SK, Bracic I, Tesic V, Kuna K, Herceg GH, Dodig D. Ultrasonographic differentiation of benign from malignant neck lymphadenopathy in thyroid cancer. *J Ultrasound Med*. 2006;25:1531–1537.

18. Leboulleux S, Girard E, Rose M, et al. Ultrasound criteria of malignancy for cervical lymph nodes in patients followed up for differentiated thyroid cancer. *J Clin Endocrinol Metab*. 2007;92:3590–3594.

19. Park JH, Lee YS, Kim BW, Chang HS, Park CS. Skip lateral neck node metastases in papillary thyroid carcinoma. *World J Surg*. 2012;36:743–747.

20. Lesnik D, Cunnane ME, Zurakowski D, et al. Papillary thyroid carcinoma nodal surgery directed by a preoperative radiographic map utilizing CT scan and ultrasound in all primary and reoperative patients. *Head Neck*. 2014;36:191–202.

21. Jeong HS, Baek CH, Son YI, et al. Integrated 18F-FDG PET/CT for the initial evaluation of cervical node level of patients with papillary thyroid carcinoma: comparison with ultrasound and contrast-enhanced CT. *Clin Endocrinol (Oxford)*. 2006;65:402–407.

22. Shie P, Cardarelli R, Sprawls K, Fulda KG, Taur A. Systematic review: prevalence of malignant incidental thyroid nodules identified on fluorine-18 fluorodeoxyglucose positron emission tomography. *Nucl Med Commun*. 2009;30(9):742–748.

23. Cancer Genome Atlas Research Network. Integrated genomic characterization of papillary thyroid carcinoma. *Cell*. 2014;159:676–690.

24. Kowalska A, Walczyk A, Kowalik A, et al. Increase in papillary thyroid cancer incidence is accompanied by changes in the frequency of the *BRAF* mutation: a single-institution study. *Thyroid*. 2016;26:543–551.

25. Kitahara CM, Sosa JA. The changing incidence of thyroid cancer. *Nature*. 2016;12:646–653.

26. Harrell RM, Bimston DN. Surgical utility of Afirma: effects of high cancer prevalence and oncocytic cell types in patients with indeterminate thyroid cytology. *Endocr Pract*. 2014;20:364–369.

27. McIver B, Castro MR, Morris JC, et al. An independent study of a gene expression classifier (Afirma) in the evaluation of cytologically indeterminate thyroid nodules. *J Clin Endocrinol Metab*. 2014;99:4069–4077.

28. Marti JL, Avadhani V, Donatelli LA, et al. Wide interinstitutional variation in performance of a molecular classifier for indeterminate thyroid nodules. *Ann Surg Oncol*. 2015;22:3996–4001.

29. Alexander EK, Kennedy GC, Baloch ZW, et al. Preoperative diagnosis of benign thyroid nodules with indeterminate cytology. *N Engl J Med*. 2012;367:705–715.

30. Nikiforov YE, Ohori NP, Hodak SP, et al. Impact of mutational testing on the diagnosis and management of patients with cytologically indeterminate thyroid nodules: a prospective analysis of 1056 FNA samples. *J Clin Endocrinol Metab*. 2011;96:3390–3397.

31. Nikiforov YE, Carty SE, Chiosea SI, et al. Impact of the multi-gene ThyroSeq next-generation sequencing assay on cancer diagnosis in thyroid nodules with atypia of undetermined significance/follicular lesion of undetermined significance cytology. *Thyroid*. 2015;25:1217–1223.

32. Nikiforov YE, Carty SE, Chiosea SI, et al. Highly accurate diagnosis of cancer in thyroid nodules with follicular neoplasm/suspicious for a follicular neoplasm cytology by ThyroSeq v2 next-generation sequencing assay. *Cancer*. 2014;120:3627–3634.

33. Elisei R, Ugolini C, Viola D, et al. BRAF(V600E) mutation and outcome of patients with papillary thyroid carcinoma: a 15-year median follow-up study. *J Clin Endocrinol Metab*. 2008;93:3943–3949.

34. Xing M, Alzahrani AS, Carson KA, et al. Association between BRAF V600E mutation and recurrence of papillary thyroid cancer. *J Clin Oncol*. 2015;33:42–50.

35. Xing M, Alzahrani AS, Carson KA, et al. Association between BRAF V600E mutation and mortality in patients with papillary thyroid cancer. *JAMA*. 2013;309:1493–1501.

36. Chen Y, Sadow PM, Suh H, et al. BRAF(V600E) is correlated with recurrence of papillary thyroid microcarcinoma: a systematic review, multi-institutional primary data analysis, and meta-analysis. *Thyroid*. 2016;26:248–255.

37. Landa I, Ganly I, Chan TA, et al. Frequent somatic TERT promoter mutations in thyroid cancer: higher prevalence in advanced forms of the disease. *J Clin Endocrinol Metab*. 2013;98:E1562–E1566.

38. Liu X, Qu S, Liu R, et al. TERT promoter mutations and their association with BRAF V600E mutation and aggressive clinicopathological characteristics of thyroid cancer. *J Clin Endocrinol Metab*. 2014;99:E1130–E1136.

39. Melo M, da Rocha AG, Vinagre J, et al. TERT promoter mutations are a major indicator of poor outcome in differentiated thyroid carcinomas. *J Clin Endocrinol Metab*. 2014;99:E754–E765.

40. Richards ML. Familial syndromes associated with thyroid cancer in the era of personalized medicine. *Thyroid.* 2010;20:707–713.
41. Sugitani I, Toda K, Yamada K, Yamamoto N, Ikenaga M, Fujimoto Y. Three distinctly different kinds of papillary thyroid microcarcinoma should be recognized: our treatment strategies and outcomes. *World J Surg.* 2010;34(6):1222–1231.
42. Ito Y, Miyauchi A, Inoue H, et al. An observational trial for papillary thyroid microcarcinoma in Japanese patients. *World J Surg.* 2010;34(1):28–35.
43. Barney BM, Hitchcock YJ, Sharma P, Shrieve DC, Tward JD. Overall and cause-specific survival for patients undergoing lobectomy, near-total, or total thyroidectomy for differentiated thyroid cancer. *Head Neck.* 2011;33:645–649.
44. Mendelsohn AH, Elashoff DA, Abemayor E, St John MA. Surgery for papillary thyroid carcinoma: is lobectomy enough? *Arch Otolaryngol Head Neck Surg.* 2010;136:1055–1061.
45. Matsuzu K, Sugino K, Masudo K, et al. Thyroid lobectomy for papillary thyroid cancer: long-term follow-up study of 1,088 cases. *World J Surg.* 2014;38:68–79.
46. Nixon IJ, Ganly I, Patel SG, et al. Thyroid lobectomy for treatment of well differentiated intrathyroid malignancy. *Surgery.* 2012;151:571–579.
47. Vaisman F, Shaha A, Fish S, Michael TR. Initial therapy with either thyroid lobectomy or total thyroidectomy without radioactive iodine remnant ablation is associated with very low rates of structural disease recurrence in properly selected patients with differentiated thyroid cancer. *Clin Endocrinol (Oxford).* 2011;75:112–119.
48. McCaffrey TV, Bergstralh EJ, Hay ID. Locally invasive papillary thyroid carcinoma: 1940–1990. *Head Neck.* 1994;16(2):165–172.
49. Chan WF, Lo CY, Lam KY, et al. Recurrent laryngeal nerve palsy in well-differentiated thyroid carcinoma: clinicopathologic features and outcome study. *World J Surg.* 2004;28(11):1093–1098.
50. Shindo ML, Caruana SM, Kandil E, et al. Management of invasive well-differentiated thyroid cancer: an American head and neck society consensus statement: AHNS consensus statement. *Head Neck.* 2014.
51. Miyauchi A, Inoue H, Tomoda C, et al. Improvement in phonation after reconstruction of the recurrent laryngeal nerve in patients with thyroid cancer invading the nerve. *Surgery.* 2009;146:1056–1062.
52. Robbins KT, Shaha AR, Medina JE, et al. Consensus statement on the classification and terminology of neck dissection. *Arch Otolaryngol Head Neck Surg.* 2008;134:536–538.
53. Randolph GW, Duh QY, Heller KS, et al. The prognostic significance of nodal metastases from papillary thyroid carcinoma can be stratified based on the size and number of metastatic lymph nodes, as well as the presence of extranodal extension. *Thyroid.* 2012;22:1144–1152.
54. Mulla M, Schulte KM. Central cervical lymph node metastases in papillary thyroid cancer: a systematic review of imaging-guided and prophylactic removal of the central compartment. *Clin Endocrinol (Oxford).* 2012;76:131–136.
55. Moo TA, McGill J, Allendorf J, et al. Impact of prophylactic central neck lymph node dissection on early recurrence in papillary thyroid carcinoma. *World J Surg.* 2010;34(6):1187–1191.
56. Shindo M, Wu J, Park E, et al. The importance of central compartment elective lymph node excision in the staging and treatment of papillary thyroid cancer. *Arch Otolaryngol Head Neck Surg.* 2006;132(6):650–654.
57. Wada N, Duh QY, Sugino K, et al. Lymph node metastasis from 259 papillary thyroid microcarcinomas. *Ann Surg.* 2003;237(3):399–407.
58. Roh JL, Kim JM, Park C. Central cervical nodal metastasis from papillary thyroid microcarcinoma: pattern and factors predictive of nodal metastasis. *Ann Surg Oncol.* 2008;15(9):2482–2486.
59. Harwood J, Clark O, Dunphy J. Significance of lymph node metastasis in differentiated thyroid cancer. *Am J Surg.* 1978;136(1):107–112.
60. Mazzaferri E, Jhiang S. Long-term impact of initial surgical and medical therapy on papillary and follicular thyroid cancer. *Am J Med.* 1994;97(5):418–428.
61. Hay ID, Hutchinson ME, Gonzalez-Losada T, et al. Papillary thyroid microcarcinoma: a study of 900 cases observed in a 60-year period. *Surgery.* 2008;144:980–988.
62. Scheumann G, Gimm O, Wegener G, et al. Prognostic significance and surgical management of locoregional lymph node metastases in papillary thyroid cancer. *World J Surg.* 1994;18(4):559–567.
63. Lundgren C, Hall P, Dickman P, et al. Clinically significant prognostic factors for differentiated thyroid carcinoma: a population-based, nested case-control study. *Cancer.* 2006;106(3):524–531.
64. Grant C, Stulak J, Thompson G, et al. Risks and adequacy of an optimized surgical approach to the primary surgical management of papillary thyroid carcinoma treated during 1999–2006. *World J Surg.* 2010;34(6):1239–1246.
65. Adam MA, Pura J, Goffredo P, et al. Presence and number of lymph node metastases are associated with compromised survival for patients younger than age 45 years with papillary thyroid cancer. *J Clin Oncol.* 2015;33:2370–2375.
66. Zaydfudim V, Feurer ID, Griffin MR, Phay JE. The impact of lymph node involvement on survival in patients with papillary and follicular thyroid carcinoma. *Surgery.* 2008;144:1070–1077.
67. Sugitani I, Fujimoto Y, Yamada K, Yamamoto N. Prospective outcomes of selective lymph node dissection for papillary thyroid carcinoma based on preoperative ultrasonography. *World J Surg.* 2008;32:2494–2502.
68. Grodski S, Cornford L, Sywak M, et al. Routine level VI lymph node dissection for papillary thyroid cancer: surgical technique. *ANZ J Surg.* 2007;77(4):203–208.

69. Kouvaraki MA, Lee JE, Shapiro SE, Sherman SI, Evans DB. Preventable reoperations for persistent and recurrent papillary thyroid carcinoma. *Surgery.* 2004;136:1183–1191.

70. Ito Y, Tomoda C, Uruno T, et al. Preoperative ultrasonographic examination for lymph node metastasis: usefulness when designing lymph node dissection for papillary microcarcinoma of the thyroid. *World J Surg.* 2004;28:498–501.

71. Chung YS, Kim JY, Bae JS, et al. Lateral lymph node metastasis in papillary thyroid carcinoma: results of therapeutic lymph node dissection. *Thyroid.* 2009;10(3):241–246.

72. Kupferman ME, Patterson M, Mandel SJ, et al. Patterns of lateral neck metastasis in papillary thyroid carcinoma. *Arch Otolaryngol Head Neck Surg.* 2004;130(7):857–860.

73. Lim YS, Lee JC, Lee YS, et al. Lateral cervical lymph node metastases from papillary thyroid carcinoma: predictive factors of nodal metastasis. *Surgery.* 2011;150(1):116–121.

74. Jeong JJ, Lee YS, Lee SC, et al. A scoring system for prediction of lateral neck metastasis from papillary thyroid cancer. *J Korean Med Sci.* 2011;26(8):996–1000.

75. Kwak JY, Kim EK, Kim MJ, et al. Papillary microcarcinoma of the thyroid: predicting factors of lateral neck node metastasis. *Ann Surg Oncol.* 2009;16(5):1348–1355.

76. Caron NR, Tan YY, Ogilvie JB, et al. Selective modified radical neck dissection for papillary thyroid cancer – is level I, II and V dissection always necessary? *World J Surg.* 2006;30:833–840.

77. Farrag T, Lin F, Brownlee N, et al. Is routine dissection of level II-B and V-A necessary in patients with papillary thyroid cancer undergoing lateral neck dissection for FNA-confirmed metastases in other levels. *World J Surg.* 2009;33(8):1680–1683.

78. Roh JL, Park JY, Rha K, et al. Is central neck dissection necessary for the treatment of lateral cervical nodal recurrence of papillary thyroid carcinoma? *Head Neck.* 2007;29(10):901–905.

79. Urken ML, Haser GC, Likhterov I, Wenig BM. The impact of metastatic lymph nodes on risk stratification in differentiated thyroid cancer: have we reached a higher level of understanding? *Thyroid.* 2016;26(4):481–488.

80. Leboulleux S, Rubino C, Bauden E, et al. Prognostic factors for persistent or recurrent disease of papillary thyroid carcinoma with neck lymph node metastases and/or tumor extension beyond the thyroid capsule at initial diagnosis. *J Clin Endocrinol Metab.* 2005;90(10):5723–5729.

81. So Y, Son Y, Hong S, et al. Subclinical lymph node metastasis in papillary thyroid microcarcinoma: a study of 551 resections. *Surgery.* 2010;148(3):526–531.

Index

Note: Page numbers followed by "f" indicate figures, "t" indicate tables and "b" indicate boxes.

Printed in the United States
By Bookmasters